DISEASE AND REPRESENTATION

Form und Funktion: Eine strukturelle Untersuchung der Romane Klabunds (1971)

The Parodic Sermon in European Perspective: Aspects of Liturgical Parody from the Middle Ages to the Twentieth Century (1974)

Bertolt Brecht's Berlin (1975)

Nietzschean Parody: An Introduction to Reading Nietzsche (1976)

The Face of Madness: Hugh W. Diamond and the Rise of Psychiatric Photography (1976)

Wahnsinn, Text und Kontext: Die historischen Wechselbeziehungen der Literatur, Kunst und Psychiatrie (1981)

On Blackness without Blacks: Essays on the Image of the Black in Germany (1982)

Seeing the Insane: A Cultural History of Psychiatric Illustration (1982)

Difference and Pathology: Stereotypes of Sex, Race, and Madness (1985)

Jewish Self-Hatred (1986)

Oscar Wilde's London (1987)

SANDER L. GILMAN

Disease and Representation

Images of Illness from Madness to AIDS

CORNELL UNIVERSITY PRESS

ITHACA AND LONDON

First published 1988 by Cornell University Press.
Second printing 1991.
First published, Cornell Paperbacks, 1988.
Second printing 1991.

International Standard Book Number 0-8014-2119-5 (cloth)
International Standard Book Number 0-8014-9476-1 (paper)
Library of Congress Catalog Card Number 87-47864
Printed in the United States of America
*Librarians: Library of Congress cataloging information
appears on the last page of the book.*

⊗ The paper in this book meets the minimum requirements of the American National Standard for Information Sciences—Permanence of Paper for Printed Library Materials, ANSI Z39.48–1984.

FOR MY PARENTS

CONTENTS

PLATES

PREFACE

The essays in this volume are the fruit of a wide-ranging inquiry into how we imagine disease and how we represent those we label as the sufferers of illness. Their sources run from the medical literature of the ancient Greeks to the most recent documents of American psychiatry; from the fine arts of the Italian Renaissance to pictures in today's newspapers and magazines. I have aimed to illustrate a relatively broad spectrum of diseases and their representations. Thus, side by side, the reader will find a study of the construction, within the literature of psychiatry, of the syndrome now labeled "schizophrenia" and an analysis of the intellectual backgrounds of Richard Strauss's opera *Salome* and its relationship to contemporary models of disease. This juxtaposition is intended to reveal the richness that the history of science, especially the history of medicine, can have for an understanding of cultural objects and the evident (but all too often ignored) importance of cultural objects for the reconstruction of the social history of science.

The creative tension that bonds these two areas, science and art, has long been sensed. Philip C. Ritterbush noted their uncanny parallels in the book based on his exhibition "The Art of Organic Form" (Washington, D.C.: Smithsonian Institution, 1968): "All images, artistic or scientific, whether they enter naively or self-consciously into our awareness, are abstractions from diverse phenomena. The abstraction of images occurs even during everyday perception, wherein the mind reduces the richness of sense to orderly pattern" (p. 9). Not merely the images' common basis in the shared perceptions of any given age but the work of art's unique ability to blend and merge images from disparate ages, levels of society, and multifaceted sources, such as "serious" and "popular" science, makes such comparative study valuable. But art is by no means primary in this relationship. For science often understands and articulates its goals on the basis of literary or aesthetic models, measuring its reality against the form of reality that art provides. I consider both perspectives essential for examining the complex cultural and social function of images of disease.

Versions of Chapters 2, 4, 5, 6, 7, 8, 9, 11, and 13 have appeared in the following sources and are used with the permission of the editors and publishers. Chapters 2 and 7: Gerald Chappel, ed., *The Turn of the Century* (Bonn: Bouvier, 1981), pp. 53–86. A German version of Chapter 2 appeared in *Sudhoffs Archiv* 62 (1978): 201–34; a Spanish version, in *Rassegna* 3 (1982): 21–24. A Spanish version of Chapter 7 appeared in *Rassegna* 3 (1982): 49–56. Chapter 4: *Modern Language Notes* 83 (1978): 871–87; a German version appeared in *Confinia psychiatrica* 22 (1979): 127–44. Chapter 5: the original English essay appeared in the *Deutsche Vierteljahrsschrift für Literaturwissenschaft und Geistesgeschichte* 52 (1978): 381–99; a German version of this appeared in *Musik und Medizin* 1977: 4:20–28; 5:23–27; 6:14–17. Chapter 6: a German version appeared in Wolfram Mauser, ed., *Phantasie und Deutung: Psychologisches Verstehen von Literatur und Film* (Würzburg: Könighausen und Neumann, 1986), pp. 40–57. Chapter 8: *Journal of the History of the Behavioral Sciences* 15 (1979): 253–62. Chapter 9: *Medical History* 30 (1986): 57–69. Chapter 11: *Critical Inquiry* 13 (1986): 293–313. Chapter 13: *Journal of the History of the Behavioral Sciences* 19 (1983): 127–35; a French translation appeared in *Spirales* 17 (1982): 58–59. All these pieces have been rewritten for publication here. I am grateful to the National Endowment for the Humanities and the American Psychoanalytic Association for grants that helped support the work done on this book.

I thank Kate Bloodgood and Howard Greier, who prepared the manuscript; Carol Betsch, who copyedited it; and Jane Marsh Dieckmann, who prepared the index. I also thank my students at the College of Arts and Sciences, Cornell University (Ithaca), and the Cornell Medical College (New York), who listened (sometimes patiently) as I worked out the ideas presented here.

SANDER L. GILMAN

Ithaca, New York

DISEASE AND REPRESENTATION

CHAPTER ONE

Depicting Disease:
A Theory of Representing Illness

Essential to the representational world are the many organized schemata
that the individual constructs during the course of his development and
that form the background frame of reference to all current processes of
perception, imagining, remembering, feeling and thinking. The representational world in all the different aspects of its organization is constantly
influenced by stimuli arising from within and without the individual, and
new schemata are constantly being created as new perceptual and conceptual solutions are being found. These schemata form the basis for future
attempts at adaptation and problem solving, although they may in turn be
modified by experience.

Joseph Sandler, *From Safety to Superego*

The Other as Diseased

In an essay entitled "What Is Schizophrenia?" Manfred Bleuler, one of
the most authentic voices in modern psychiatry, commented:

For nearly 100 years, the group of schizophrenic psychoses have been
intensively studied, yet they appear to many to be totally baffling and
insufficiently researched. A shocking antithesis! Too little thought has
been given to how much this antithesis results from our own prejudiced
thinking. We conceive ourselves, our personalities, and our own egos as
being steady and firm. The fact that we could disintegrate mentally by
way of natural processes—as the schizophrenic does—is a monstrous,
uncanny concept.[1]

It is the fear of collapse, the sense of dissolution, which contaminates the
Western image of all diseases, including elusive ones such as schizophrenia. But the fear we have of our own collapse does not remain internalized. Rather, we project this fear onto the world in order to localize it
and, indeed, to domesticate it. For once we locate it, the fear of our own
dissolution is removed. Then it is not we who totter on the brink of
collapse, but rather the Other. And it is an-Other who has already shown
his or her vulnerability by having collapsed.

It is in these artificial structures that we build for our fear—the representations of what Mary Douglas has called the "yearning for rigidity in us all"—it is in these fictions of a whole world, that we find solace.[2] Some of the structures we employ to exorcise the fear that we may lose control—indeed, that we are not really in control at all—are the rigid forms of art. For art, whatever form it is given, is an icon of our control of the flux of reality.[3] It is therefore within a very specific aesthetic tradition, the tradition of imagining and portraying disease, that we project our sense of eventual (indeed, inevitable) loss. The portrait of the sufferer, the portrait of the patient, is therefore the image of the disease anthropomorphized. Our examination of the image of the sufferer provides us with rigid structures for our definition of the boundaries of disease, boundaries that are reified by the very limits inherent to the work of art—the frame of the painting, the finite limits of the stage, the covers of the book, the perspective of the photograph, or the narrative form of the novel. In placing such images within culturally accepted categories of representation, within "art," we present them as a social reality, bounded by a parallel fantasy of the validity of "art" to present a controlled image of the world. I echo here the view of W. J. T. Mitchell, who introduces his first-rate study *Iconology* with the observation that he is "not arguing for some facile relativism that abandons 'standards of truth' or the possibility of valid knowledge." Rather, he supports "a hard, rigorous relativism that regards knowledge as a social product, a matter of dialogue between different versions of the world, including different languages, ideologies, and modes of representation."[4] I would add that this relativism, present within all systems of representations, can tell us little about the underlying realities but much about the construction of our understanding of those realities. It is not that syphilis is as phantasmagoric as masturbatory insanity, but that the social reality of each (the "real" disease and the "imagined" one) is constructed on the basis of specific ideological needs and structured along the categories of representation accepted within that ideology.

The fixed structures of art provide us with a sort of carnival during which we fantasize about our potential loss of control, perhaps even revel in the fear it generates within us, but we always believe that this fear exists separate from us.[5] This sense of the carnivalesque provides us with exactly the missing fixity for our understanding of the world which the reality of disease denies. For illness is a real loss of control that results in our becoming the Other whom we have feared, whom we have projected onto the world. The images of disease, whether in art or in literature, are not in flux, even though they represent collapse. They are solid, fixed images that remain constantly external to our sense of self. Thus an inherent tension exists between the world of art representing disorder, disease, and madness and the source of our anxiety about self-control. This tension provides the ambiguity inherent in the creation and reception of images of disease. It also provides the basic reference against which all images of disease, whether literary or visual, are measured.

Lillian Feder, in a magisterial study of madness in literature, has shown that the tradition of representing madness within literature is continuous and only marginally influenced by shifting popular or medical views of the nature or scope of madness.[6] I will extend this argument here: the image of all disease, the very face of the patient, is a continuous one, and through a study of its continuities comes a sense of the interrelationship of all our projected fears of collapse. This continuity, however, reflects changing functions that the image of disease has within an age's or an individual's overall sense of control. In some cases, the fearful is made harmless through being made comic; in some cases it looms as a threat, controlled only by being made visible. How we see the diseased, the mad, the polluting is a reflex of our own sense of control and the limits inherent in that sense of control.

Thus the relationship between images of disease and the representation of internalized feelings of disorder is very close. In this matrix the references to collapse (or to the needed sense of control) draw upon the historical pattern of the images found within aesthetic traditions. A free play exists between the uses of these images—whether they are altered and reproduced as visual images, incorporated as descriptive devices or metaphors in texts, or whether their presence haunts the presuppositions of "scientific" nosologies used in medical classification. Yet each presentation reflects the social constraints and implications of the medium selected. We can turn to those paradigmatic shifts in the history of imagining disease—to the Renaissance rediscovery of the body, for example, or the professionalization of the treatment of the mentally ill during the late nineteenth and early twentieth centuries—and see how clearly contradictory icons of the patient exist simultaneously within certain images.[7] Leonardo and Freud thus have much more in common than one would, on first glance, suppose!

The Other's Sense of Disease

The idea of representing the diseased through visual images reaches back through the ages. The act of "seeing disease" (as well as "seeing works by the diseased," whether mad or tubercular) is socially coded in many complicated ways. To decipher this code one must be able to reconstruct the patterns that dominated and shaped the perception of the patient, the sufferer of disease. There are, however, at least two different levels on which this codification of illness functions: first, on the level of the social construction of categories of disease; but then, perhaps even more important, on the level of the internalization of such images in groups who are labeled as being at risk. In this book we shall examine both the construction of fictions about disease and the acceptance of these fictions as realities about the self.

The understanding of the patient as a vessel holding disease and, therefore, an extension of the disease, is determined by the norms of the society in which the observer and the observed are present. The basic structure is that of all stereotyping, the inherent and universal fantasy made between the "good" mother (whom we can control) and the "bad" mother (who lies outside of our potential for control). Rooted in the pre-Oedipal development of all human beings, this internalized fantasy provides us with a simple but compelling model to separate all those factors that reflect our own fear of chaos, of the disruptive, of the inchoate, and locate them in a specific point in the world.[8] Disease, with its seeming randomness, is one aspect of the indeterminable universe that we wish to distance from ourselves. To do so we must construct boundaries between ourselves and those categories of individuals whom we believe (or hope) to be more at risk than ourselves. These bounded categories are invested with all of the raw intensity of our pre-Oedipal selves. Thus in contemporary America there is an assumption among physicians that the diseased and the beautiful cannot be encapsulated in one and the same category. Young physicians often see beautiful patients as exemplary or "good" patients, patients who will follow doctor's orders and therefore will regain health.[9] The aged or poor patient, on the other hand, is seen, even by the trained physician, as one who is a "bad" patient, a patient who will probably "make trouble" and whose health will not improve. Indeed "lower-class" patients were often diagnosed as being more gravely ill and were given poorer prognoses than those of other social classes when, in fact, they differed from those patients only in terms of the visible (or stated) criteria of class.[10] Cultural differences concerning gender also play a major role in constructing those groups understood as being more at risk. Obesity, while statistically more frequent in males than females, was used as a diagnostic criterion twice as often for women as for men.[11]

Such categories of difference determine the construction of the idea of the patient in a direct and powerful manner, drawing the boundaries between the "healthy" observer, physician or layperson, and the "patient." The construction of the image of the patient is thus always a playing out of this desire for a demarcation between ourselves and the chaos represented in culture by disease.[12] But we are all at risk—we will all be ill, will fail, will die. What happens, however, when our sense of ourselves as "the patient," of ourselves as existing on the wrong side of the margin between the healthy and the diseased, becomes salient to our definition of self?

The mode of approach is equally complex. While one can speak of the general attempt of society to localize and therefore limit the source of pollution, when one is oneself at risk, much more convoluted images are generated. In the present study I will examine the internalization of the cultural presuppositions of disease using the model that I outlined in my recent book on Jewish self-hatred.[13] There I proposed that whenever an image of difference projected onto a group within a society has sufficient salience for an individual in the stereotyped group as to be completely internalized, the individual acts as if the image is a pattern for self-definition whatever the validity or implications of the charge of difference or the image imposed.

The basic structure is the reactivation of the fantasy of psychological wholeness that existed in all of us before we distanced ourselves from our first caregiver. It is this fantasy of wholeness which lies at the root of all of the bipolar images of difference (health vs. disease; good vs. bad; white vs. black) which comprise our constructions of all stereotypes, including those of health and disease.[14] Our internalized sense of difference is a product of that primal moment in everyone's experience when we first became aware that we were different—different from the caregiver, unable to control our world. We need to project the fantasized source of our anxiety about our original loss of control. The individuals who comprise the screen onto which group fantasies are projected likewise share this internalized, universal sense of difference. This sense of difference is triggered by any deep-seated sense of ontological insecurity, such as that created by a double-bind situation in which one must rationalize one's sense of self with the image of the Other projected upon a group with which one is identified. This moment of insecurity reproduces the repressed anxiety of that primal moment.

When we are in such a state we desire to overcome it by reconnecting ourselves with that force, society, which has replaced the mother as the prime determiner of our sense of self. We thus actively seek to accept society's sense of our own difference in order to recreate our sense of oneness with the world. Thus anyone who is labeled as "Jewish" in times of crisis concerning the Jews, or as being "ill" at all times, whatever the objective reality behind that label, reacts by internalizing the image of "Jewishness" or "the diseased" projected by the dominant group that it fears and thus wishes to emulate. Anna Freud observed this pattern of action among the Jewish children evacuated to her London clinic during World War II when they played Nazis and Jews.[15] All of the children identified with the power of the aggressor as an apotropaic gesture to preserve their own sense of power. They projected those qualities of

"Jewishness" ascribed to themselves onto an appropriate subgroup of "Jews," the victims in their games, as a means of preserving their own sense of control over their identity. So do we all play at being "well," denying our sense of our own fragility.

Individuals who internalize such images projected by the dominant society must respond to this type of self-stereotyping. They respond either by denying it (and proving to the dominant group the validity of its perception of the inherent difference of the Other) or affirming it (while projecting the negative associations about "being Jewish" or "being ill" onto specific subgroups among those labeled as "Jewish" or "diseased"). Thus whenever an individual accepts the charge of being different, he or she also accepts all of the negative associations that accompany that image. The image of the Jew possessing a damaged or damaging discourse has made those writers who were labeled as Jewish and accepted the assigned label (rather than an internally generated one) need to prove that their discourse is unimpaired. The image of the diseased makes those so categorized need to prove their basic healthiness. Thus anyone can be labeled as a Jew or as diseased and can accept the implications of this category—being Jewish or being ill is not merely an attribute of the self but, more important, is the agreement of certain internalized images of the self with the projections of difference by the dominant group. The reality behind the image (and there are real diseases behind these images), whether it is the reality of the Jew or of the patient, is not at the heart of the matter. Rather it is the acceptance, for any number of reasons, of the projection of the Other as at least an aspect of self-definition with which we shall be concerned.

One examines this type of internalization best by turning to those tangible creations, texts in the widest sense of the word, that directly refer to the code of difference to be internalized and are created in those media that have immediate and evident salience for the given individual. These texts fix the world and provide an illusion of immutability which denies the abyss of difference in which those stigmatized as different perceive themselves. For Jewish writers one turns to those of their writings which fix their references to Jews and Judaism. In terms of our fantasies about disease, since we are all at risk all of the time, the works of art that represent, that fix, the image of the patient are a key to an understanding of our structuring (and distancing) of our own sense of fragility and mortality.

Models of Disease and Their Realities

It is not trivial to understand how such labels of disease are created and internalized, how the ill are (and have been) perceived. For it is the perception of the patient that structures the patient's treatment, the patient's status, the patient's self-understanding, as well as the patient's response to that complex interaction of social and biological forces that we call "disease." The infected individual is never value-neutral, that is, solely a person exhibiting specific pathological signs or symptoms. Like any complex text, the signs of illness are read within the conventions of an interpretive community that comprehends them in the light of earlier, powerful readings of what are understood to be similar or parallel texts. In every social group there are those catastrophic diseases that so deeply influence the self-understanding of the members of the community as to evoke images of past catastrophes. The medical profession, as well as society in general, incorporates such sets of symbolic readings of these signs of pathology in its understanding of the disease, giving these symbolic meanings a status parallel to the original signs and symptoms within our cultural and social context.[16] These communal interpretations of the disease, the signs and symptoms, construct the image of the illness and the patient suffering from that illness. It is this set of symbolic readings and their historical context which provides the set of associations which we, as doctors, patients, or observers, subconsciously apply to the idea of specific diseases.

The visual images of the diseased, and their verbal parallels, form the subject of our study. In this book, I have sketched histories of some of these images. Some of these fictions about disease are spun about "real" illnesses, such as syphilis or AIDS; some of them are spun about fantasy illnesses, such as masturbatory insanity (where there is a physical act that is interpreted as pathological). Whatever the "reality," I have focused on the myth-making about the disease and the historically determined responses of writers and artists to such constructions of disease. Then I have examined some of the echoes and parallels of these images in a series of diverse representations. From private correspondence through scientific monographs and illustrations to fictions, all of these representations create images of the patient, of the sufferer, which present variations on the act of "seeing the patient."

The association between the discourse about disease and the representation of this discourse is in the psyche of the generator of the images examined. All of these essays are attempts to decode their underlying structures of representation. The act of seeing is the act of the creation of historically determined (and therefore socially acceptable) images that permit a distinction to be made between the observer and the Other. On the one hand, this distinction can be simply the line between the observer as "healthy" and the Other as "diseased."[17] But this dyad can be articulated in a much more complex manner. For the late nineteenth-century avant-garde accepted (indeed, reveled in) the label of "degenerate." (This can be seen in Chapter 12, where I discuss how the language of aesthetics is used to describe the syndrome now labeled "schizophrenia.") Here the ill and corrupt became the positive pole; the staid and stolid—the healthy—the negative pole. The glorification of the art of the mentally ill (as well as its abnegation) had its roots in this dichotomy, as do many late nineteenth-century representations of the mentally ill. For the image of the patient can be a depiction of the Other as diseased, but it can also serve as the alter ego of the observer, an alter ego that is the glorification of difference. Dickens's image of the asylum as the extended family echoes to no little degree the positive virtues he projects into the stable family. He accepted the rhetoric of the reformed asylum and saw the stability of the world of the asylum as a positive microcosm. Darwin, on the other hand, saw the insane as the antithesis of the civilized, as the picture of regression. For Dickens, the effect is comic; for Darwin, it is to no little degree frightening. Both "see the insane," but each sees them through his own construction of madness. When one turns to other contexts, such as the creation of Richard Strauss's opera *Salome*, one can observe how a careful and meticulous artist can manipulate his audience by playing upon certain expectations concerning disease and its location in society.

Model Theory and the Construction of Disease

According to Miriam Siegler and Humphry Osmond, modern medicine postulates eight clearly differentiated models for mental illness alone. Ranging from the "medical" model, in which the patient is the object of treatment, through the "conspiratorial" model, which denies the existence of the concept "patient," these views circumscribe the complex ways in which various groups define their relationship to the mentally ill. Models, as Siegler and Osmond are at pains to point out, are "abstractions. They are inventions of the human mind to place facts, events, and theories in an orderly manner. They are not necessarily true or false."[18] They are ordering principles, nothing more or less. They are the structures generated by the mythopoesis of disease. But the ordering principles described by Siegler and Osmond do not exhaust the often imperceptible differences between models. For rather than being eight self-enclosed structures, they are eight major nodes on a continuous spectrum of interlocking definitions. Each model, through an infinite series of submodels, flows into other related models. This continuum is illustrated by the subtle analysis provided by Paul R. McHugh and Phillip R. Slavney in their study of "the perspectives of psychiatry."[19] It holds true in the construction of all diseases, whether "real" or "invented," whether emotional or somatic. And these models of perception shift when the models of science upon which they are based shift. One can speak of contrastive models only after a certain mass of differentiation is obtained.

This synchronic manner of observing the existing models of describing insanity is, however, inherently incomplete. For, just as there is a continuum of models that exist contemporaneously, so too are there innumerable historical models from which these models stem or against which they react. Indeed, as in Chapter 9, in which we trace how Western models of disease are absorbed into Chinese medicine, one can see how powerful systems can (and do) displace other systems understood as weak. This process can also be seen in the involved history of one of the most controversial psychiatric diagnoses, that of schizophrenia, where various models of disease interact and replace one another. A diachronic view of Siegler and Osmond's eight models would show a latticework of models from every time and level of historical development present in residual form within their synchronic view of disease. Some models have been reduced to the folkloric, others exist only in Western general historical consciousness, while still others possess all of the status given by society to the healing arts. Thus the critical reader understands not only the contemporary manner of viewing insanity as an exemplary disease but also the evolution of the models employed. For more often than not the historical development of a given model or set of models reveals hidden preconceptions that have been masked or mutilated through the passage of time. They reveal how the discourse of power uses (or generates) images of illness for many ends, drawing on this wide repertory of images to isolate, stigmatize, and control.

"Madness" is often the test case for those who claim that there is nothing but the social construction of disease, that these models of mental illness exist independent of any reality. They believe that no such entity as mental illness exists; therefore, any history of madness is, in truth, a representation of only a socially constructed (and therefore, in their minds, "unreal") category of difference.[20] If one considers the ideas of disease—all disease, including mental illness—as realities, but as realities mirrored in and conceptualized through the pressures of social forces and psychological models, then the question becomes much more complex and, indeed, much more interesting. For realities are interesting to all of us at risk (and we are all at risk, or so we understand ourselves). If the ideas were only part of a complex system of representation without any reality present, we who pride ourselves on our "insight" and "rationality" would know that this was a world that could not threaten us. Those who deny the reality of the experience of disease marginalize and exclude the ill from their own world. Pure fantasy is much easier to understand; it would be totally protean and distanced. Fantasy constrained by realities, whether the realities are of physical or mental illness, is much more complex and therefore perhaps (in an odd reversal of Occam's razor) more believable. For the palpable signs of illness, the pain and suffering of the patient, cannot be simply dismissed as a social construction, even though this pain may be understood by patient and health care practitioner alike in a socially determined manner.

In order to make the social construction of the various images of disease more visible, and to illustrate how various levels of historical consciousness are present in a given model for disease, a heterogeneous series of representations of disease has been chosen for this book. Rather than using the historical background of these categories of disease merely to illustrate the prejudices of present models, as has been the case, for example, with the exercises in the history of psychiatry by such critics of contemporary psychiatric practice as Michel Foucault and Thomas Szasz, the texts and images under consideration will be examined without negative preconceptions of their place in the development of categories of disease, including those of mental illness.[21] Early modern as well as contemporary models of disease, including aspects of mental illness, have been selected as the objects of my analysis, since, while the distance that time provides seems to help clarify the construction of categories of disease, we can examine our contemporary constructions of illness with much the same approach. I have not avoided the most complex contemporary problems in the construction of models of disease, such as schizophrenia and AIDS, since I believe that the web of my argument provides sufficient cross-references to make the historical roots of the models of disease in these cases clear.

A Test Case: The Construction of Violent Insanity

Earlier investigations of models of diseases which examined the historical evolution of such structures chose to ignore the distancing effect of historical material. Instead, they used earlier texts to criticize models that evolved later. Such post facto approaches to the history of disease are possible, of course, but they tend to offer a simplistic parallel between prior and existing models rather than the subtle and complex interplay of models that actually exists. The simultaneous presence of multiple models of a disease, such as insanity, can often be the explanation for seeming inconsistencies within systems built upon these models. Such complexity is evident within contemporary models, but it is present in all models of disease, from those of the ancient Greeks to those of contemporary America.

The analysis of representations of disease illuminates the function of such models as means of social control. One can turn to a specific problem in the interrelated history of madness, violence, and the body—the construction of the image of the insane as violent—for illustration. One of the structures that emerges in examining such popular images of the insane is the dichotomy perceived by the general public between two basic states of "madness"—the passive state and its active antithesis. Both are understood to be highly exaggerated states of being and therefore indicative of "madness." The first state, while of interest historically, plays little role in the present study. The image of the mad person as suffering from the sin of lethargy, call it melancholy or depression, is of interest only because it reappears today in some of the charges brought by the opponents of contemporary diagnostic categories who see madness as simply shamming illness. Melancholy, depression, lethargy, one of the ten deadly sins in the medieval canon, categorizes the "mad" simply as lazy. This perceived exaggeration of a normal state has permitted the antipsychiatric movement to use the popular image of the lethargic mad person as the basis of its view that all one has to do to cure the mentally ill is to motivate them. What is striking is that the iconography associated with melancholia infiltrates other categories of disease, such as syphilis and AIDS, as will be shown in Chapter 14.

The other state is of considerably more interest through its construction of the image of the violent insane. It is the "mad" as maniacal, out of control, running amok. In this state the mad are perceived as unable to control their own actions, limbs wildly waving, slavering, and, most important, violently aggressive. It is the popular image of the mad, found everywhere from medieval religious art depicting the objects of Christ's cure to contemporary comic strips illustrating uncontrolled rage, and underlies the paradox inherent in understanding the popular notion of the mad as criminal.

How are "mad-dog" criminals supposed to look, how are they supposed to behave? In the public eye they are the epitome of the hyperactive, aggressive, "mad" person. Let us stop for a moment and consider why this is. The mad, especially in the incarnation of the aggressive mad, are one of the most common focuses for the general anxiety felt by all members of society, an anxiety tied to a perceived tenuousness of life. If I am afraid that I am to be attacked, have my goods stolen, lose my status in society, I do not want this fear to be universal, pervading every moment of my life. I want to know who is going to rob me, who is going to attack me, who is going to steal my hard-won status. So each society selects a certain number of categories onto which it projects its anxieties. Because of the very limitations on the number of outsiders in Western society, we can tabulate these categories. We are afraid of Jews, Blacks, Women, Homosexuals, Madmen, Gypsies, and others we designate as "different." But this liturgy of Otherness can be extended or expanded by the needs of any given society. The nineteenth century's fixation with the Otherness of redheads is one example that today strikes us as comic. And yet such an example, because of its inappropriateness (or seeming inappropriateness), can help us understand the implications and strength of the image of the aggressive mad. Redheaded people are dangerous. They are not in control of their emotions. They are visibly different. Now, whatever the antecedent of the image of the fiery redhead is, whether or not it comes from a Celtic inheritance as perceived by the dark-haired or light-haired inhabitants of central Europe, redheadedness signaled that one should have an appropriate sense of anxiety. If you see someone who is redheaded, you can be assured that he or she may well act in an aggressive and dangerous manner. Aggressiveness, especially aggressiveness perceived as out of the control of the individual (for we do not determine the natural color of our hair) is confined to those individuals who bear specific signs.

To see how this operates in regard to the mad as perceived in contemporary society, let us take another example, one that will be immediate and direct, since it is one that I am sure each of us has experienced at one time or another. As is evident, with the increasing deinstitutionalization of the mentally ill, it is becoming more and more frequent that the casual observer encounters on the street someone who is both behaving oddly and looking odd. On the streets of our cities we see the "bag-lady." We register her as different because she looks bizarre. Her appearance and her collection of shopping bags mark her as an individual who does not fall within the range of what we have been taught to perceive as normal— either in dressing or in comportment. And worst of all she is arguing, screaming at an unseen, internalized adversary. How do we react? Well, one of our initial reactions is anxiety. Perhaps she will "turn" on us, make us the brunt of her "insane" rage, hurt us, involve us. We cross the street, avoiding her.[22] Now, the "bag-lady" and "bag-man" live in their own world. Their demons are within them. Their behavior is erratic and perhaps dangerous, but dangerous only for themselves. We perceive this as an attack on our order, on a world that must be held in check for us to function in it. Such anxiety is higher in cities than in rural areas.[23] The mentally ill can function in less stressful and demanding environments, such as rural areas, at a level of impairment which would make them nonfunctional in cities. "The insane" are thus marked by their actions, and these actions generate responses that are dictated by the context of the observer.

Our response to the perceived aggressiveness of the mad (as well as of all the other outsiders) reassures us. We have localized the source of our fear. We know who is dangerous. We respond correctly in such situations and thus we have control over our world. But what happens when, as one might well expect, our preprogrammed, stereotypical perception of the "mad" comes into violent conflict with the realities of mental illness, which do not signal themselves in the expected manner? What happens when it is not the identifiable "mad person" who turns out to be aggressive, but the "normal, nice kid next door?" We have a pattern in twentieth-century America of evident public surprise when the "mad bomber" turns out to be a retired, meek little man living on a pension, or the "son of Sam" turns out to work for the post office and live in a high-rise apartment. Such a context is not appropriate for the "mad-dog killer." The banality of real mental illness comes into conflict with our need to have the mad be identifiable, different from ourselves. Our shock is always that they are really just like us. This moment, when we say, "they are just like us," is most upsetting. Then we no longer know where lies the line that divides our normal, reliable world, a world that minimizes our fears, from that world in which lurks the fearful, the terrifying, the aggressive. We want—no, we need—the "mad" to be different, so we create out of the stuff of their reality myths that make them different. Madness, now in the concrete form of the "mad-dog killer," must still be understood as inherently different and identifiable.[24]

We have been talking in fairly broad abstractions about the popular understanding of madness and the function of this understanding in our daily lives. Let us for a moment turn to a specific problem in forensic psychiatry and see how this myth-building has continued into the present (and perhaps will continue into the future). Let us consider the myth of what makes a "mad-dog killer." Perhaps the best place to begin is with the quintessential "mad-dog killer" of nineteenth-century fiction, Raskolnikov, the murderer of the old moneylender in Feodor Dostoevski's *Crime and Punishment*. Now, no one is going to confuse Raskolnikov and Dostoevski's Petersburg with the real world. The novel is clearly a fictional creation, the ground for examining a series of intellectual and philosophical problems, and in which the "mad-dog killer" is used as the focus of this investigation. Why does Raskolnikov kill the old woman? Well, one of the suggested reasons was that his poor food and vile lodgings ruined his health. He then read a number of dangerous books, the power of which overwhelmed him while he was in this debilitated state. His pattern is one that meshes well with a nineteenth-century understanding of the basis of psychopathology. Wilhelm Griesinger, the most influential German psychiatrist at mid-century, coined the phrase: "Mind illness is brain illness," and Raskolnikov's sociopathic act was explained, at least in part for his contemporaries, by the basic alteration to his somatic state. It isn't the mind that's sick, it's the body (and in the case of the "mad-dog killer" Raskolnikov, the cause of this illness rests in the basic sickness of the state itself). This may work well in fiction. A specific illness is attributed to a specific limited cause, which lies outside the control of the individual, so that the actions are, in truth, those of an automaton. In the real world, or at least in the world of the courts, this fiction persists, in spite of the major insights into the nature of psychopathology acquired during the twentieth century. One could begin with the 1904 German trial of Wilhelm Fischer, accused of having murdered his girlfriend.[25] He was shown, through physical evidence, to have suffered some type of "congenital epilepsy" which made him fall prey to the baneful influence of his readings of the German avant-garde philosopher Friedrich Nietzsche. He was tried and found to have been suffering from diminished capacity. By 1924 the myth that links faults in human biology with sociopathic acts reappeared in Clarence Darrow's claim that the murder of Bobby Franks by his clients, Richard Loeb and Nathan Leopold, Jr., might well have been the result of some type of endocrinological fault. One of Darrow's defense witnesses, Dr. H. S. Hulbert, even intimated that perhaps the baneful influence of "congenital epilepsy" might be at cause: the cause of what?—not the crime itself, but of the fact that Leopold and Loeb fell prey to their reading, also, in this case, of Nietzsche. Darrow's summation was brilliant. He pointed out that there had to be some fault within his clients which predetermined their weakness and their unnatural response to their reading. For, Darrow stated, "I have read almost everything that Nietzsche ever wrote. . . . More books have been written about him than about all the rest of the philosophers within a hundred years. More college professors have talked about him"—and, Darrow implies, none of them went crazy and killed a little boy.[26] By 1924 the myth of a purely biologically determined etiology for irresistible impulse had become so entrenched in popular fancy that Leopold and Loeb, like Walter Fischer twenty years before, received lesser sentences than their crimes would have otherwise called for. This is not to say that Fischer, Leopold, and Loeb were not mentally ill. Most probably all three, by the best views of their and our age, could be understood to be. But more important, their attorneys were able to persuade those who judged them that they were "crazy." That is, that they fulfilled the public's expectations to be seen as "madmen." The biological evidence was introduced to provide them with "identifiable signs," much like red hair, which would label them and make them different.

For this is the center of our popular understanding of madness: madness must express itself in a way that is inherently different. When in the 1960s there seemed to be evidence that sociopaths all showed similar genetic errors, a great sigh of relief was heard in society. Here was a clear, irrefutable marker that provided a specific sign and a direct etiology for sociopathic and psychopathic acts. That this genetic pattern proved to be chimerical surprised few who thought about it in any depth. For how could all of those acts labeled by society as psychopathic or sociopathic possibly be reduced to a single root cause? The desire to divide the sane from the mad, the criminal from the normal, had been at the basis of the most successful forensic psychiatric system in nineteenth-century Europe, that of Cesare Lombroso.[27] Lombroso, in studies of criminal men and women, saw the criminal as a specific subtype, a throwback, who possessed specific stigmata, signs, which identified his or her madness. Lombroso, who was a professor in Turin in the north of Italy, found most of his signs through his study of criminals from the south of Italy. Signs of madness were closely related to signs of social inferiority in Lombroso's system!

The broad spectrum of mental illness must be understood as resulting from a broad spectrum of causes, which, as in somatic illness, play themselves out over time but which, unlike some somatic illnesses, may manifest different constellations of symptoms. While we need a specific cause and pattern for "madness," this need is society's and mirrors society's desire to control and to isolate those elements that it perceives to be uncontrollable. A differentiated understanding of mental illness, not a reductive one, is needed in law, when the desire is to evaluate and treat those designated as mentally ill.

The case against John W. Hinckley, Jr., accused (and then acquitted) of the attempted assassination of Ronald Reagan, illustrates the dichotomy between societal understanding of "madness" and a workable definition of mental illness.[28] One is struck in looking back over the case by the demand of the defense to introduce evidence by Dr. Marjorie Lemay, a radiologist, that computer-assisted brain scans showed that Hinckley's brain had "shrunk." The debate concerning the admission of this evidence revolved about the question of whether or not it was "relevant," and the court finally decided that it was. But relevant to what? There is certainly no link between brain size and schizophrenia shown by psychiatry at this time. Even the defense acquiesced to this fact. Why then was it necessary to introduce this material? Because it showed that there was a potential physical cause of Hinckley's action, a cause that lay outside of his own control, that lay buried deep within his biology, not his psyche. Hinckley's illness was linked, none too subtly, with the repetitive viewing of the movie *Taxi Driver*, viewings that showed an innate susceptibility, because he, unlike the millions of others who saw the movie, acted upon his viewing.[29] This was, by the way, the gist of the testimony given by Dr. Ernest Prelinger during the trial—never, of course, in such a blunt, clearly mythopoetic manner, which returns us to Raskolnikov's reading anarchist's pamphlets in his hovel, but cast in the most up-to-date language of medical science. As with the earlier case, such evidence, which draws not on competent medical knowledge but on the world of myth, corrupts the language of science. While it plays to the stereotypical perception of the public and has its desired effect, the mitigation of the sentence of the accused, it is bad medicine. For it is the reification of our need to be shown how, in the most specific detail, the "mad" are different from us, and different in a way in which we can never be. For we do not harbor the hidden curse of "congenital epilepsy," neither are our brains "shrunken." These are the signs that make the "mad" different from us, but they are signs read only by the observer and bear little resemblance to the realities of mental illness.

Now a caveat. What I have been speaking about is the popular understanding of the "mad." There are specific physical alterations which may precipitate sociopathic or psychopathic acts. One need but remember the University of Texas sniper with his brain tumor or the "crocodile man" with his faulty limbic system.[30] These are illnesses that exist within individuals and that are specifically localizable. What I am writing about is the *need* to see such a pattern at work behind all "madness." This is an important distinction, since it influences the way that the public sees all mentally ill people. The fear of aggression from the mentally ill is not limited to the fear of the "bag-lady." Once we have explained to ourselves that Fischer, Leopold, Loeb, or Hinckley have specific markers that can be recognized and that set them off against the normal world, we may contain our anxiety and limit it to the "mad" as its cause. But our category of the "mad" has been radically expanded. The reaction to the Tylenol (and related) murders of the 1980s is indicative. We are all afraid of these "mad people," as they have been called over and over in both the media and official pronouncements. They are aggressive, and we must defend ourselves. But against whom? Against the "mad." But the mentally ill are not all aggressive; they do not all demand to be feared by their actions, their external or their internal signs. Most of the mentally ill in no way correspond to our stereotype of them, but the perception of the small number of the mentally ill as the embodiment of our image of the "mad" causes us to place all of the mentally ill into the greater category of the "dangerous lunatic," to use a good nineteenth-century label. The result is one that is seen every day: the suppression of information about mental illness, since it is perceived as a stigma in our society; the isolation of the mentally ill as if they had contagion or the avoidance of them if they present themselves in public view; the sense that the mentally ill form another world that is beyond, or below, or outside of our own. And the mentally ill do respond to this stereotyping of themselves. Mental illness is part of the potential of the human condition. It has many possible manifestations, many causes, many outcomes. But society does not respond to this differentiation. The mentally ill are simply "mad," and the stereotype of madness dominates and shapes their realities since they must live in our world, no matter if we say that they live in their own world. The danger with such cases as that of John Hinckley, Jr., is not that Hinckley was found to be mentally ill. It is that the idea of madness which ran like an undercurrent through the trial was rooted in the stereotype of the aggressive madman and the specific and limited nature of his illness. Hinckley's benign appearance initially puzzled the public. How could a nice young man do a thing like that? When the evidence of his "shrunken" brain was finally introduced, it could well have been seen as proof enough. The public's stereotype of the mad was reified by the twists and turns of the Hinckley case. When we are next confronted by one who is mentally ill, whether within the family or on the street, this reification will have the effect of heightening the anxiety caused by and directed at that person. It is not the confusions raised by the Hinckley trial which are over the long run dangerous within our society, but rather the perpetuations of the stereotypes concerning the mentally ill.

It is indeed the social implications of the construction of stereotypes of disease, society's image of the patient as well as the internalized response of the patient, which is the reason for any study of these structures of perception and representation. In this book our ongoing attempt to categorize (and, therefore, to distance) ourselves from those we label as different (and their response) will be examined.

Madness and Representation:
Toward a History of Visualizing Madness

Representations of Madness

What does art show us? Certainly not the "real" world. The images of Bosch or Van Gogh, of Warhol or Escher may reflect the mental representations of some inner world, but not the mundane one in which we live. And yet these private constructions are real. They are expressions of myths about the world, the ideas that we project onto it and that shape our understanding of the realities that we experience.[1] The central reality for the health care practitioner is illness. One rarely questions that physical illness is real, that it is part of the world. We see the signs and symptoms of illness, and they tell us something about the state of the patient. Not so evident is that this process of "seeing" is highly charged by the qualities that we ascribe to illness. Indeed, we can create "diseases" that have a life quite independent of any biological, emotional, or psychopathological source. When Adolf Hitler spoke of the Jews as a "cancer in the body politic," the phrase was not merely a metaphor; it was charged with all of the fear that we associate with that illness. When the doctor or nurse wishes to avoid the AIDS patient, all of the anxiety associated with sexually transmitted diseases surfaces. In no area of medicine is the problem of reading the hidden message buried in our perception of the patient more difficult than in the treatment of mental illness.

Following World War II there were major swings in the perception of mental illness. First there was a radical reaction to the models of mental illness held by traditional psychoanalytic psychotherapy. Such writers as Thomas Szasz and R. D. Laing began to see mental illness as an artifact of society. Then the resurgence of a biologically oriented psychiatry in the past decade has led to the illusion that mental illness is simply an artifact of biology. Both views ignore the fact that the *idea* of mental illness structures both the perception of disease and its form. To illustrate this mixture of the "seeing" of an illness and its reality, we can begin in the late Middle Ages. The illness melancholy was viewed as the result of the imbalance of the humors; black bile, a mythic entity, dominated the melancholic. The model is given to us by the medieval German poet Walther von der Vogelweide:

> I sat down on a stone,
> and crossed my legs
> and set my elbows on them;
> I rested my chin and cheek in my hand.
> Then I pondered very earnestly
> how one ought to live one's life on earth.
> I could not find the solution.[2]

But Walther did not see himself as "mad" or even as "melancholic." He had taken the classical pose of the pensive philosopher, a pose analogous to figures of grief in scenes of the Crucifixion. How do these images of philosophic thought and grief relate to the image of the melancholic madwoman (Plate 1)? Both are understood to be states of the disruption of balance, and when this imbalance is exaggerated, it slips into melancholy. Madness is thus extreme states of imbalance. But why are these images female? The superficial reason is grammatical: *melancholia* is a feminine noun. But this is only the point of departure. The female is perceived as being especially prone to the exaggeration of emotional states; thus she becomes the icon of melancholia. When male characters in the medieval epic were portrayed as melancholic, they were given passive, "female" characteristics. When the mentally ill define themselves, in reality or in fiction, it is in the same passive relationship to society as the woman's. Myth-making usually surrounds fictive signs and symptoms, like black bile, as a means of representing an invisible state—mental illness. The entire tradition of the "cutting of the stone of madness" presumes such a stone as the cause of madness. But like the position of the melancholic woman and her black bile, the stone of madness is merely the visualization of some unknown state (Plate 2).[3]

During the Middle Ages and the Renaissance, this manner of seeing the insane resulted from the need to separate out and identify those who were perceived as different. Indeed, as early as the thirteenth century the face of the madman embellished a transept corner on the cathedral at Reims, joining the other visual parodies of humanity (Plate 3). The "cut-

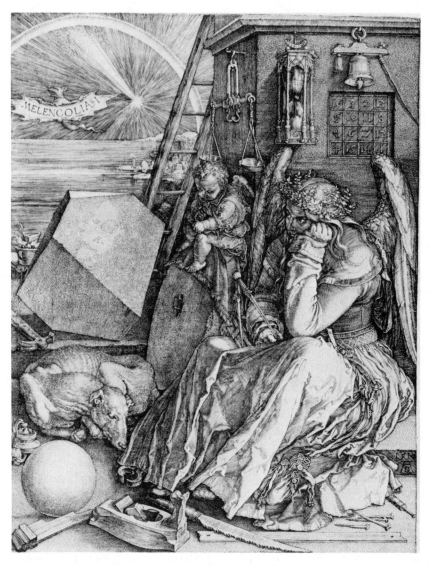

1. Albrecht Dürer, *Melancolia I* (1514) (Herbert F. Johnson Museum of Art, Cornell University; Bequest of William P. Chapman, Jr.).

ting of the stone of madness," however, is not an image of the correct mode of treatment. It is not a Renaissance trepanning, but rather the mocking of those who needed to see madness as rooted in some sort of objective physical cause. The Renaissance simultaneously used and suspected the older theory of the humors. Such thinkers as Paracelsus and

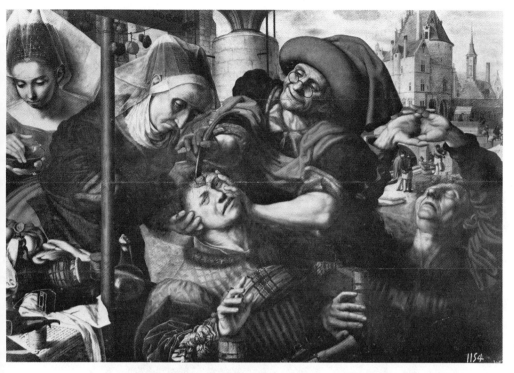

2. Jan Sanders van Hemessen, *Cutting of the Stones of Folly* (c. 1530) (Prado, Madrid).

Fracastoro began to doubt the idea of imbalance, and the artist reflected and augmented that doubt. The physicians in that tradition were quacks, indicated by their garments and tools; the patients were usually shown as rustics in much the same way. These portraits, then, are pictures of the rube as fool being taken by the big-city slicker.

The stone of madness is the web of falsity that convinces both patient and physician of the efficacy of such treatments of mental illness. But the artist knew his audience: he portrayed the stone of madness as if it were real in order to point out to his viewers their own involvement in this deception. We do not merely sit back and laugh at the gullibility of the poor rube; we are part of the action. We too believe, even if on a more sophisticated level, that all we have to do is localize the root of the illness and then—magic!—it will vanish, leaving the ill like the evil spirits Christ drove from the swine.

Up to this point in history we see the myths about madness as contained within the frame of the works of art. The frame literally draws the line between the woodcut or painting and the realities of the world. But this framing was no longer felt to be safe enough. A new myth arose out of the need to contain the mentally ill within some structure that would isolate them from the world—the image of a ship on which representative mad people are confined. Beginning with Sebastian Brant's *Ship of Fools* in 1494, this image became a standard means of separating the outsider from the world of the "sane" observer. Some versions have sexual references. In Hieronymus Bosch's, there are icons of immorality—the eating of cherries and the hazel branch tied to the mast (Plate 4). These parallel the icons of insanity. Here, the most prominent is the fool seated in the position of the melancholic, his fool's stick clutched in

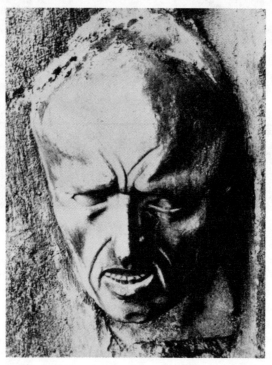

3. The mask of the madman, transept corner, Reims Cathedral (thirteenth century) (Warburg Institute, London).

his hand. He is perched on a desiccated, divided branch, which serves as the icon of madness for the entire ship. The power of this image—the floating world of the fool—rests to no little degree on the myth of the mad as travelers, an image still with us in R. D. Laing's patient Mary Barnes and her "journey through madness." In the sixteenth century the mad were the explorers, such as Columbus, and they were condemned for disrupting the stable image of society.

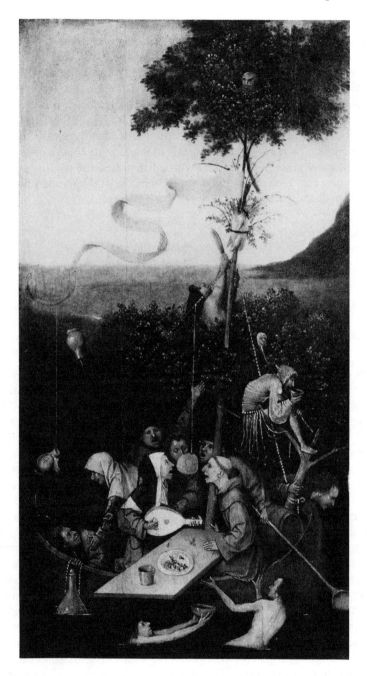

4. Hieronymus Bosch, *Ship of Fools* (late fifteenth century) (Louvre, Paris).

The confinement of the insane in asylums, the real world's counterpart to the ship of fools in art, began in the Renaissance.[4] By the eighteenth century, the mad were portrayed in the state-run asylum, an image closely associated with other images of confinement such as prison. William Hogarth's work, especially his series of prints *The Rake's Progress* (1735), continued the tradition of Brant by showing how society confined all those forces that threatened social order (Plate 5). Hogarth's hero, Rakewell, is portrayed in exactly the same manner as the statue of "raving" madness which adorned the portals of Bedlam, the Bethlem asylum. Under the final plate in the series, which illustrated the decline and fall of the young fop, Hogarth penned these lines, so no viewer would miss the import of the image:

> O Vanity of Age! here
> See The Stamp of Heaven effac'd by
> Thee—The headstrong Course of Youth thus run,
> What comfort from this darling Son!
> His rattling Chains with Terror hear,
> Behold Death grappling with Despair;
> See Him by Thee to Ruin Sold,
> And curse thyself, and curse thy Gold.[5]

Rakewell inherited his money rather than earned it, and the curse on money unearned in the struggles of the world led him to the madhouse. It is a madhouse populated by the entire spectrum of the insane, from the melancholic lover seated on the stairs to the religious zealot in the cell to the far left. As in *Ship of Fools*, these represent the entire range of the outsider. But Hogarth's contemporaries, unlike those of Bosch, saw this image of Bedlam, in the words of the German philosopher Lichtenberg, as an "extended Macro-Bedlam, the world itself; not all the madmen are chained, and even the chains have their degrees."[6]

The mad can be identified by the myths of their external appearance, as in melancholy, their signs of illness (the stones of madness) or their setting. In the eighteenth century, Swiss preacher-author Johann Lavater introduced a new way of seeing the insane—physiognomy. Lavater, drawing on a tradition as old as Babylon, began to examine human beings not on the basis of external appearance, clothing, or position, but on inherent qualities—the shape of the nose, the color of the eyes, the structure of head and frame. All these characteristics predetermined character and thus the predisposition to mental illness, which he believed to be merely a reflection of character. Skin color, shape of the face, the length of the nose—all played a role in his system. Just as Lavater's portrait of two cretins captures the idiocy of the subjects in their "sloping

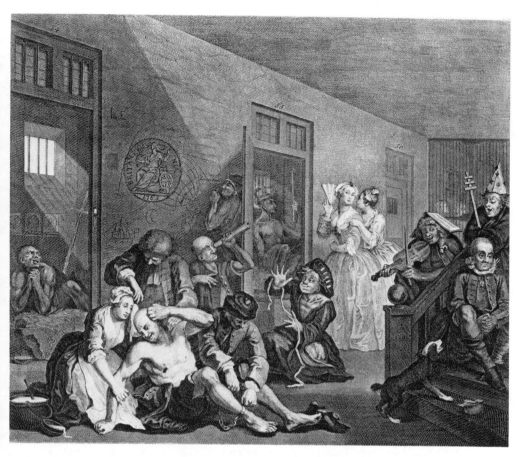

5. William Hogarth, *The Rake's Progress*, Plate VIII (1735/1763) (National Library of Medicine, Washington, D.C.).

foreheads," his melancholic is characterized by the (Saturnian) "unequal forehead," depressions in the temples, and sunken eyes; the blackness of aspect and disheveled hair complete the classic image. From the Renaissance, line drawings of the heads of typical human types were employed to present inherent typologies of appearance.[7]

While the tradition of physiognomy continued unabated from the Renaissance through the eighteenth century, it was only in the 1770s that this mode of description and illustration captured the popular fancy of all Europe. In that decade Lavater's works on physiognomy were an immediate success throughout the continent. In Lavater's programmatic work *On Physiognomy* of 1772 there is an outline of a physiognomy of illness which, however, is not proportionally represented in his major, four-volume *Physiognomic Fragments,* published between 1774 and 1778. Lavater's impressionistic analysis of physiognomy postulated a strict relationship between physical and spiritual traits. Rooted in Leibniz's view that the source of human identity lies in the individuality of the body, Lavater saw the monist relationship of body and mind as the key to the personality. His illustrations of this relationship are rooted in the simplistic visual analogies found in the Renaissance. His influence, however, was intense and immediate. In the second volume of *Physiognomic Fragments* there are two plates illustrating mental pathologies of the most diverse nature, under the general heading "weak, mad humans" (Plate 6). Lavater rhapsodized about the nature of mental pathology in his introduction to the fragment. He drew from these cases of mental illness proof of the efficacy of his method.[8]

The difficulty of the medium used to illustrate the cases presented in Lavater's *Fragments* was evident to his collaborators on the work, especially to the twenty-six-year-old Johann Wolfgang von Goethe. Commenting on the added complexity introduced by the nature of the illustrations into his physiognomic analysis of one of the plates, Goethe wrote to Lavater: "Thought a bit yesterday about the four mad ones and Brutus. Brother, Brother—how difficult it is to bring the dead etching to life, where character only glimmers through misunderstood lines, where one is in doubt what has meaning and what doesn't. How different is life!"[9] Goethe concerns himself with the shortcomings of the medium rather than the validity of the method. This view is later echoed in Immanuel Kant's comment concerning the nature of physiognomic analysis. In his *Anthropology from a Pragmatic Point of View* (1798) Kant compares the line drawings of the Renaissance with the fashionable silhouettes employed in part by Lavater and concludes that it is the medium that determines the observer's analysis.[10]

The Medical Semiotics of Insanity

By the end of the eighteenth century it was commonplace that forms of insanity, such as melancholy, could be identified by the physical appearance of the person afflicted. Shortly following this period, this cultural commonplace begins to appear in technical medical descriptions of insanity in the form of illustrations of the mentally ill. Thus if one looks at the medical literature on insanity during the eighteenth century one is struck by the paucity of graphic material. Even in the most avant-garde writings on mental illness these visual presentations are lacking. In Vincenzo Chiarugi's *On Madness in General,* published in three volumes in 1793 and 1794, there are but two plates. In the first, modes of treatment

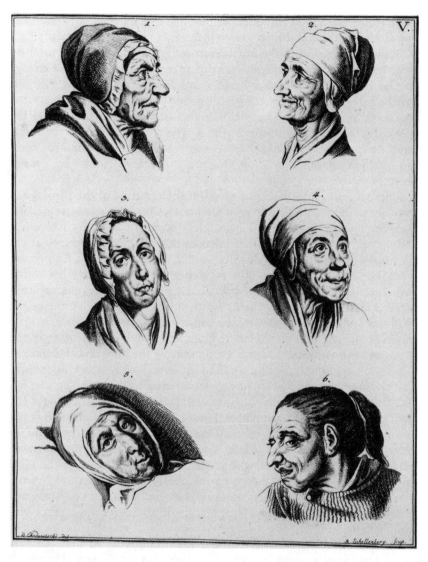

6. One of Daniel Chodowiecki's plates of the insane for Lavater's *Physiognomic Fragments* (1774–78) (Olin Library, Cornell University, Ithaca, N.Y.)

are illustrated, the patients serving as objects, and in the second, the patient as such vanishes completely, the illustrations being anatomical studies of brain structures.[11]

It is therefore even more striking that when Philippe Pinel published his *Medico-philosophical Treatise on Mental Alienation, or Mania* in

27

1801 he accompanied the publication with a plate that illustrated the appearance of mental illness in two patients, an idiot and a maniac (Plate 7).[12] By the first year of the nineteenth century, illustrations of insanity were introduced into medical works on mental illness through a change in the philosophy of the scientific description of insanity. Philippe Pinel's role in the introduction of humane means of treatment for the insane is well known. That he was also instrumental in altering the mode of observing the insane is less so. His study of medical classification, *Philosophical Nosology or Analytic Method as Applied to Medicine*, which appeared in 1798, described diseases in order to classify them.[13]

Pinel's approach to medicine stood in the tradition of the *Idéologues*, who, founding their philosophy of science on Condillac's sensationalism, developed a strictly empirical approach to scientific facts. For Helvétius, Condorcet, Pinel, and the other Idéologues, systematic description was an impossibility; only single cases could be observed and limited inferences made from them. This radical empiricism directly led to the introduction of illustrations of psychiatric patients in the medical literature. The illustrations in Pinel's study of insanity permitted the reader to observe the cases described. The confrontation between the scientific observer and the observable fact is heightened by the immediacy of the medium of illustration. In his plate presenting the idiot and the maniac, Pinel compared the size of the skull to the overall body size. He contends that the maniac, who was subject to only sporadic attacks of insanity, has a skull better proportioned to the overall size of the body than does the idiot and closer to the ideal proportions of the Apollo Belvedere. (It is not surprising therefore that the maniac's disability is not as constant or great as that of the idiot.) While Pinel did not make any further comparisons, he created an analogue to the relative appearance of the ideal and the pathological. He presented the observer with a series of visual clues of two forms of mental illness (idiocy and mania) in contrast to a classical ideal of expression. Thus a scale of normative appearance was established.

While Pinel's introduction of the illustrations of mental patients seemed to create an even greater sense of objectivity, the actual nature of the graphic art employed revealed the preconceptions inherent in them. The desired objectivity of Pinel's method can be seen as inherently biased once the parallels to his mode of illustration are known. For the visual structure of Pinel's plate is borrowed from the tradition of Lavater's physiognomy. The immediacy (as well as the difficulty) of observing the uniqueness of the insane lies behind both Lavater's and Pinel's visual presentation of the mentally ill. While departing from two generally different models of insanity, they both use illustrations to indicate the

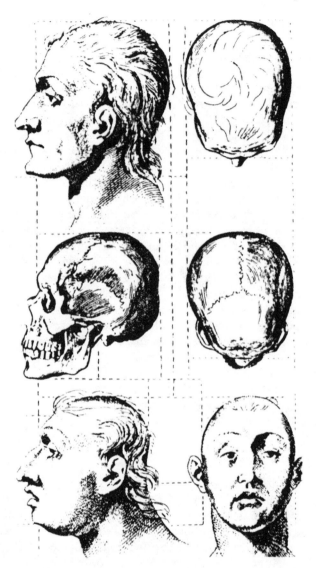

7. The head of a maniac contrasted with the head of an idiot, from Philippe Pinel's *Traité médico-philosophique* (Paris: Richard, Caille et Ravier IX [1801]) (private collection, Ithaca, N.Y.).

pathology of insanity as reflected in the physiological structure of the heads of patients. Secondarily, both qualify the heads presented as those of the mentally ill by the fixed expressions on their faces.

These two approaches merge quite naturally in the French edition of

Lavater edited by Jacques Louis Moreau (de la Sarthe). Moreau de la Sarthe was one of the most influential psychiatrists of his day, having written the essay "Mental Medicine" in the *Methodological Encyclopedia* (1816).[14] In 1807 he brought out a seven-volume translation of Lavater's *Fragments* supplemented by a series of appendices, the first of which concerned itself with the "physiognomy of the insane." The major plate in this section reprints the heads of the maniac and the idiot from Pinel as well as the head of Victor, the feral child from Jean Marc Gaspard Itard's *On the Education of the Wild Man of Aveyron* (1801). But Moreau is much more interested in the expression of the faces presented by Pinel and Itard. Concerning the appearance of the maniac, Moreau extrapolates the following: "His state of deep, melancholy madness is unmistakable. One can easily see that the characteristic traits are present in the constant expression of his physiognomy rather than in the configuration of his head." Of the feral boy, who was also assumed to be mentally ill, the portrait "needs no commentary, and one cannot overlook the dominant expression of ferocity, of amazement, mixed with agitation and the excessive mobility of the face."[15]

Here the transferal of radical objectivity from the measurable (i.e., Pinel's measurement of relative skull size) to the impressionable (i.e., the analysis of the expression of the mentally ill) has been completed. While studies of expression, such as Johann Jakob Engel's *Ideas on Imitation* (1785–86), became popular at the end of the eighteenth century, pathologies of expression were not central to their scope. It is with the blending of physiognomy and the new psychiatry that such questions were raised for the first time on the continent.

Medicine and Art

In 1806 Sir Charles Bell, one of the pioneers in describing the physiology of expression, had turned to the question of the expression of the emotions in art with the publication of a work that never went completely out of print during the entire course of the nineteenth century, his *Essays on the Anatomy of Expression*.[16] Illustrated by Bell himself, the work, which would certainly have been known to any professional (or, indeed, amateur) artist in Great Britain during the nineteenth century, provides an extended commentary on what the artist was supposed to be representing when depicting the insane (Plate 8). First "you see him lying in his cell regardless of everything, with a death-like fixed gloom upon his countenance. When I say it is a death-like gloom, I mean a heaviness of the features without knitting of the brows or action of the muscles." Here the madman is the passive image of insanity, even though clearly

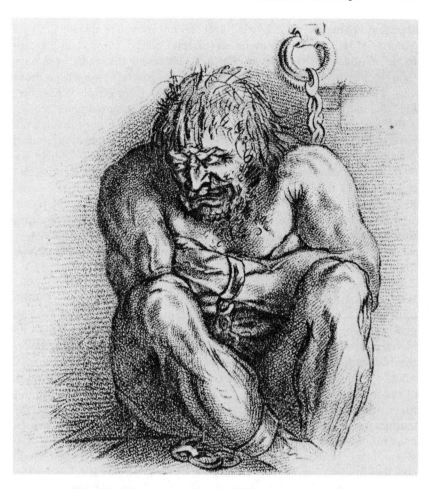

8. Charles Bell's "Madness," from his *Essays on the Anatomy of Expression in Painting* (London: Longman et al., 1806) (private collection, Ithaca, N.Y.).

masculine. (Bell uses the pronoun "he" throughout his description of "madness.") Second, "his inflamed eye is fixed upon you, and his features lighten up into an inexpressible wildness and ferocity." The madman has a "human countenance . . . devoid of expression, and reduced to the state of brutality." To understand it "we must have recourse to the lower animals; and as I have already hinted, study their expression, their timidity, their watchfulness, their state of excitement, and their ferociousness. If we should happily transfer their expression to the human countenance, we should, as I conceive it, irresistibly convey the idea of madness, vacancy of mind, and mere animal passion." With his visualization of the insane as bestial, Bell has not moved much further than Moreau de la Sarthe, who included the feral boy of Aveyron in his catalogue of images of the insane. For Bell, however, the image was more than documentary, for when one portrays the insane "it is with a moral aim, to show the consequence of vice and the indulgence of passion": Bell understood the iconographic implications of his madman.

Bell's portrait of the "madman" stands in the tradition of juxtaposing passive and aggressive madness as well as within the new science of physiognomy. In the early eighteenth century Caius Gabriel Cibber had sculpted two statues for the portal of Bethlem Hospital (Bedlam) which depicted melancholic and raving madness. These full-length figures came to represent, in the British public's mind, the visual image of the insane (and here, too, the moral implication was evident). A similar representation appeared in the final plate in Hogarth's series *The Rake's Progress,* where the mythic qualities ascribed to the mentally ill were rarely so manifest.

William Blake, one of the artists involved in preparing the first English version of Lavater's physiognomy, reversed the poles. For him the mythic image of madness was that of the biblical king Nebuchadnezzar, who ate grass like an animal in his madness (Plate 9).[17] But Blake presented his Nebuchadnezzar with the specific physiognomy that Lavater ascribed to the melancholic. The hidden message in his work is that of the new science of physiognomy, which persuades the viewer of the truthfulness of the mythic image taken from the Bible. By looking at this figure, not merely at his animallike "claws" but at his physiognomy, we can see his madness. Thomas Rowlandson's somewhat earlier portrait of a maniac used much the same device. The face of the maniac was based on Lavater's views of the violent, animallike physiognomy of the maniac. Blake and Rowlandson, as well as Lavater, also drew on yet another mythic overlap: the visual analogy between human beings and animals, with specific qualities ascribed to the animals used for comparison. Charles Bell's views, rather than heralding a new approach to the pictorialization of the insane, summarized a traditional British manner of visualizing the insane.

The Phrenologists and the New Psychiatry

After Blake engraved his *Nebuchadnezzar,* a new tradition of visualizing the insane was introduced into England from the continent. Franz Josef Gall, the founder of phrenology, had fled Vienna in 1801, settling in Paris, where from 1810 to 1818 he published his massive four-volume study *Anatomy and Physiology of the Nervous System in General and*

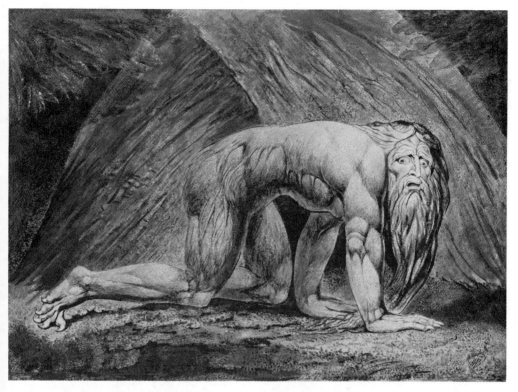

9. William Blake, *Nebuchadnezzar* (1795) (Tate Gallery, London).

the Brain in Particular. In 1819 there appeared a supplemental atlas of illustrations depicting the structure of the brain and various human types.[18]

Many of these latter plates were taken from Moreau de la Sarthe's translation of Lavater, but in addition there were eighteen plates illustrating the skulls and/or visages of the mentally ill. Gall's collaborator on this project was Johann Gaspar Spurzheim, who coined the term *phrenology.* In 1817 Spurzheim, who was practicing medicine in London, published a monograph entitled *Observations on the Deranged Manifestations of the Mind, or Insanity.* For Spurzheim (and for later phrenological interpretations of insanity, such as that by Andrew Combe) there existed a clear relationship between shape and size of the skull and the potential for insanity: "We continually repeat that the brain is an organic part . . . subject to the same considerations as any other organ. Now, every part of the body, whatever its configuration may be, can become diseased." For him "the configuration of heads is neither to be overlooked nor to be over-rated." Spurzheim's illustrations again equated the appearance of the mentally ill (here three idiots) with their skull shape and size. He cites Pinel's overly cautious refusal "to draw any inference, not even from the small heads of idiots."[19] But in Spurzheim's illustrations too the same implicit emphasis is placed on the face and expression of the idiots as in Pinel's plate. While Spurzheim is not primarily concerned with the expression of the mentally ill, it did serve as the visual proof for their debility and, therefore, as a partial proof of the accuracy of his equation between skull size and mental pathology. This tradition of representing the physiognomy of the insane became popularized in the phrenological literature of the nineteenth century, where the mentally ill are often portrayed.[20]

In the phrenologists' work the notion that observation enhances the validity of the analysis is present. At approximately the same time that Gall and Spurzheim were using illustrations of insanity to support their view of the physiological origin of madness, a student of Pinel began to expand the concept of psychiatric illustration. Jean Etienne Dominique Esquirol, in a series of articles in the *Dictionary of Medical Sciences* (1828–30), incorporated simple line drawings of patients (see Plates 15, 16). What is unique is that many of these illustrations were full-length studies of the attitudes as well as of the expressions of the insane. When Esquirol's collected papers appeared in 1838, these illustrations were appended in a full-fledged atlas. These twenty-seven plates, drawn from life at the Salpêtrière, were but a small fraction of the actual number of studies commissioned by Esquirol: "The physiognomic study of the mentally ill is not merely an exercise in curiosity. This study enables one to decipher the character of the ideas and affects which compose the madness of these patients. What fascinating results could be had from such a study! I have had more than two hundred of the insane sketched. Perhaps I shall one day publish the results of my observations on this theme."[21]

Esquirol introduced a manner of viewing the insane which, while consciously rooted in Pinel's implied philosophy of psychiatric illustration (and counter to the phrenologists), is much more sophisticated than either approach. The stark portraiture, the absence of any background, the detail of position and expression all add dramatically to the total image of the insane. Esquirol's innovation in psychiatric illustration was, however, not without precedent. Blake's *Nebuchadnezzar* is a full portrait of that demented monarch. Indeed, his position is as expressive of his madness as is his face. Other artists of the early nineteenth century also presented full-length studies of the insane in which the total figure is expressive of madness. Blake's friend Henry Fuseli, in his painting *Mad Kate* (1806–7), and Thomas Barker of Bath, in his *Crazy Kate*, based their work on a character in William Cowper's *The Task* (1785) and employed the full-length figure of the insane servant girl to exemplify her insanity.[22] Esquirol's illustrator Desmaison carries on this tradition. His drawings and Ambrose Tardieu's etchings of them created a sense of isolated verisimilitude—a reality dissociated from any general context, as in the portraits by Fuseli and Thomas Barker of Bath.

One of the difficulties of tracing the history of psychiatric illustration in the nineteenth century is that the original drawings of psychiatric patients used as the basis for the illustrations in medical works are usually not preserved. In one major case the reverse is true. When Etienne Jean Georget, one of Esquirol's disciples at the Salpêtrière, was in the process of revising his first work on the nature of insanity, he commissioned a series of pictures of his patients. Several of these paintings have been preserved, but the death of the author prevented their realization as illustrations. Georget's *On Madness* of 1820 was one of the major works of the school founded by Pinel. In his study Georget comments on the need to observe the appearance of patients as an aid in diagnosis:

It is difficult to describe the physiognomy of the insane. One must observe their physiognomy in order to capture its image. The patients cannot be recognized from their normal state. Their physiognomy is distorted, fully deformed. The physiognomies are different from individual to individual. They vary according to the illness, the various ideas, which dominate or motivate them; according to the character of the insanity; the stage of the illness, etc. In general the idiot's face is stupid, without meaning; the face of the manic patient is as agitated as his spirit, often distorted and cramped; the moron's facial characteristics are dejected and without expression; the facial characteristics of the melancholic are pinched, marked by pain or extreme agitation; the monomaniacal king has a proud, inflated facial expression; the religious fanatic is mild, he exhorts by casting his eyes at the heavens or fixing them on the earth; the anxious patient pleads, glancing sidewards, etc. I will stop this rather simple listing of patients, for only the direct experience of them can give one an idea of the rest.[23]

Georget emphasized the fleeting nature of the expression of the insane. Here, a major critique of the physiognomy of the insane is rooted not in its difficulty or impossibility, but again, as in Pinel, in the need for direct observation to achieve an understanding of it. It is also evident that Georget's opinions on the nature of psychiatric illustration, while similar to those of the phrenologists, also departed from their views. He was interested in capturing the momentary, typical physiognomies for further study. To this end he requested his friend Théodore Géricault, one of the greatest of the French Romantic painters, to paint pictures of ten patients at Salpêtrière between 1821 and 1824. In the course of events they would have served as the basis for etchings. Therefore, the patients are portrayed, as in the illustrations to Esquirol's work, without backgrounds. However, they are also painted as portraits, and thus, unlike many of Esquirol's illustrations and unlike other contemporary illustrations of symbolic states of madness by such painters as Fuseli, Géricault's paintings serve to capture the uniqueness as well as the universality of each mental state in each individual patient. Likewise, because they were painted as portraits, the paintings all capture passive states. His portrait of the "monomaniacal assassin" is described in the *catalogue raisonné* of his works as "an intelligent head with the expression of audacity and perversity" (Plate 10).[24] These qualities, however, are read out of the totality of his expression. Here the observer has the rare opportunity to judge how the artist, who had immediate contact with a patient, interpreted the physiognomy of the insane. It is evident that Géricault employed many portrait techniques to fix the individuality of each patient. However, as contemporary representatives of the genre of portrait painting, they are all half-length studies, stressing the visage of the sitter as the source for any interpretation of his or her mental state. In England the break with the moral or symbolic presentation of the insane occurred under the direct influence of the French tradition.

In 1825 Alexander Morison published his *Outlines of Lectures on Mental Diseases.* The next year this work was expanded in a second edition through substantial additions to the text and an appendix of thirteen engravings. While some of these plates were taken from Esquirol's work, Morison's illustrations exclusively emphasized the face. He writes in the "explanation of the plates" that the repetition of the same ideas and emotions and the consequent repetition of the same movements of the muscles of the eyes, and of the face, give a peculiar expression, which in the insane state is a combination of wildness, abstraction, or vacancy, and of those predominating ideas and emotions that characterize the different species of mental disorder. Morison opposes the purely materialistic views of Gall and Spurzheim and sees "the following series of Plates as conveying an idea of the *moveable* physiognomy in certain species of mental diseases."[25]

Morison thus postulates expression as a result, not of any inherent fault in the patient, but of the acquisition of patterns of expression through constant repetition. In 1840 Morison brought out a self-contained atlas of the mentally ill, his *Physiognomy of Mental Diseases*, which contained ninety-eight illustrations (Plate 11). The supplemental portraits reveal an abandonment of the sharp lines of the engraving for

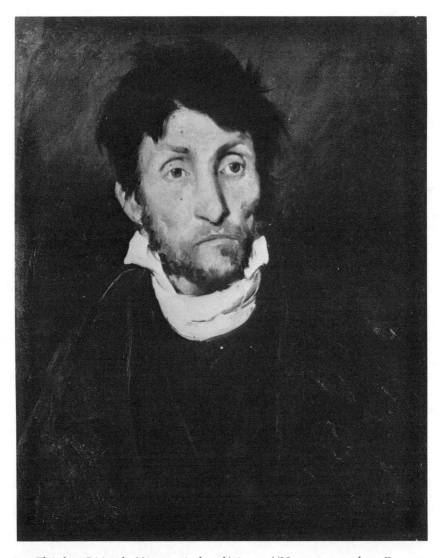

10. Théodore Géricault, *Monomanie du vol* (1821–24) (Museum voor schone Kunsten, Ghent).

the more impressionistic use of the lithograph. The intent in these sketches seems to have been to catch the momentary states of the mentally ill. Here a major shift has been undertaken in the technology of illustration, which also seems to add a greater sense of the movement of the patients. Morison still concentrates on their faces, but the general emphasis is shifted to the overall attitude of the figure. Esquirol's influ-

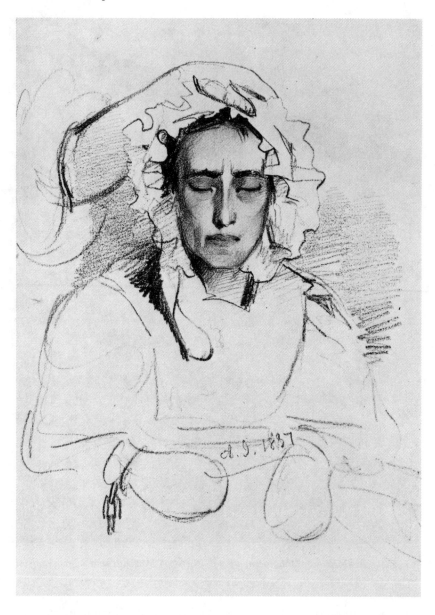

11. The original drawing upon which Alexander Morison was commissioned for his 1840 atlas on the mentally ill; a case of "puerperal mania at onset" (Royal College of Physicians, Edinburgh).

ence is apparent in the initial use of illustration by Morison; in the larger collection the contrast between these earlier portraits and the lithographs done in 1838 indicates Morison's own major contribution to the tradition of psychiatric illustration.

One additional tactic in the early attempts to increase the verisimilitude of psychiatric illustration is to be found in the second edition of Karl Heinrich Baumgärtner's *Physiognomy of Illness* of 1842. Baumgärtner presents a wide range of illustrations of the appearance of patients suffering from disease, including various forms of mental illness; all of them in color. Géricault's paintings would have been reduced to black-and-white etchings; Baumgärtner takes the etching based on sketches by Sandhas and heightens their immediacy by having them colored. But the basic philosophy behind Baumgärtner's seven illustrations of forms of mania still reflects a simplistic understanding of the relationship between the body and the mind: "The mind dominates the motor nerves. Its condition is reflected in the movement of the body."[26] (And as a result, he portrays gestures and positions as well as appearances.)

The tradition of Baumgärtner's presentation of human physiognomy is echoed in Karl Wilhelm Ideler's (1841) *Biographies of the Mentally Ill Presented in Their Development.* The eleven clinical histories discussed by Ideler are accompanied by lithographs by C. Resener. Much more sophisticated in their analysis than Baumgärtner's case studies, Ideler's portraits nevertheless reflect the same monist view of the relationship between mind and body.

Photography of the Insane

By the 1850s psychiatric illustration was enhanced by a major technological breakthrough: the application of the newly invented art of photography to the visual representation of the insane. Photography had developed more or less contemporaneously in Great Britain and France beginning in the 1830s. Although one of its first uses was in fixing of scientific subjects, it was only in the 1850s that a systematic approach was undertaken for applying the camera to psychiatric cases, by Hugh W. Diamond, resident superintendent of the Female Department of the Surrey County Lunatic Asylum (Plate 12). On 22 May 1856, Diamond read a groundbreaking paper, "On the Application of Photography in the Physiognomic and Mental Phenomena of Insanity," before the Royal Society. The paper outlined three major areas in which the photograph could be used to aid in the diagnosis and treatment of the insane. First, the photograph "speaks for itself with the most marked pression."[27] It is an objectively accurate record of the physiognomy of the insane. Second,

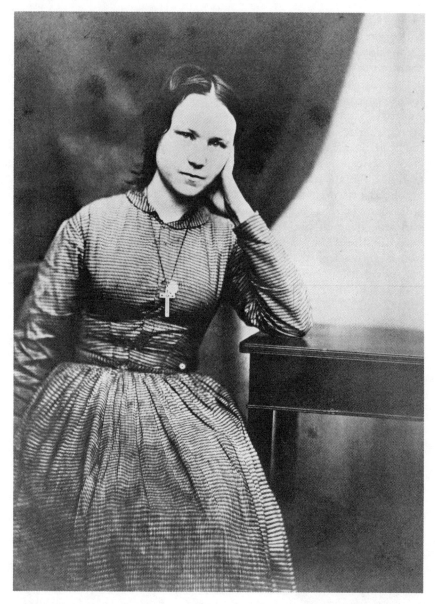

12. Hugh Diamond's photographic portrait of "religious melancholy" (c. 1856) (Royal Society of Medicine, London).

because of this accuracy it can be used in cataloging the development of psychopathologies. Third, it can reveal to the patients, in the most direct manner, their own pathological state. Therefore, the photograph is for Diamond a substantial improvement on the older forms of psychiatric illustration. The same thought occurred to the anonymous writer in the *Cornhill Magazine* for 1861:

> It is equally true that with such portraits and engravings of portraits as we have had, it has been utterly impossible to get beyond the nebulous science of a Lavater. We required the photograph. Certainly it looks a hard thing to say that the great portrait-painters are not to be trusted. Is it to be supposed that these masters did not know their business, and have failed to give us correct likenesses of the persons who sat for them? It must be remembered that to give a general likeness is one of the easiest strokes of art. With half-a-dozen lines the image is complete, as anyone may see in the million wood-engravings of the day; while at the same time it would be difficult to gather from these rough sketches, where two dots go for the eyes and a scratch for the mouth, what is the precise anatomy of any one feature. So while we can accept as in the main truthful the portraits that have come down to us, it is impossible to place perfect reliance on any particular lineament.[28]

In viewing Diamond's photographs today it is clear that the supposed objectivity of the medium is suspect. Diamond's images of the insane are rooted in the portrait photograph of the period as well as in the general tradition of Esquirol. The photographs, because of the long exposure time needed in calotype prints, are static. The new technology proscribes the recording of anything but fixed expression. The importance of Diamond's theory and practice of psychiatric illustration was nonetheless seen almost immediately. Bénédict-Auguste Morel in the atlas to his *Physical, Intellectual, and Moral Degeneracies of the Human Species* published in 1857 has at least one plate based upon a photographic representation of a mental pathology. Here, however, the difficulties inherent in this first generation of photographic illustration are illuminated.[29] For while the basis of Morel's illustration was a photograph, it is reproduced by means of a lithograph. This substitution of one medium for another led to subtle but meaningful changes. A contemporary, H. G. Wright, observed that a lithograph "is entirely destitute of all those minute points of expression which alone could give any value to such an illustration."[30] His comment, however, was directed not to Morel but to the reproduction of a selection of Hugh W. Diamond's photographs in a series of essays by John Conolly.

Conolly, one of the most important figures in mid-nineteenth-century British psychiatry, published this series, "The Physiognomy of Insanity," in *The Medical Times and Gazette* in 1858. Conolly believed that the study of scientific representations of the insane could lead to an understanding of "the peculiar expression and the general external character of mental suffering, or derangement of mind, and of structural changes, or of congenital or induced peculiarities in the brain." He believed that neither Esquirol nor Morison had achieved a truly scientific representation of the moods of insanity because of the limits in "graphic skill or . . . the painter's art." Photography, however, can do so: "There is so singular a fidelity in a well-executed photograph that the impression of very recent muscular agitation in the face seems to be caught by the process, which the engraver's art can scarcely preserve. This peculiarity seems to produce part of the discontent often expressed when people see the photographic portraits of their friends or of themselves. It gives, however, peculiar value when, as in the portraits of the insane, the object is to give the singular expression arising from the morbid movements of the mind; and thus, instead of giving pictures which are merely looked at with idle curiosity, furnishes such as may be studied with advantage."[31]

Here the problem of the transition from photograph to lithograph becomes apparent. For although photographs of the insane were available as the subject of scientific study, they were not as yet used as illustrative material owing to the difficulty and expense of reproduction. While Isaac Newton Kerlin does use a series of photographs to illustrate his *Mind Unveiled; or, A Brief History of Twenty-two Imbecile Children* in 1858, his work remains a rare attempt to use the medium of photography directly.[32]

Medical textbooks of the fifties and sixties are concerned with the question of the visualization of insanity. Wilhelm Griesinger's *Pathology and Therapy of Mental Illness* (1845), the most popular textbook of the mid-nineteenth century, discusses the issue in detail but does not have any illustrations.[33] Griesinger, however, was instrumental in establishing the *Archive of Psychiatry and Neurology* in 1868, which, beginning with its first volume, published lithographs of psychopathologies. In Max Leidesdorf's *Textbook of Mental Illness* of 1865, the author presents a series of "the most evident forms of psychopathology from melancholy to idiocy," based upon photographs taken at the asylum at Hall.[34] Thus as late as the 1860s, interpretive lithographs were still being employed to illustrate medical texts. The concept of the visualization of the insane had become a commonplace in the medical literature. Indeed Leidesdorf does not even need to justify his use of this visual material. The transitional period of psychiatric illustration ended in the 1870s.

Complicated theories of the relationship between the mind and the body had begun to appear in the 1850s, contemporary with the introduction of photography into the study of psychiatric pathologies. It was only in the 1870s, however, that the theoretical trend and the new medium met. Alexander Bain, in *The Senses and the Intellect* (1855) and *The Emotions and the Will* (1859), had redefined, in the wake of John Stuart Mill, the nature of consciousness.[35] The mechanistic relationship between mental pathology and its unique expression, which so overshadowed earlier theories of the visualization of the insane, would have to be altered as the relationship between expression and insanity came to be seen as rooted in normal modes of expression. Bain does not discuss this question directly. In 1873, however, there appeared a volume that on its surface should not have been a major addition to the development of psychiatric illustration, but which in fact altered its concept completely.

Charles Darwin's *Expression of the Emotions in Man and Animals* is generally acknowledged as the seminal work on the universality of human and animal expression (see Plates 33, 34).[36] While Darwin's volume is seen as the first important study of expression, little attention has been given to it as one of the key texts in the evolution of psychiatric illustration. Darwin's use of posed photographs and interpretive engravings (based on photographs) sanctioned the older tradition of representing the insane as the "wild man" by placing it within the confines of a scientific text. Chapter 8 presents a detailed study of Darwin's perception of the insane and its background.

Authors of many medical works refused to rely on such engravings as those used by Darwin for their illustrations, seeing the "unmediated" nature of the photograph as proof of the special nature of the insane. Between 1877 and 1880 Desiré Magloire Bourneville and Paul Regnard, both attached to the asylum at the Salpêtrière, published the *Photographic Iconography of the Salpêtrière* (Plate 13).[37] This collection of illustrated studies relied on the direct reproduction of medical photographs of the insane. In 1888, under the leadership of J. M. Charcot, the head of Salpêtrière, the periodical *New Iconography of the Salpêtrière* was founded. Among the founders was Albert Londe, head of the photographic service at the asylum. This periodical, devoted both to illustrating studies of mental pathologies and to studies of the representation of the insane in the visual arts, numbered twenty-eight volumes, the last of which was published in 1918. Charcot and Londe presented an image of the insane as the hysteric, an image that dominated the visualization of the insane well into the twentieth century. In creating a pattern by which the stages of the newly fashionable disease could be described in detail, they found a disease that lent itself to being recorded in still photographs. Their classificatory system was as fictive as were the actions of their "pet" patients who quickly learned to act out the stages of hysteria expected by the head of the hospital and were then photographed.

Freud and Following

Charcot's student Sigmund Freud rejected the visualization of the patient as an aid to analysis. In doing so he centered psychoanalysis on the

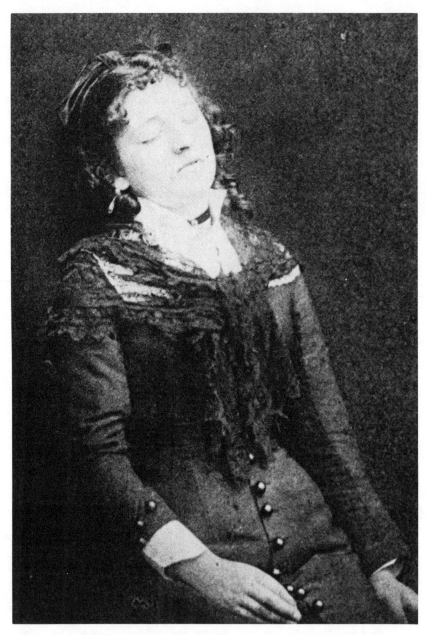

13. Albert Londe's photograph of Blanche Wittmann, Charcot's "pet patient," from the *Iconographie photographique de la Salpêtrière*, vol. 3 (1879–80) (Oskar Diethelm Historical Library, Cornell Medical College, New York).

analyst's listening to the patient. Listening, parallel to seeing the patient, necessitated ground rules for interpretation. One of the most orthodox of Freud's followers, Theodor Reik, stressed the need for the analyst to "follow his instincts" while listening to his patient:

> Young analysts should be encouraged to rely on a series of most delicate communications when they collect their impressions; to extend their feelers, to seize the secret messages that go from one unconscious to another. To trust these messages, to be ready to participate in all flights and flings of one's imagination, not to be afraid of one's own sensitivities, is necessary not only in the beginnings of analysis; it remains necessary and important throughout. . . . We need not fear that this approach will lead to hasty judgments. The greater danger (and the one favored by our present way of training students) is that these seemingly insignificant signs will be missed, neglected, brushed aside. . . . The voice that speaks in him, speaks low, but he who listens with a third ear hears also what is expressed almost noiselessly, what is said *pianissimo*. There are instances in which things a person has said in psychoanalysis are consciously not even heard by the analyst, but nonetheless understood or interpreted. There are others about which one can say: in one ear, out the other, and in the third.[38]

The pattern of interpretation suggested by Reik is equivalent to the manner by which the nineteenth-century psychiatrist interpreted the appearance of his patients. But for both Freud and Reik, representations of the patient, whether tape recordings or transcripts, could not stand as surrogates for the patients themselves. Psychoanalysis did not, however, reject the visualization of the analysand because of the limitations inherent in observing the patient. Indeed, Reik continued his argument with an example concerning his observation of one of his patient's abnormal reactions in passing before a mirror. Rather, psychoanalysis, in rejecting the rigid representationalism of nineteenth-century theories of understanding mental processes, also rejected their basis of empirical proof.

Here Reik's choice of metaphor is important. Borrowing the image of the "third ear" from Nietzsche (where it has a totally different implication), Reik emphasizes the aural aspect of psychoanalysis to the exclusion of the visual, as well as stressing intuition as opposed to cognition. While Kant, in his *Critique of Practical Reason*, had divided the senses between empirical and cognitive functions, he maintained the view that knowledge was based on some type of innate ideas.[39] Freud and Reik stressed the "intuitive," that is, a priori, nature of knowledge, rejecting the sensory, the visual, for a global understanding of the patient represented in their system by the aural. The visual aspect of diagnosis has certainly not vanished from contemporary clinical psychiatry. Even though modern clinical psychiatry is heavily indebted to psychoanalysis for many of its basic theoretical premises, the idea of seeing the insane has not been banned from its manner of presenting psychopathologies.

An excellent example is the standard handbook of psychiatry by Alfred Freedman, Harold Kaplan, and Benjamin Sadock. In its massive multivolume form it is devoid of illustration, in line with "serious" contemporary work in psychiatry. When the publishers provided a student edition of selections from this handbook, however, it was heralded as an "illustrated edition." The illustrations ran the gamut from gynecological diagrams to pictures of brain localization. Included are the traditional photographs of the "chronic schizophrenic woman showing characteristic mannerism and facial grimacing," the "chronic catatonic patient," and the "hebephrenic patient." These photographs stress position and expression. They are direct descendants of the psychiatric atlases of the nineteenth century.

Also included in the text is a plethora of photographic material that shows the same influence of the atlas but emphasizes an entirely new area of perception. The reader is confronted with the image of the seemingly dismembered body of a clothes mannequin lying in an open space, with two miniscule figures running in the background. The caption refers to the fact that "paranoid patients are often unable to separate the thought from the deed and fear that their angry impulses can kill others or themselves." The image of a female hugging three children while a male sits apart in the background is introduced to illustrate "a patient's relationship to his parents and siblings."[40] These illustrations no longer represent the external aspect of the human being, but rather mental life and history. Here the older model of representing the insane is linked to the Freudian model of explanation. This combination, in a teaching aid, is somehow not only accepted but expected. The corollary to the continued interest in seeing the insane in clinical psychiatry is the rich literature on the psychology of expression. This area has flourished in the twentieth century.[41]

Studying expression in works of art or photographs as a source for interpreting expression has been undertaken without comprehending the historical and cultural bias inherent in such a procedure. While many recent studies in the psychology of expression have claimed to focus not on the object but on the nature of perception, there has been a naiveté present concerning the representation of such perception. An understanding of the implications of the representational function of art works or photographs would have been helpful in comprehending what the subject was actually responding to or what the investigator was recording. The introduction of abstraction in art, parallel to the introduction of psychoanalysis, removed

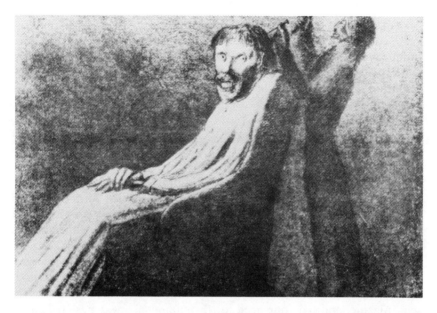

14. Alfred Kubin, "Madness," from his *Dämonen und Nachtgeschichte* (Dresden: Reissner, 1926) (private collection, Ithaca, N.Y.).

the actual representation of the mad and the asylum from the focus of the fine arts, although some artists such as Edvard Munch, Robert Riggs, George Bellows, and Alfred Kubin carried this tradition into the twentieth century (Plate 14). It was only in the 1970s that the photographic representation of the insane assumed the status of the work of art. Mary Ellen Mark's photographs from the Oregon State Hospital were widely seen as a breakthrough in perceiving the insane through the artistic means of the camera.[42]

Julio Cortázar, the famed Latin American author, provided the text for a series of photographs taken at the Hospicio Hecha por los Internados in Buenos Aires.[43] This sensitive literary reaction to the asylum and its inhabitants is introduced by a short three-page survey of the physiognomy of insanity by a Buenos Aires psychiatrist. Here the connection between the aesthetic and the medical modes of seeing the insane is retained. The visualization of the insane maintains its own vocabulary of images. These images are linked to the various manifestations of mental illness in much the same way that psychiatric nomenclature relates to that same spectrum. The selection of a specific representational system is related to the entity described but is not interchangeable with that entity. It is the means by which observers can order their perception of reality.

47

Each age uses bits and pieces of existing systems to reorder the universe for itself. It may restructure these systems to appear new and unique, yet, since it is always relating to the reality in the world, basic communalities of description and perception remain constant. The representation and perception of the insane continues and will continue throughout society's dealing with those it has designated as the mentally ill.

The Implications for Therapy

The tradition of visually representing madness in the form of various icons, whether physiognomy or body type, gesture or dress, points toward the need of society to identify the mad absolutely. Society, which defines itself as sane, must be able to localize and confine the mad, if only visually, in order to create a separation between the sane and the insane. Thus the strength of the visual stereotype is in its immediacy. One does not even have to wait for the insane to speak. The mad are instantly recognizable, and it is our need for instantaneous awareness (which is often based on our construction of images of "madness" rather than the illnesses themselves) which is the rationale for the visual stereotype of the insane. The power of this need to create such delimiting images should be noted. For however much clinicians (not to mention the lay public) believe themselves to be free of such gross internal representations of difference, they are present, and they alter the relationship with the patient or client.

Let us take one salient example. One of the most striking problems of contemporary clinical treatment of the mentally ill is the often debilitating side effects, extrapyramidal syndromes (EPS), of the neuroleptics prescribed for the treatment of the major psychoses. EPS is a major problem in all hospitals where there is any long-term treatment of the mentally ill. The gross disruption of motor skills in some of these side effects, such as tardive dyskinesia (TD), with its Parkinson-like symptoms, should make the recognition of the patients in the hospital setting simple. And yet the most recent presentation of work on this question at the 1986 American Psychiatric Association meeting in Washington showed that clinicians were "significantly less able" to identify such patients than specially trained researchers.[44] (In the sample studied the researchers were able to diagnose a quarter of the patients as significantly impaired; the clinicians identified only about 10 percent as having TD.) And this happened even though the symptoms are gross enough to warrant a paper in the previous year's meeting asking "Is there an epidemic of tardive dyskinesia?"[45]

The clinicians were unable to *see* the gross movement disorders in their patients because their patients were supposed to "look crazy." The historical materials presented in this chapter point toward a strong subliminal understanding of the idea of difference in the appearance of the mentally ill. Clinicians are aware of patients "sounding crazy"—they are trained to be aware of the lapses in discourse and language which indicate the presence of psychopathology. What is missing is an equal awareness of the visual stereotyping of the mentally ill. Especially in the hospital setting, patients are supposed to "look crazy." This "look" is what often sets them apart from the clinicians, at least in the clinicians' subconscious awareness. It is therefore of little moment that the patient actually does "look different" (and that that difference is caused by the patient's response to medication). The inability to see the movement disorders in patients is a direct result of the visual patterning through the age-old tradition of representing the insane. The clinical implications of such a set of visual stereotypes are therefore direct. They are also an indicator that the patterns described in this chapter are not merely historical but are operative today.

CHAPTER THREE

The Rediscovery of the Body:
Leonardo's First Image of
Human Sexuality and Disease

Leonardo's World and Ours

On 9 April 1476 "Leonardo di Ser Piero da Vinci" was anonymously accused of having had carnal relations with the "soddomitare" Jacopo Saltarelli. Tried for this crime with two others, Leonardo was released, evidently through the interposition of one of the leading families in Florence, the Tornabuoni, one of whose members was also accused.[1] The charge of homosexuality brought against Leonardo has traditionally led to detailed speculation about the roots of his homoeroticism and its significance for his aesthetic production. In this chapter I shall be departing from quite another point than did Sigmund Freud, for I shall be examining neither the nature nor the roots of Leonardo's sexual orientation but rather the question of what being gay in Renaissance Florence could have signified for Leonardo.[2] I shall assume not that homosexuality is a psychopathology but rather that any neurosis present in the homosexual is the result of the cultural conflict that arises between the individual's sense of self and society's image of the homosexual, against which this self-image is constantly measured. It is the presence of a society's construction of the Other—here the Other as defined by one of the salient markers of difference in the West, human sexuality—which shapes and focuses the image of the self.

It is important to contrast the internalized myths and their self-representation to the realities of Florentine daily life. Had Leonardo been publicly convicted of sodomy, he would most probably only have been fined about ten florins.[3] This was a very different world from that of Rome under Paul IV, where sodomy was one of the capital crimes punished by the Inquisition.[4] Indeed, many of the younger generation of artists and artisans in the circle in which Leonardo found himself were overtly gay, and little social ignominy seemed to result from the awareness of their sexual orientation. But in direct contrast to this social acceptance, homosexuality was marked by the culture in which Leonardo lived as a sign of the loss of control of an individual over those inner forces that human beings must harness. Homosexuality was understood as a form of "lust" and was condemned in a general condemnation of lustfulness as a sign of the absence of rational control over the self. This view was embedded in the signifiers of culture, in the books and tracts in which was represented the society's mirage of difference. This mirage was of great importance, since it denoted, as much by its status as by its acceptance, the importance of sexual difference as a marker of Otherness, a marker rebutted by social practice but reified by cultural (and theological) definitions of difference. Here the basic distinction is between practice, exemplified by daily reality, and theory, exemplified by the book. Thus the homosexual became one of the cultural signs of Otherness in the world of the book, an individual inherently different from the ideal state in which the body is dominated by the rational mind. It is within the cultural world of books, of images, the world of religious as well as secular texts written about homosexuality, which were available to Leonardo, that the image of the homosexual as deviant was present. And thus it is in the world of texts and images that we shall seek the source of Leonardo's internalization of the implications of that label applied to his sexual orientation. The juxtaposition of Leonardo's sense of self and the greater culture's understanding of the homosexual is mirrored in Leonardo's images of sexual difference.[5]

Leonardo's Anatomical Drawings and Freud

The image I shall be examining in this chapter, while not as well known a work as those images analyzed by Freud—the *Mona Lisa* and the *Virgin and Child with St. Anne*—is a work of immense power. It was not created as a work for the public sphere but is rather from a more private source of images, Leonardo's notebooks.[6] The image is, however, not unknown. It was the first page from Leonardo's anatomical drawings to be engraved and was circulated in a number of impressions as early as the late eighteenth century.[7] Indeed, Johann Friedrich Blumenbach, in one of the classic studies of Enlightenment racial biology, cites this engraving as existing in 1795 (Plate 15).[8]

All of the engraved versions of Leonardo's image of human sexuality reproduce only one set of figures, the hemisected figures in coition. And

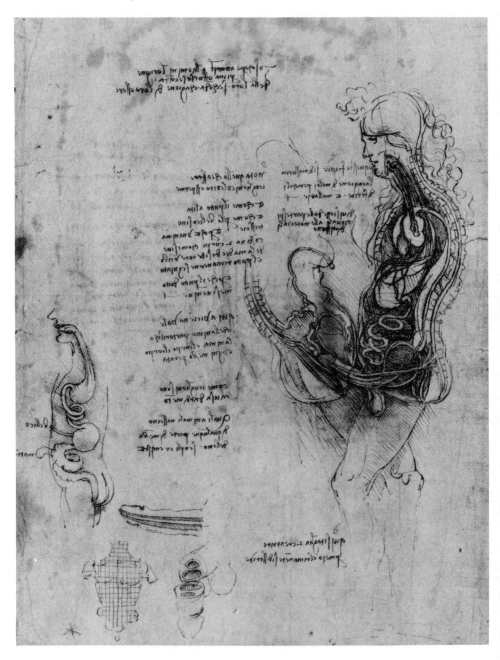

15. Leonardo's first drawing depicting human sexuality (Queen's Collection, Windsor).

all of them tend to "improve" upon Leonardo's original. Indeed, it is one of these "improved" versions which led Sigmund Freud to his citation, in the notes to the 1919 revision of his essay on Leonardo, of a particularly damaging misreading by Rudolf Reitler of this very anatomical drawing, and to his embarrassed retraction of it in the 1923 version.[9] The irony is that Reitler's misreading of Leonardo's image of coition is based on the same type of error of transmission as Freud's own misreading of Dmitri Mereschkowski's account of Leonardo's childhood dream about the bird introducing its tail into the infant Leonardo's mouth.[10] Reitler used a version of Leonardo's image which had been "completed" and thus distorted in the nineteenth century; Freud used Mereschkowski's novel with its mistranslation of the bird's name. (Freud's primary source, in addition to the novel, seems to have been the German translation of Edmund Solmi's monograph on Leonardo, which also mistranslated the bird's name.)[11] Each of these confusions has a specific importance for the story that it tells. Freud's reliance on the novel about Leonardo's life was in no little part due to the confluence of two facts: Freud read the life of Leonardo, the creative genius as outsider, in Mereschkowski's account (which begins in medias res) at the very point in his own life that Leonardo's biography begins (in middle age and at the sensed highpoint of his creativity), and Mereschkowski's novel was a world bestseller, giving its author a high status as a creative genius, a status sought after by Freud from the time of his contact with Wilhelm Fliess. Freud sees himself both as Leonardo and as the author of the novel about Leonardo and thus identifies completely with the validity of Mereschkowski's point of view (and the language of its representation).

Reitler's perspective is a bit different. He sees the Leonardo anatomical drawing only through the eyes of the engraver, who, like Mereschkowski, has altered it for his or her own ends. But the alterations are not merely those of completion, for the engraver in adding the feet of the figures adds them incorrectly. Reitler falls into the trap of centering his analysis on these added features, and thus Freud, who quotes Reitler extensively in the notes to the 1919 edition, repeats Reitler's error. What is most interesting is that the anonymous engraver selects only the hemisected coitus figures from the sheet, ignoring the other figures and the commentary. This omission is, unbeknownst to Reitler, the source of his central error of interpretation. For once the hemisected figures are restored to their context within Leonardo's anatomical notebooks, and once the central principle for their interpretation is elucidated, then the preselection of these hemisected coital figures as the central focus of Leonardo's earliest representation of human sexuality can be judged to be biased. One must examine the entire page, all of the figures in relationship to each other, as well as understand the implications of Leonardo's internalization of the idea of sexual difference in this first set of images of sexuality.

Leonardo's Representation of Heterosexuality

The general principle for the elucidation of this early anatomical plate, created between 1493 and 1500, was stated in the first modern history of anatomical drawing, that of Ludwig Choulant, published in 1852.[12] Choulant, in his essay on Leonardo, stresses that in these early plates Leonardo was creating visual images out of his reading on anatomy. That is, he was transposing one type of representation, the verbal, into another, the visual. And indeed, if we read the entire historical literature on Leonardo's anatomical drawings, these very early drawings are all understood as attempts by Leonardo to translate the verbal imagery of the medieval anatomists into his own repertoire of visual images. This baseline is important since it determines the relationship between text and image, both within the confines of the page taken from Leonardo's anatomical drawings and between these early drawings and the literary tradition in which they stand. Leonardo's primary source for his early anatomical drawings is the work of the fourteenth-century anatomist Mondino (Raimondo de' Luzzi). The edition of Mondino which Leonardo evidently used was either the first printed Latin one, published in 1478 and unillustrated, or the 1493 Italian translation that appeared while Leonardo was beginning to record his study of human anatomy.[13] This need, therefore, to move from the printed word to the image will be the guideline for our study of Leonardo's representations of human sexuality.

Let us begin by examining the hemisected coital figures that so confused Reitler and Freud. The sexual anatomy of these figures seems to be that imagined by the medieval anatomist. The figures are joined completely, the "key and lock" fantasy of the structure of the genitalia which even certain contemporary biologists see as the source of the relationship between the shapes of male and female genitalia. "According to this theory females avoid having their eggs fertilized by the males of other species by evolving complicated genitalia that permit insemination only by the corresponding genitalia of males of their own species; the male has the 'key' to fit the female's 'lock.' "[14] This can also be stated in terms that would have appealed directly to Leonardo, the image of the genitalia as part of the *machina mundi*, the universal machine in which all of the segments have their proper fit.[15] The joining of the male and female in the image is complete, following the ideology of the "key and lock" metaphor—the cervix opens to receive the glans penis. But there is a second level of implication present in the "key and lock" image of the genitalia in Leonardo's representation. For not only does the structure of the "lock" preclude contact with any except those who have the correct "key," but the "key and lock" are so structured that they complement each other exactly. This image of the inherent perfection of human anatomical structures is important to the understanding of the implications of the "key and lock" structure of the genitalia.

The representation of the penis reflects the fantasy existence of a second canal that transmits the animal spirit from the spinal cord to the embryo. Medieval anatomists needed to create a boundary between the urine, which was viewed as polluting (at least to the degree that it reflected pathology), and the semen, the source of a new soul. It was a boundary between the material and the spiritual. In addition, the uterus residually reflects the medieval idea that it was divided into seven cells. The breasts are directly linked to the uterus, as in conception the retained menses are carried, by means of the epigastric veins, to the breast and there form milk. According to Kenneth Keele, the most insightful contemporary historian of science to deal with Leonardo's anatomical drawings, "Leonardo visualises conception arising from the act of coitus, according to the ideas of Plato and Hippocrates, in which the semen flowed from the spinal cord to the penis. Here [in the coital figure] the imagined nerves necessary for such transmission are displayed."[16] Now, Leonardo is himself quite doubtful about the nuances of this model of coitus and conception. In the notes to this figure, he questions the truths of Mondino's repetition of Avicenna's views on the nature of conception and wonders what role the testicles (the "first cause" of the sperm) played in relationship to the "second cause of the sperm," the spinal cord. All of these errors in anatomical representations and relationships can be traced back to specific literary sources; indeed, Leonardo provides them for us in the notes on this page.

Leonardo's source is the verbal image of human sexuality, but it is not only that found in the medieval anatomies. His primary source is Plato, who in his *Timaeus* saw the spinal marrow as containing " 'the universal seed stuff' of mortals." Keele states quite directly that "the drawing of Leonardo follows Plato's description so literally that it is difficult to avoid the conclusion that Leonardo was illustrating what he read in the *Timaeus*." He repeats that this plate has figures that are "composed almost entirely of visualized structures as gleaned from the literature" and are "representations of the literature he had read in preparation for his own anatomical explorations." But Keele does not proceed quite far enough, for it is in *Timaeus* that the verbal source of the image that dominates all of the figures on this page is to be found.

It is the ideology of the function of the testicles, in Leonardo's question appended to the hemisected figures, "How are the testicles the cause of ardor?" which leads us back to the text, *Timaeus*. It is not merely the question of the "primary" or "secondary" sources of sperm but rather the nature of the human sexual drive which is central. Plato observes:

> And the seed, having life, becoming endowed with respiration, produces in that part which it respires a lively desire of emission, and thus creates in us the love of procreation. Wherefore also in men the organ of generation becoming rebellious and masterful, like an animal disobedient to reason, maddened with the sting of lust, seeks to gain absolute sway, and the same is the case with the so-called womb or matrix of women. The animal within them is desirous of procreating children.[17]

It is the idea that the semen creates within the rational individual, for Plato both men and women, the "animal within" which dominates the image of human sexuality for Leonardo. We are helpless, manipulated by this "animal within," unable to act except to engage in intercourse. The human being, at that point, becomes the vessel that holds sexuality and is dominated by it.

But for Leonardo, this is not all that is involved in the act of heterosexual coitus. For Leonardo appends one further note to the description of the hemisected figures: "By means of these figures, the cause of many ulcers and diseases will be demonstrated." While both Mondino and, indeed, Plato speak of the diseases attendant to the genitalia (either in terms of the ulcers which may result from the medication applied after a hernia operation or the repression of the semen with its resultant illness), Leonardo's choice of vocabulary ("per queste figure sidjmosstere / lacagiche dj moltj pericholj / dj ferite e mallattj") points to one very specific disease, the yet unnamed syphilis. It is possible that this reference is the earliest recorded anatomical/medical reference to the new disease. Leonardo's reference appears at the very moment when the disease was first spreading throughout Italy and records the telltale signs of the illness, the genital ulcers that are its most prominent feature.[18]

The iconography of disease permeates the hemisected coital figures. Not the image of the hemisected figures themselves, for they exist in more primitive form in the anatomical illustration of the Middle Ages, but rather an iconographic feature that is almost lost to the contemporary observer. Let us again observe the figures. The virtual disappearance of the female figure was already commented on by Reitler. She is but womb and breasts. There is nothing about her which seems to point to pathology. Her breasts are pendulous, but they are quite different from the breasts of the natives of the New World which are portrayed in Theodor de Bry's plates, where, according to the insightful work of Bernadette Boucher, the breasts serve as a sign of primitive bestality.[19] They are not flat, aged, and worn; rather, they are the milk-laden breasts of the pregnant woman. The woman is seen as but the potential container of the embryo. And pregnancy is understood from the Middle Ages on as a potentially pathological situation.

The male figure is drawn with much more detail. What is striking in his representation in terms of the clearly drawn head and face is the cascade of hair which dominates. Here we have an iconographic reference that is clear only when slightly later images appear of the male as the sufferer from syphilis. Albrecht Dürer, in 1496, engraved the first broadside (by Theodoricus Ulsenius) that directly represented the syphilitic. What is striking about Dürer's figure is that he is dandified, his clothes and hair signify his role as a fop. He is covered with the visible signs of his illness, with the "boils, ulcers and crusts" described in Ulsenius's Latin hexameters (see Plate 39).[20] With the cascade of hair Leonardo is pointing to the image of the syphilitic.[21] It is the fop, the young male, who is at risk from the new disease with its evident sexual origin. He is paralleled to the other individual, the pregnant woman, who is represented as being at risk. Thus sexuality is not merely the release of the beast within, it is also the characterization of this "beast" as polluted and polluting. Coitus points toward defilement and illness.

These analogies to the hemisected image, as I have noted, are taken from the anatomy of the late Middle Ages. Yet the position of the act of coitus, upright, is unusual even for such hemisected figures, and it too has iconographic significance. When Leonardo's corpus is examined it is clear that there is a set of visual analogies to this upright position. Leonardo's images of "pleasure and pain" and "virtue and envy" use the classical model of the self divided against itself as the image of irreconcilable differences. Clearly, the Platonic antithesis between the masculine and the feminine would fall into such a set of dichotomies for the Renaissance mind. But one other representation of sexuality from Leonardo's iconographic storehouse should be introduced here. For in the tradition of the representation of Leda and the swan, from Greco-Roman art through Leonardo, the sexual act is performed with two upright figures.[22] Thus the upright position points toward the existence of antithesis as well as to the existence of a type of sexual contact which exemplifies the male as possessing the "beast within"—Zeus in the form of the beast raping Leda. Leonardo's *Leda* combines, in the sense of sensuality in the female, both attraction to and repellence by the aggressive male, a sensuality that also mirrors the "beast within."

Leonardo's Representation of Homosexuality

In terms of their historical suppression, the more interesting set of images is that on the left side of the page. Here too we have the translation of verbal images into visual ones. For we have an image here of what Leonardo calls in a reference to the hemisected figures the "material" (i.e., alimentary) parts as opposed to the "spiritual" (the thoracic) parts. Here we have a figure who represents only the "material" parts, the alimentary canal from the mouth to the anus. Leonardo's literary source for this image is Aristotle's essay on the parts of animals. In this image Leonardo represents the jejunum as lying between the upper and lower stomachs, after which the gut becomes narrower and convoluted, ending in a straight portion running to the anus. This is the representation not of a human alimentary canal but of that of a specific type of ruminant, those beasts that Aristotle calls "horned animals." The alimentary canal of these "horned animals" runs "in a straight line to the place where the residue is discharged, which is called the anus." And these parts have only one function, according to Aristotle, the "treating of food and . . . [the] dealing with the residue produced."[23] The human alimentary canal, which has but one true stomach and which ends with its sigmoid flexure leading to the rectum, is unrepresented.

The other figures on the left side of the page are of equal interest. The small torso, which is represented so that it can be easily enlarged, seems to represent a sexless figure, as does the more detailed hemisected figure of the alimentary canal. There are two figures of the penis, a transverse section (with testicles, the source of ardor) and a longitudinal section that represents the penile passages, one for the urine, the other for the animal spirit derived from the spinal cord. The image of the penis, here erect and functioning quite independent of any external control, is represented as an autonomous force. This view that the genitalia, both male and female, can assume a life of their own, has already been quoted from Plato. Leonardo subscribed to this view, at least for the male organ, as he observed in his notebooks:

This [the penis] disputes with the human intellect, and sometimes has an intellect of its own. And though the will of man may wish to stimulate it, it remains obstinate and goes its own way, sometimes moving on its own without the permission or intention of a man. Thus be he sleeping or waking it does what it desires. Often a man is asleep and it is awake, and many times a man is awake and it is asleep. Many times a man wants to use it, and it does not want to; many times it wants to and a man forbids it. Therefore it appears that this animal often has a soul and intellect separate from a man; and it appears that a man who is ashamed to name or show it is in the wrong, always being anxious to cover it up and hide what ought to adorn and show with solemnity like a minister of the human species.[24]

What is striking in the figures on the lefthand side of Leonardo's page is the visual relationship between the longitudinally represented penis and the anus of the alimentary figure. It is posed for entrance, at least visually. Here we can return to the ideology of the "key and lock" metaphor for the depiction of the genitalia. The vagina and uterus match perfectly to the form of the erect penis; but so do the rectum and anus, as represented by Leonardo. The ambiguity of such a fantasy about the structure of the body, a fantasy that grows out of the ideologies associated with sexuality, presents a parallel case to Leonardo's image of heterosexuality. For Leonardo the relationship between the anus and the penis is parallel in form (and therefore in function) to the relationship between the vagina and the penis. But the anus is clearly that of the "horned beast" of Aristotle's text.

The idea of anal intercourse, here between a figure with a ruminant digestive system (and without any overt sexual signifier) and a penis without a body, returns us to the image of the bestial, the link between Plato and Aristotle, between the two texts translated into images by Leonardo. In the Church tradition the term "bestial" is one of the encoded terms for homosexuality. (Clement of Alexandria quotes Plato in this context: "It seems to me on this account that Plato in the *Phaedrus* deprecates pederasty, calling it 'bestial,' because those who give themselves up to [this] pleasure 'take the bit' and copulate in the manner of quadrupeds, striving to beget children [thus]."]25 Indeed, Leonardo himself, in a passage quoted from his notebooks (1488, *Fiore di Virtù*), refers to the fact that the "bat, owing to unbridled lust, observes no universal rule in pairing, but males with males and females with females pair promiscuously, as it may happen."26 This passage is indicative of one view of the nature of the animal. Homosexuality was understood as the result of unbridled lust, and was therefore a quality ascribed to the beast.27 Traditionally, the animals that served as the icons of homosexuality were the hare, the weasel, and the hyena, all of which were understood to be deviant within the animal kingdom.28 But, by the Renaissance, all sexuality outside the control of reason had become suspect in this model. Indeed, all sexuality outside the bounds of the sacrament of marriage and the intent of conception was lustful, and therefore bestial, according to the standard authorities such as Thomas Aquinas. (Aquinas lists four categories of sexuality which are "lustful" and therefore sinful, ranked from the least serious to the most serious offense: masturbation; intercourse in an unnatural position; homosexuality; bestiality).29

One further problem arises in examining Leonardo's set of images, which by their juxtaposition represent anal intercourse as a visual parallel to the heterosexuality of the hemisected figures. It is evident from Leonardo's notes that heterosexuality is associated with disease, with syphilis and pregnancy. What is not evident is that anatomists writing contemporaneously with Leonardo commented on the diseases of the anus and related them to "lustful" living. One of the most important Renaissance commentators on Mondino, Jacopo Berengario de Carpi, in his *Isagogae Breves* (1522), observed that the "anus suffers all kinds of ills, which are hard to heal. . . . Sometimes a lascivious shamelessness of riotous living and burning lust in either sex by seeking low retreats or byways cause these ills."[30] This reference to anal intercourse, both heterosexual and homosexual, makes it evident that the anus could be pathologically influenced by "misuse." The anatomists whom Leonardo knew condemned anal intercourse on much the same ideological grounds as did the Church, but also indicated that such acts led to disease. The parallel between Leonardo's sense of the nature of heterosexuality and his internalization of his culture's image of homosexuality, as present in its authoritative written texts, did not, however, originate only in the written works of the theologians and the anatomists.

It is in *The Divine Comedy*, that text which was central to Leonardo's understanding of his own culture, the quintessentially Italian text by which Italian culture even in the Renaissance defined itself, that a vocabulary of verbal images (and their visual realizations) is provided which Leonardo could have drawn upon to comprehend the image of sexuality as bestial.[31] Twice in *The Divine Comedy*, Dante uses the term *sodomite*. The first time, in the *Inferno*, it is used as a term of political opprobrium, as Richard Kay has shown in his essay "The Sin of Brunetto Latini."[32] In the *Purgatorio*, however, Dante describes the lustful, those dominated by bestial forces, and he calls upon an image that is visually extraordinarily powerful. In Canto Twenty-six Dante refers to the poets Guido Guinicelli and Arneut Daniel as those consumed by the lust of the beast. What Dante first hears when he approaches them and those condemned with them is their muttering:

There I see on either side each shade make haste, and one kiss the other without staying, satisfied with short greeting:

even so within their dark battalions one ant rubs muzzle with another, perchance to spy out their way and their fortune.

Soon as they break off the friendly greeting, ere the first step there speeds onward, each one strives to shout loudest;

the new people, "Sodom and Gomorrah," and the other: "Pasiphaë enters the cow that the young bull may haste to her lust."[33]

Here two models of bestial lust (the lust of the antlike figures), the heterosexual and the homosexual, cross. The rhetoric of "Sodom and Gomorrah" points toward the sins of the bestial in the form of the homosexual with a generally accepted biblical reference; the reference to Pasiphaë, the mother of the Minotaur, is perhaps less well known.[34] The legend is one of the standard repertoire of literary images of sexual transformation and perversion, having its best-known retelling in Ovid and Apuleius. Minos, king of Crete, calls upon Poseidon to send a bull from the sea for a sacrifice in order to confirm his right to rule. Pasiphaë, his wife, falls in love with the bull and contrives to have Daedalus disguise her as a cow to have carnal relations with the animal.

The alimentary figure, the figure with the viscera of the "horned beast," Leonardo's realization of Aristotle's anatomy of the beast, is the image of the beast within. This figure, Leonardo's "material" figure, however, seems sexless. Leonardo draws on it two labels. One is "umbilicus," which relates to the caecum; but from the gut stems an appendage unknown in anatomy and labeled with a term likewise unknown, "matron." This is indeed *metron*, Greek for "womb," placed outside the figure for, like Pasiphaë, the figure is a reversed image. Such a reversal also has a long tradition in classical anatomical thought. In Galen's anatomy the genitalia of the male and female were understood as being constructed as mirror images. If the woman were turned inside out, if "the uterus [were] turned outward and projecting [w]ould not the testes then necessarily be inside it? Would it not contain them like a scrotum? Would not the neck, hitherto concealed inside the perineum but now pendant, be made into the male member?"[35] What prevents this inversion in most women is the absence of the excess heat of the male, that which drives the male to "lust." It is the wellspring of the bestial and is represented by the figure of the inverted woman, driven by the heat of the male, her uterus projecting like a penis. It is the man-woman, the sexual being who is simultaneously penis and uterus.

It is the woman, Pasiphaë, hiding within the image of the beast, who waits to assuage her lust; and it is the bestial within the human being which drives her to this action. It is an image with the bestial internalized, with the uterus, the sign of reproduction as a sign of the reversal of the roles of the sexes, externalized. The condemnation of the passive homosexual, the male as female, in Church law is reflected in this image.[36] The Church condemned any male taking the "female" role, condemned homosexuality as a reversal of the "natural order" of the world. The significance of the placement of the uterus, the organ of reproduction, outside of the body is Leonardo's sign of the "bestial" in his fantasy of role reversal within the traditionally accepted model of human sexuality.

The body itself becomes the vehicle for his critique of the irrational forces of sexuality, of the internalized sense of his own sexuality as condemned by the world in which he lives. This critique is a result of the double bind in which Leonardo finds himself, between his sense of his own sexual identity, a sense reified by the attitudes of his peer group in Florence, and the mythic images of the homosexual present in the books that dominate his world, texts from the world of science as well as literature.

Leonardo's Rejection of Sexuality

Leonardo's bodies are transparent. We see the bestial forces within, which move the individual in ways that are contrary to the teachings of the Church and the directives of the State. The result of the double bind that condemns both heterosexual and homosexual activity is mirrored in Leonardo's rejection of all sexuality as grotesque, as documented in the famed passage inscribed on one of the later anatomical plates: "The sexual act and the members employed therein are so repulsive, that if it were not for the beauty of the faces and the adornments of the actors and the pent-up impulse, nature would lose the human species."[37] It is not any specific form of sexuality but all sexuality that Leonardo condemns, repressing any sense of his own sexual identity, at least within the confines of the anatomical notebooks. Leonardo has internalized the negative image of sexuality which has salience for him. Accused of homosexuality he converts the image of the condemned sexual act into the literal representation of bestiality. All sexuality is dangerous, it is sinful. It is the loss of consciousness and identity which leads to public humiliation, as he observes in a text written at about the same time that he created the plate representing coitus: "Of Lust: And they will go wild after the things that are most beautiful to seek after, to possess and make use of their vilest parts; and afterwards, having returned with loss and penitence to their senses, they will be greatly amazed of themselves."[38]

It is thus within this internalized matrix that Leonardo, when he first attempts to represent human sexuality in a direct manner, understands his own Otherness. But this internalization is also ambiguous. For Leonardo condemns both homosexuality and heterosexuality as the conquest of the ugly, of the pathological, as the bestial, but he also equates them as natural, that is, as being sanctioned by his fantasy about the structure of human anatomy. The inherent ambiguity of this position is reflected in this first translation of images from texts into representations of sexuality. Here we have the moment of creative fantasy of Leonardo looking to the body of the Other and finding there his own body represented.

CHAPTER FOUR

Masturbation and Anxiety: Henry Mackenzie, Heinrich von Kleist, William James

On Models of Seeing

How we "see the insane" is determined by our psychological need for coherence and consistency, for a boundary between ourselves and the Other. But the images that we select and the forms in which we cast them also reflect the historical needs (and models) of a culture and an age. Through such images we differentiate between ourselves—the sane, in control of our world—and the mad. We employ various modes of representation, words or pictures, to accomplish this differentiation. However closely related such images are, the shift from visual to verbal is often not an insignificant one. The literary image of the insane may often be the embodiment of the visual image; literary icons may seem to be the verbal equivalent to the icons of visual art. And yet they are different because of the social and cultural significance of the literary medium. It is not that one system structures or influences the other system. While they share a set of signs that signify "madness" as opposed to sanity, the means by which the two systems present these signs may alter their meaning. For example, the special signification of words, of the act of writing as the sign of the rational in our society, means that the shift from the visual to the verbal image is not gratuitous. It presents us with yet a further level of meaning in the act of representation which we can explore.

One of the central myths embodied in the representations of madness in our society is the necessary relationship between the diseased mind, symbolized by an individual no longer in command of language, and the irrational forces of human sexuality. But as Michel Foucault has amply shown in his *History of Sexuality*, sexuality, or at least the discourse in which it is represented, also has its history.[1] To illustrate the historical alteration of representations of the fantasy of sexuality, as well as our unique individualization in perceiving the world, I have selected three texts spanning almost one and a half centuries. These texts all reflect the subtle interaction of historical models and personal perspective in regard to a specific moment, as well as the confrontation of the author with a madness rooted in the individual's sense of the body. The texts are as varied in their genre as in their dates of composition: Henry Mackenzie's sentimental novel of 1771, *The Man of Feeling*; Heinrich von Kleist's letter of mid-September 1800 to Wilhelmine von Zenge; and William James's Gifford Lectures on Natural Religion given at the University of Edinburgh in 1901 and published under the title *The Varieties of Religious Experience.*

These works present individual confrontations with the image of the insane as perceived through specific root-metaphors of sexuality. Each text demonstrates the individual use of such root-metaphors in shaping the experience and its expression in literary form. The variety of texts adds to an understanding of the function of such perception of the insane in the past two centuries. Each also reflects dominant concerns of the "Enlightenment," or at least the post-1700 world, the nature of sexuality as the corruption of the rational and the powerful image of "self-abuse" as the ultimate icon of sexual collapse. Not seduction by the Other but seduction by the hidden forces within the self is the ultimate sign of the domination of sexuality over rationality for the post-Enlightenment world. What is striking is the powerful association of masturbation with madness, which lasts well into the twentieth century.

Mackenzie and Hogarth's Asylum

Harley, the sentimental hero of Henry Mackenzie's novel *The Man of Feeling*, is persuaded by an acquaintance to visit one "of those things called Sights, in London, which every stranger is supposed desirous to see,"[2] the asylum officially called the Bethlem Royal Hospital but better known as Bedlam. After initial humane objections to exposing "the greatest misery with which our nature is afflicted, to every idle visitant who can afford a trifling perquisite to the keeper," he accompanies his friend "and the other persons of the party (amongst whom were several ladies)" to the asylum. The path taken by this party through the asylum is marked by the inmates they see. First they are led "to the dismal mansions of those who are in the most horrid state of incurable madness." Here "the clanking of chains, the wildness of their cries, and the imprecations which some of them uttered, formed a scene inexpressibly shocking." The company is horrified and wishes to flee, much to the chagrin of their guide, who, "as he expressed it in the phrase of those that keep wild beasts for a shew, [thought they] were much better worth seeing than any they had passed."

The group then moves to that part of the asylum set aside for those "not dangerous to themselves or others," and Harley leaves his companions to observe the inmates by himself. He first sees a man "making pendulums with bits of thread," marking "a segment of a circle on the wall with chalk." He is a mathematician gone mad trying to plot the orbit of comets based on Newton's conjectures. Harley then sees a figure scrawling numbers on a slate. He is a stock speculator reduced "to poverty and to madness." A schoolmaster "of some reputation" also is not lacking from Mackenzie's Bedlam, gone mad attempting to discover "the genuine pronunciation of the Greek vowels." All forms of discourse are in collapse in the asylum, all are bizarre (see the discussion in Chapter 13), and they signify madness.

Harley rejoins his companions in the women's wing, where he spies "separate from the rest . . . one, whose appearance had something of superior dignity." Mackenzie devotes the other half of this chapter to a recounting of the tale of this melancholic figure represented as different, as noble. Separated from her true love, who went to the West Indies to seek his fortune and died, she was almost forced "to marry a rich miserly fellow, who was old enough to be her grandfather." She was reduced to madness. Harley, who converses with the poor mad girl, leaves "in astonishment and pity! . . . He put a couple of guineas into the man's hand: 'Be kind to that unfortunate'—He burst into tears, and left them."

Mackenzie's image of Bedlam quite clearly conforms to the traditional bounds of the understanding of madness in the eighteenth century. Madness is the product of a congenital inability to deal with the vicissitudes of life. But more than this, Mackenzie offers his reader a manner of seeing the insane. The initial contact is vague, distant, not really describing, rather giving the reactions of the observers. The second level is more detailed, giving capsule descriptions of the history and present state of the scientist, speculator, and schoolmaster. The most detailed presentation, that of the melancholic lover, is presented at the conclusion of the chapter. Mackenzie adapts a specific visual model for his portrayal of Bedlam. It is three-tiered and, like the literary sketch in *The Man of Feeling*, has an inherent moral lesson.

In 1735 William Hogarth published his series *The Rake's Progress* (see Plate 5). This sequence of eight plates was so popular that a retouched version was reissued in 1763. It contains, in its final plate, the most influential visual representation of the asylum in European art of the eighteenth century.[3] It presents a selection of inmates, among them the lunatic scientist figuring longitudes on the wall, a mad astronomer observing the heavens through a tube, and a mad tailor, driven insane by pride. The plate, the culmination of the degeneration of Rakewell, moves from the dark cells at the top and back to the prostrated figure of Rakewell in the foreground. Here too the figures of the female visitors, so randomly introduced into Mackenzie's image of Bedlam, appear. The influence of Hogarth on Mackenzie's description of Bedlam is in itself not unexpected. Swift had used what can be described as a Hogarthian technique in his analogy to a madhouse in "The Legion Club" (1736), directly referring to Hogarth's plate.[4] What Mackenzie accomplishes is to transfer both the visual presentation of Hogarth's Bedlam and its moral message into a fiction of the insane.

Hogarth's message of dissolution punished by madness and Mackenzie's appropriation of that image have their roots in an understanding of the absolute link between the physical body, represented by the individual's sexuality (or passion), and the mind. For Hogarth the sign of Rakewell's corrupt decay is Rakewell's sexual activities, exemplified by Hogarth's presentation of the brothel scene at the Rose. Rakewell's madness is linked to physical excess, specifically to his unbridled sexuality. In Mackenzie's novel moral dissolution is punished by madness. In his portrait of the young girl driven mad by her father's unnatural demands, insanity results from a similar disruption of the natural order of sexuality. However, while Rakewell's madness is his punishment, the girl's is her escape. Her father, however, is punished: "God would not prosper such cruelty; her father's affairs soon after went to wreck, and he died almost a beggar."

Here is the link between Rakewell's world and that of Mackenzie's asylum. For in Rakewell's world his moral (and sexual) dissolution is the direct result of his inherited (rather than earned) wealth. Hogarth is certainly not offering the viewer an anticapitalist message—quite the contrary, he sees earning a living as the highest goal. Living on acquired wealth, at least in the dissolution of London, leads to sexual adventures and eventual madness. This is quite a different path from that taken by his protagonist in the *Harlot's Progress*, whose dissolute end is not of insanity but of physical disease and decay. In the asylum visited by Harley, the beautiful woman's madness is the result of "love sickness" (erotomania); her father's punishment is bankruptcy, the economic parallel to insanity. Madness and wealth are linked in these two models in an overt manner. "Natural" actions—the earning of wages, the correct, fatherly attitude toward the daughter—are violated, and the result is an overturning of the world, which dissolves into madness or financial ruin. These are parallel signs of dissolution which link the basic economics of the worlds in which they are found with the representation of the "rational."

Both the artist and the writer put their moral fable center stage. While the fictions are different, their presentations are identical. Each is surrounded by similar casts of characters to give the sense of the world of the asylum. In both there is an intrusion of the observer who sees the events. He also sees the other observers but distances himself from their curiosity. The origin of the madness that forms the centerpiece, and in a sense defines the asylum, is the madness of passion, of human sexuality. The observer remains distanced from those whose lives have been destroyed by passion. In the plate his is the artist's eye, his voice that of the moral poem appended to the plate; in the novel, his eye is that of the sentimental hero. Unlike the early eighteenth-century reaction of moral outrage, Harley's reaction is physical, is that of a man of feeling: he bursts into tears and leaves the asylum. In Mackenzie's representation of the asylum, the appropriate response to those destroyed by sexuality is a passionate one, but one that results in the observing "eye" leaving the place of the confinement of passion.

Kleist and the Iconography of Onanism

In the fall of 1800 the young Heinrich von Kleist journeyed to Würzburg.[5] Two days after his arrival he visited the Julius-Hospital, an asylum founded by the Prince-Bishop Julius Echter von Mespelbrunn in 1576. Kleist's description of his tour through the asylum begins with a description of the physical buildings, but soon his interest and eye turn to the inmates. The first patients observed by the writer "lay upon one another, like blocks, totally without sensation."[6] They are without features, shadows about whom one could wonder "whether they were human." As in Mackenzie's portrait of the asylum, Kleist's madmen take three-dimensional shape in the eye of the observer when he is actually approached by one of the patients. Harley's guide can talk sensibly about the other inmates, can intelligently observe that "the world, in the eye of a philosopher, may be said to be a large madhouse," while at the same time he believes himself to be the "Chan of Tartary." With Kleist it is the mad professor who "asked so quickly and casually and spoke such a correct, coherent Latin, that we truly wondered how to answer him, as if he were a rational man." A black-cowled specter, a monk, suffers from the delusion that, having once mumbled in delivering a sermon, "he falsified God's word." Here too we find a merchant "who went mad out of chagrin and pride, because his father was nobled and did not bequeath his title to his son." But these background figures, with their confused and garbled discourses, are dismissed in a few lines. Central to Kleist's portrait of the asylum is the final figure, "whom an unnatural sin had driven mad." Kleist describes him in considerable detail:

An eighteen-year-old youth, who had shortly before been extremely handsome and still bore some signs of this, hung above the unclean opening with naked, pale, desiccated limbs; hollow chest; powerless, sunken head,—his dead white face, like that of a tubercular patient, became florid, lifeless, veined. His eyelids fell powerlessly over his dying, fading eyes; a few dry hairs, like those of an old man, covered his prematurely bald head; his dry, thirsty, parched tongue hung over his pale, shrunken lips; his hands, bound and sewn in restraints, lay behind his back. He could no longer move his tongue to speak, he had hardly the strength even for his piercing breaths. His brain-nerves were not mad but exhausted, completely powerless, no longer able to obey his soul. His entire life was nothing but a single, crippling, eternal swoon [*Ohnmacht*].

Kleist's presentation of the Julius-Hospital is indebted to the visual image and the attendant root-metaphor of the tableau of the insane as found in Hogarth and Mackenzie. *The Man of Feeling* had been translated into German in 1794 (with subsequent editions and translations in 1802, 1803, and 1808). Hogarth's unabated popularity can be seen in the continued posthumous publication of Lichtenberg's commentary. Lichtenberg's extensive interpretation of the Bedlam scene in *The Rake's Progress* appeared first in 1808. While it is not certain that Kleist knew either the illustration or the novel, it is evident from his text that he had been exposed to this eighteenth-century visual model of the asylum. His description thus reflected the figures and their arrangement as found in Hogarth's asylum as well as its root-metaphor. The view of the asylum as a microcosm of the rational world is the external structure by which Kleist organizes his comprehension of the madman. It also, however, provides him with the key in placing aspects of his personal, unresolved struggles within the fictional world of an asylum that serves as a metaphor for the world.

Kleist expands and transcends the eighteenth-century function of the visual image of the asylum because he uses a model of madness, that of masturbatory insanity, from which he cannot distance himself even through projection. Although he selects figures from the actual population of the asylum for inclusion in his description in such a way as to reflect his visual model, he enlarges upon the implications and function of the figures he employs. Much like Mackenzie, Kleist restructures the representations of "madness" as a result of sexuality to fulfill his own needs and to reflect a specific construction of the idea of madness which dominated his own time. But Kleist's use of the model of masturbatory insanity also alters the point of observation of the decay of the rational into madness. The natural link is made between the decay of the rational and, as shall be shown, the question of earning a living. For Kleist the central figure in his panorama is the youth, with whom he clearly identifies. Anton Müller, who functioned as the second medical officer in the Julius-Hospital after 1798, describes one of the patients present during the period from February 1798 to October 1801 (i.e., during the period when Kleist visited the asylum): "a young man from Saxony, idiotic because of the sin of self-pollution, here not the cause but rather the result of the earlier manifestation of idiocy, brought him ever more to the level of the bestial."[7] While it is evident that the description of the youth owes much to Hogarth's image of the prostrate Rakewell, Kleist's description of his disease and its appearance provides a key to his incorporation of this figure in his representation of the asylum in the light of the altered implication of the somatic origin of madness.

While Rakewell's state is the result of a life of dissolution, Kleist's youth is brought into the asylum through "an unnatural sin," "self-pollution." To understand this reference and its importance in this letter, the nature of Kleist's trip to Würzburg must be understood. Kleist had resigned his commission in the Prussian army in April 1799. During the following two years he became engaged to his pupil Wilhelmine von Zenge, undertook the still puzzling trip to Würzburg, and decided to become a writer. His voyage is therefore a voyage of self-definition, not only in terms of his "calling" but in terms of his economic redefinition of himself as an author. (It had only been since Friedrich Gottlieb Klopstock's successful career, beginning in the 1760s, that writing was understood in the German states as an economically independent, i.e., middle-class, profession.) Elaborate theories concerning the rationale for the trip to Würzburg have been proposed, most dealing with some physical malady that prevented Kleist from consummating his relationship with his fiancée.[8] However, the best explanation for the Würzburg trip has been proposed by Heinz Politzer, who views it as the means by which Kleist resolved the crisis in his identity which had resulted from his moving from the world of the military to that of the literati. But Politzer overlooks a central point in his analysis of the description of the Julius-Hospital, in that Kleist in this description creates his first work of fiction. Politzer dismisses the description of the Julius-Hospital as "projections of the charges against the self. . . . The 'unnatural sin,' this 'weakness' . . . assumes a major place in them. Whatever this is to be identified as—whether masturbation, homosexuality, or an unknown third cause—it stood for one who had gone against the will of nature and represented Kleist's status before his trip to Würzburg." Here the attempt to avoid the question of Kleist's own source of self-doubt causes Politzer to miss one of the strongest arguments in support of his thesis. For Kleist is describing a case of masturbatory insanity in his portrait of the youth, and the implications of this directly reflect the nature of his identity crisis.

The hypothesis that masturbation was a cause, if not the prime cause,

of insanity was first promulgated in the anonymous English moral tractate *Onania; or, The Heinous Sin of Self-Pollution* (1700).[9] But it was not
until the publication in 1758 of Samuel Auguste André David Tissot's
*L'Onanisme, ou Dissertation physique sur les maladies produites par la
masturbation* (translated into German in 1785) that the idea of masturbatory insanity became commonplace in the lay as well as the medical
community. By 1784 Germany's most respected educator, Christian
Gotthilf Salzmann, had published for the broadest possible audience his
essay *On the Secret Sins of Youth*, which appeared in a fourth edition in
1819.[10] With Kleist's interest in popular medical and psychological questions it is most probable that he knew the general tenor of the literature
on insanity *ex onania* whether directly or indirectly.[11] Central to all of
the literature on masturbation was the image that the masturbator
ceased to be a productive member of society and became dependent,
often institutionalized.

Kleist's description of the eighteen-year-old youth reflects, in all of its
ramifications, the contemporary understanding of the economics of masturbatory insanity in the tension between the rational, "natural" world
of sexuality and the world of sexual abuse. According to the eighteenth-
century view, masturbation dissipated the vital essence of natural spirit
and therefore led to insanity. Benjamin Rush, the most important figure
in eighteenth-century American medicine, reports the following case
study in 1812: "A.B. aged seventeen, of a cold phlegmatic temperament
of body, of a sedentary life, and studious habits, in consequence of indulg-
ing in the solitary vice of onanism, has lately become very much diseased. His vision is indistinct, and his memory much impaired, and he
now labours under much muscular relaxation, prostration of strength,
atrophy, and depression of spirits."[12] The potentially productive member
of society becomes mad and institutionalized simultaneously. A further
case study from the original tractate *Onania*, which was translated into
German as early as 1765 and widely read and cited, stressed the collapse
of the nerves and the loss of feeling in the limbs.[13] This "weakness in the
entire body," or "loss of feeling,"[14] as described by G. W. Becker in his
Prevention and Healing of Onania with All of Its Results in Both Sexes
of 1803, leads to "weakness [*Ohnmacht*] and epilepsy."[15] The weakness
that leads to or is part of madness is the overt sign of the link between the
physical and the rational, the strength of body and therefore of mind,
mens sana in corpore sano. But it is also a sign of the exclusion of the
masturbator from the world of commerce, of competition, for which he
or she is not fit.

Indeed, the very mode of treatment of the patient leads the reader to
understand the nature of his illness. Totally catatonic, sewn into restraints that fix his hands behind his back to prevent further masturba-

tion, he sits in a "tranquillizer," a chair that, among other things, "relieves him, by means of a close stool, half filled with water, over which he constantly sits, from the foetor and filth of his alvine evacuations."[16] The stool is described by Kleist as "the unclean opening" (Plate 16). But central to Kleist's image is the silence of the masturbator. He has lost all use of speech. He is not only without sensation, but without language. Language, the means by which the author defines his or her role in the world, the tool through which the author attains economic independence, is lost. The masturbator cannot be a writer. Thus Kleist uses the commonly understood description of insanity *ex onania*, of a madness rooted in the abuse of the body, in creating the central fiction for his presentation of the Julius-Hospital. Where Mackenzie and Hogarth sought to present the relationship between sexuality and madness as central, in Kleist's world the model for that relationship was no longer heterosexuality, but masturbation. The images have remained constant; their implications have changed markedly.

Kleist uses the young man suffering from all of the symptoms that Voltaire ascribes to the masturbator.[17] And Kleist lists these in the context of an exchange of letters with his fiancée. This was a correspondence standing at least partially within the dual tradition of the philosophical and travel epistles. This fictional form, so beloved in the eighteenth century, placed its emphasis on the didactic nature of prose. To this point Kleist's use of the image of the asylum is in keeping with the form of the philosophical correspondence. But this correspondence is also the exchange of letters between two lovers, one tormented by emotional problems concerning both his private and his public lives. Kleist's image of the masturbator *sans* language is thus embedded in a complex verbal construction. For he is using language to represent one without language while addressing a passive reader. How much more complex a presentation than is first suspected. For the didactic nature of the metaphor of the asylum as found in Hogarth and Mackenzie is also embedded in language. Hogarth appends a long verbal explanation to his engraving (which is absent in the painting upon which it was based), and Mackenzie translates Hogarth's image and text into a verbal account of his visit of Bedlam. The destruction of the language of the central figures, condemned to madness because of their sexuality and their passions, is illuminated by the author/engraver's command of language.

If Kleist's fear was the prospect of insanity brought about by his earlier sexual practices, it was also closely linked with his potential choice of a career. Not only are the prime symptoms of masturbatory insanity fatuity and the loss of language, but language is also the cause of masturbatory insanity. While little space is given in eighteenth-century studies to the cause of masturbation, most authorities of the time place the

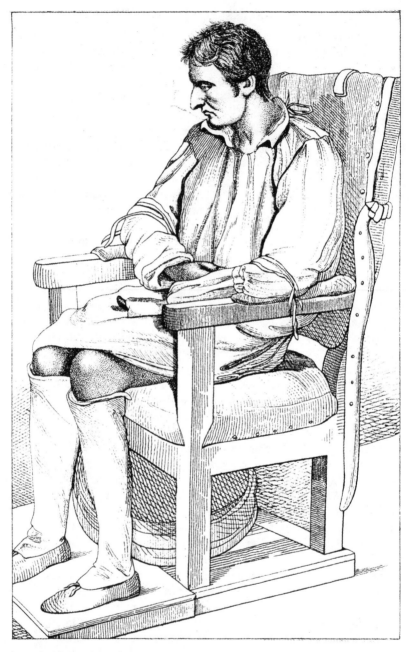

16. The retaining seat described by Kleist, from the atlas to J. E. D. Esquirol, *Des maladies mentales* (Paris: Baillière, 1838) (private collection, Ithaca, N.Y.).

blame squarely at the door of "evil books, bad society, novels, and love stories."[18] Becker makes his Rousseauian charge even more specific:

Many writers, especially the French, have made the effort to present in such glowing colors all types of physical sensuality, both natural and unnatural, so that their works are purchased by many usually properly educated and well-to-do individuals of both sexes and read with unbelievable zeal. These works tickle the fantasy and the imagination with the most voluptuous representations, which are expanded in the imagination. The readers observe with unmistakable pleasure the copperplate engravings, and believe that such a means of achieving pleasure is without detriment for the body, and is more readily permitted than the satisfaction of the sexual drive outside of marriage.[19]

Thus it is the reading of fiction which is the primary cause of masturbation, of which the central symptom is the loss of language. (This type of parallelism is found consistently within European medicine and is codified by C. F. S. Hahnemann's homeopathic medicine of the nineteenth century with its motto "similia similibus curantur.") Here Kleist's dilemma becomes clearer. Having overcome his earlier struggle with masturbation, still haunted by the prospect of insanity because of it, he is considering beginning a new career as a writer. Fiction as the source of the masturbatory impulse is also an element in the root-metaphor of mental illness that he applied to his reality. Writing is somehow associated with madness; the act of creating language, with the silence of the inhabitant of the madhouse. Thus in composing his description of the Julius-Hospital Kleist moves from the traditional didactic model to a representation based on the model of masturbatory insanity which he uses to exorcise the specter of his own madness. Here the creation of a world of words (the letter with its image of the figure of the youth) is used to destroy a fiction (the coupling of madness and writing).

The externalization of his fear in the fiction of the young man destroys the fear by making it palpable. Kleist's horror at the conclusion of the description ("O better a thousand deaths, than a single life like this!") is his reaction to the fiction he himself has created. The passage ends with his awareness that he has created a work of art: "O away with this horrible image—." The image is that of Hogarth's asylum modified by an early nineteenth-century construction of mental illness which is used to present Kleist's internal conflict. In using the association between the madness that he felt and its implied somatic cause to his own ends, Kleist manages to distance his own fear of collapse and change. The act of writing banishes this fear, reducing it to comprehensible form. With the act of creating this image of madness he achieves the first stage in his new identity as an author.

William James and the French Patient

In Edinburgh, the home of Henry Mackenzie, some hundred years after Kleist's visit to the Julius-Hospital, the American philosopher and psychologist William James delivered the Gifford Lectures on Natural Religion.[20] James included ample discussion of the psychopathic aspects of religious experience. It is, however, not so much his discussion of this aspect of religion which is of interest, but his examples. In the segment of the lectures entitled "The Sick Soul," James quotes extensively from Tolstoy and Bunyan in describing the nature of the melancholic mind. The conclusion of this chapter in the printed version of the lectures presents "the worst kind of melancholy," that "which takes the form of panic fear."[21] To illustrate this ultimate form of the sick soul he cites the following anonymous account:

> Whilst in this state of philosophic pessimism and general depression of spirits about my prospects, I went one evening into a dressing-room in the twilight to procure some article that was there; when suddenly there fell upon me without any warning, just as if it came out of the darkness, a horrible fear of my own existence. Simultaneously there arose in my mind the image of an epileptic patient whom I had seen in the asylum, a black-haired youth with greenish skin, entirely idiotic, who used to sit all day on one of the benches, or rather shelves against the wall, with his knees drawn up against his chin, and the coarse gray undershirt, which was his only garment, drawn over them inclosing his entire figure. He sat there like a sort of sculptured Egyptian cat or Peruvian mummy, moving nothing but his black eyes and looking absolutely non-human. This image and my fear entered into a species of combination with each other. *That shape am I*, I felt, potentially. Nothing that I possess can defend me against that fate, if the hour for it should strike for me as it struck for him. There was such a horror of him, and such a perception of my own merely momentary discrepancy from him, that it was as if something hitherto solid within my breast gave way entirely, and I became a mass of quivering fear.

The passage goes on to chronicle how the author was able, only after months, to overcome his anxiety. This "melancholia" had, according to the writer, "a religious bearing," and he was able to transcend it through clinging to scripture.

The source of the vision of the insane youth is given by James in the following manner: "Here is an excellent example, for permission to print which I have to thank the sufferer. The original is in French, and though the subject was evidently in a bad nervous condition at the time of which he writes, his case has otherwise the merit of extreme simplicity. I translate freely." Indeed, James's translation is free, for the source is none other than William James himself. James's son recorded that his father stated that the incident had actually happened to him, and the son dated this vision to the spring of 1870.[22]

The vision of the madman has a specific function in *The Varieties of Religious Experience*. Coming as the final example in James's discussion of "the sick soul," it serves for the author as his ultimate statement of "the fear of the universe" and "the real core of the religious problem: Help! help!" James's cry for help is focused in his presentation of his own experience. But the use of the fictional mode of expression and its form is inherent not in the vision, usually equated with the "great dorsal collapse" of January 1870, but in James's models.[23] It is vital to understand that James's fantasy came at that moment in his own life when he was confronted with a series of life choices as to his career path. Here again is the link between images of madness (and as we shall see, a madness understood as the result of "self-abuse") and the question of career choice and economic definition of the self.

Within the fictional structure surrounding the invented quotation there exist two clues to the origin and nature of the models employed by the author. The primary one is explicit. In a footnote to the passage, William James refers to his own father's work, *Society, the Redeemed Form of Man*, "for another case of fear equally sudden." The elder James recorded his hallucinatory experience near Windsor Castle when William was an infant. He experienced his crisis after a "comfortable dinner" with his family: "To all appearance it was a perfectly insane and abject terror, without ostensible cause, and only to be accounted for, to my perplexed imagination, by some damned shape squatting invisible to me within the precincts of the room, and raying out from his fetid personality influences fatal to life."[24] For the elder James the source of this vision is "the curse of mankind, that which keeps our manhood so little and so depraved . . . its sense of selfhood." This manifests itself in the fruitless search for truth, and the elder James's experience proved to him that "truth must reveal itself if it would be known. . . . For truth is God, the omniscient and omnipotent God, and who shall pretend to comprehend that great and adorable perfection?"

While ignoring his father's Swedenborgian theology, William James makes use of the external structure of this experience when, shortly after the beginning of the twentieth century, he looks back to record his experience of some thirty years earlier. The general structures of the two passages are remarkably similar. The sense of anxiety appears suddenly, it is conceived of as a being, it destroys all sense of equilibrium, and it resolves itself in a form of religious awareness. But the specific nature of the vision is different. The amorphous "damned shape" takes on a definite form for the younger James in his vision of the madman.

Here the question of the second model becomes of great importance. How does James see the insane? For his image is quite unlike the asylum scenes of the late eighteenth and early nineteenth centuries with their Hogarthian root-metaphor. He sees a solitary figure, without background or context, seated, his knees drawn up to his chin, an idiot, "looking absolutely non-human." James's portrait reflects a nineteenth-century understanding of how the insane are to be seen. For James's description is an almost literal portrait of one of the plates in Jean Etienne Dominique Esquirol's monumental *Des maladies mentales considérées sous les rapports médical, hygienique, et médico-legal* (1838). This standard work contained the first atlas containing full-length portraits of the mentally ill. Plate twenty-four presents a figure seated on a low shelf, his knees drawn up to his chest, his coarse singlet drawn over his knees (Plate 17). His gaze is directed straight at the observer. In his text Esquirol notes that this figure represents an idiot named Aba in the asylum at Bicêtre. He can say only "ba ba ba," and is so simple that he can only feed himself. He has no memory. And finally, "Aba is a masturbator."[25] James's vision of the insane is filtered through Esquirol's image of Aba. This explains, at least to a certain degree, why James creates a French source for his vision. It is not so much that James is describing Esquirol's plate, but that he conceived of his image in terms of a nineteenth-century visualization of the insane.

When the final piece of information, James's contemporary account of his vision, is sought, the reader is stymied. For while it is evident that James underwent a period of severe depression in the winter of 1870, no reference is made during this period, either in his diaries or in his letters, to such a vision. One is led to the inescapable conclusion that James first recorded this vision during his writing of the Gifford Lectures. At this point he looked back at his earlier experience through the description in his father's text, which was not published until 1879, and through his scientific reading concerning the physiognomy of the insane. One might imagine that a scholar of James's reputation would avoid an overtly autobiographical presentation in a series of university lectures. But James's vision had an even more deeply personal bias, which is revealed in his text.

In James's text the existential anxiety that generated and was generated by the vision had a specific personal relationship. Why does James visualize a madman when his father sees nothing, only sensing the presence of evil? Taking into consideration the struggle between the elder Henry James and his sons, William and Henry Jr., one might assume that the use of the structure of his father's vision may lead to a solution to the

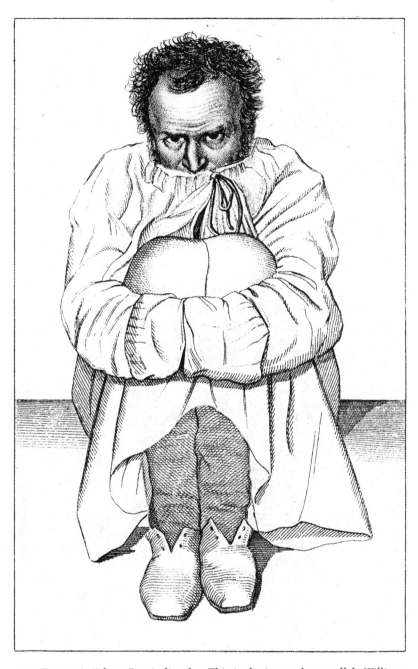

17. "Dementia," from Esquirol's atlas. This is the image that parallels William James's representation of his own madness.

enigma of the vision.[26] However, James's use of the image of the madman provides the final clue. For James's vision, which so frightened him, with which he so identified, portrayed a victim of masturbatory insanity. James's soul-sickness of 1870 was indeed philosophical in its manifestation, but the evil "inherent in the universe's details" was of a personal nature. James's fear of madness was not an abstract fear, such as that portrayed by his father. It was a direct fear of receding into madness as a result of his own behavior.

The extensive entry in James's diary on February 1, 1870, describes his fear in a direct manner: "Hitherto I have tried to fire myself with the moral interest, as an aid in the accomplishing of certain utilitarian ends of attaining certain difficult but salutary habits. I tried to associate the feeling of Moral degradation with failure. . . . But in all this I was cultivating the moral . . . only as a means and more or less humbugging myself."[27] James's sense of inadequacy, his recently concluded medical studies, the success of his friends (such as Charles Peirce) could all be laid at the door of his personal life. James was confronted with a choice of what he was to do with the rest of his life. Coloring this choice was James's inner sense of his own sexual inadequacy, which stemmed from the condemnation of masturbation as a sign of a "weak personality."[28] Contemporary writers, such as Henry Maudsley, emphasized the relationship between diffuseness of character and masturbation: "The patient becomes offensively egotistic and impracticable; he is full of self-feeling and self-conceit; insensible to the claims of others upon him and his duties to them: interested only in hypochondriacally watching his morbid sensations and attending his morbid feelings. His mental energy is sapped; and though he has extravagant pretensions, and often speaks of great projects engendered by his conceit, he never works systematically for any aim, but exhibits an incredible vacillation of conduct, and spends his days in indolent and suspicious self-brooding."[29] This pattern eventually leads to insanity.

In looking back at his experience of 1870, James frames his vision to incorporate the structure of his father's sense of dread. The conflict between father and son, the guilt felt in his personal life, his sense of inadequacy especially in regard to his father, all merge in the vision. In structuring his "vision" some thirty years after it occurred, James is able to externalize these feelings in his fiction recounting his earlier vision of his fear of masturbatory insanity. Here purgation is accomplished through the description of an earlier purgation.

Madness and Sexuality

The three texts that have been examined present three different constructions of the image of the insane. Mackenzie's novelistic treatment is indebted to Hogarth's model, transferring it from the realm of art to that of literature. He preserves Hogarth's didactic model of the asylum as a moral microcosm, simply replacing Hogarth's fable of *The Rake's Progress* with his own tale of unrequited love. He preserves the somatic explanation for madness, stressing its sexual origin. Mackenzie assumes the parallel between "natural" and "unnatural" actions as the cause of madness. He continues, within another dimension, Hogarth's view of the "economic" source of madness. On one level Kleist does much the same thing. He uses the didactic root-metaphor of the asylum to present a lesson about the world to his fiancée. He incorporates this lesson into a model of somatic madness, that of masturbatory insanity, a model that had a special implication for him. However, he projects onto the central figure in the tableau of the insane his own persona. Unlike Mackenzie's hero, who can leave the asylum, Kleist feels himself trapped within its walls.

Here is the basic difference between Mackenzie and Kleist. Whereas for Mackenzie (and Hogarth) the object of the work is to teach the reader (or observer) a moral lesson, Kleist provides a private rationale for the use of this motif. Kleist's text contains a second level of imagery, grounded in the personal implications of masturbatory insanity for him. He externalizes his inner search for identity in the writing of this text. Externalization, according to Karen Horney, is "an active process of self-elimination." It manifests itself in "the tendency to experience internal processes as if they occurred outside oneself and, as a rule, to hold these external factors responsible for one's difficulties."[30] It can also serve as a means of coming to terms with such processes by dissociating oneself from them. Kleist presents a moral lesson concerning human nature to his fiancée while at the same time using the act of writing as a means of liberating himself from his inner conflicts. He permits himself to become a writer through this act of externalization.

With William James's vision of the mad, the image of the insane passes from the eighteenth-century model of masturbatory insanity to a type of psychologization of that model in the nineteenth century. No longer is there the overtly didactic overlay found in Hogarth (and by implication in Kleist). The madman is seen as an individual psyche, not as an inhabitant of the asylum. While James draws on Kleist's second root-metaphor, that of masturbatory insanity, it is the psychological conflict between father and son present in the model of his father's own vision of doom which structures James's text. The conflict between parent and child over career choice now understood in the concept of masturbatory insanity is played out by James in his recounting of his own earlier experience. He remembers his vision through the filter of these two modes of presenting experience. The biological aspect exists, indeed, is central, but it recedes as the psychological qualities of James's image dominate.

With these three images it is clear how older representations of madness (and its relationship to the body) are replaced by other paradigms. The older models are retained but are invested with a new function. Thus while the external image may remain the same, its signification is quite often radically altered. Seeing the insane means apprehending these shifts in representation.

CHAPTER FIVE

Images of the Asylum:
Charles Dickens and Charles Davies

Visiting the Asylum

On 17 January 1852, Charles Dickens's periodical *Household Words* brought an anonymous contribution entitled "A Curious Dance round a Curious Tree," intended to make its readers appreciate their bounty during the holiday season. The essay was substantially by Dickens, as the manuscript shows, with, however, some passages by Dickens's subeditor, William Henry Wills.[1] The "Curious Dance" was the Boxing Day festivity held annually at St. Luke's Hospital for the Insane (Old Street, London); the "Curious Tree," the Christmas tree, the lighting of which ends the essay. The essay was felt to cast such a positive light on the asylum that the directors of St. Luke's reissued the essay as a pamphlet, with Dickens's permission, in 1860.[2]

The essay, certainly appropriate as a moral lesson in counting one's blessings, begins with a description of the reformed asylum at the close of the eighteenth century. It had replaced the proverbial Bedlam, Bethlem Hospital, where "lunatics were chained, naked, in rows of cages that flanked a promenade, and were wondered and jeered at through iron bars by London loungers." The benevolence of the new institution was "mixed, as was usual in that age, with a curious degree of unconscious cruelty." Dickens proceeds to quote at some length and in detail from John Haslam's *Observations on Madness and Melancholy, Including Practical Remarks on Those Diseases* of 1809. Haslam, after a parliamentary inquiry in 1815 revealed such practices at Bedlam, was dismissed from his post there. Dickens sees the forced feeding of patients who refused to eat, the manacles shackling the violent, as signs of the older model for insanity: "These practitioners of old, would seem to have been, without knowing it, early homeopathists; their motto must have been, *Similia similibus curantur;* they believed that the most violent and certain means of driving a man mad, were the only hopeful means of restoring him to reason." It was, however, not in the "chambers of horrors" of the old Windmill Hill Asylum that Dickens actually found himself on that Boxing Day, Friday, 26 December 1851, but in an asylum where "on that night there would be . . . 'a Christmas Tree for the Patients.' And further that the 'usual fortnightly dancing' would take place before the distribution of the gifts upon the tree." The asylum into which Dickens entered bore little resemblance to the "chambers of horrors." Vestiges of the old manner of treating the inmates are present only in the alcoves in "which the chairs, which patients were made to sit in for indefinite periods, were, in the good old times, nailed." This sign of the past, a past ironically characterized as "the good old times," is contrasted with "a niche in which . . . stood a pianoforte, with a few ragged music-leaves upon the desk. Of course, the music was turned upside down."

These observations are made while Dickens is walking through the asylum, toward the "Curious Dance" to be held in a farther gallery: "As I was looking at the marks in the walls of the Galleries, of the posts to which the patients were formerly chained, sounds of music were heard from a distance. The ball had begun, and we hurried off in the direction of the music." The polar structure of the essay can be seen in these passages. The past is the age in which torture dominated the asylum; today, the asylum is the world of civilization. Dickens consciously chooses the image of music and the dance as his metaphor for the new asylum. By the time Dickens reaches the gallery in which the dance is taking place, he (and his readers) have passed through the length of the asylum.[3]

His eye casts itself about the "brown sombre place, not brilliantly illuminated by a light at either end, adorned with holly," and fastens itself on the dancers:

> There were the patients usually to be found in all such asylums, among the dancers. There was the brisk, vain, pippin-faced little old lady, in a fantastic cap—proud of her foot and ankle; there was the old-young woman, with the dishevelled long light hair, spare figure, and weird gentility; there was the vacantly-laughing girl, requiring now and then a warning finger to admonish her; there was the quiet young woman, almost well, and soon going out. For partners, there were the sturdy bull-necked thick-set little fellow who had tried to get away last week; the wry-face tailor, formerly suicidal, but much improved; the suspicious patient with a countenance of gloom, wandering round and round strangers, furtively eyeing them behind from head to foot, and not indisposed

to resent their intrusion. There was the man of happy silliness, pleased with everything. But the only chain that made any clatter was Ladies' Chain, and there was no straiter waistcoat in company than the polka-garment of the old-young woman with the weird gentility, which was of a faded black satin, and languished through the dance with a love-lorn affability and condescension to the force of circumstances, in itself a faint reflection of all Bedlam.

Among the dancers were to be found not only the patients but also the staff, who no longer consisted of the sadistic torturers of the old asylum but had become an extended family. The master, Thomas Collier Walker, and his wife are described as the parents of this family. His wife, Charlotte Eliza Walker, is described as one "whose clear head and strong heart Heaven inspired to have no Christmas wish beyond this place, but to look upon it as her home, and on its inmates as her afflicted children."

The lighting of the Christmas tree climaxes Dickens's visit. In this moment the shades of Christmas past are once and forever exorcised from the asylum:

The moment the dance was over, away the porter ran, not in the least out of breath, to help light up the tree. Presently it stood in the centre of its room, growing out of the floor, a blaze of light and glitter; blossoming in that place (as the story goes of the American aloe) for the first time in a hundred years. O shades of Mad Doctors with laced ruffles and powdered wigs, O shades of patients who went mad in the only good old times to be mad or sane in, and who were therefore physicked, whirligigged, chained, handcuffed, beaten, cramped, and tortured, look from Wherever in your sightless substances, You wait—on this outlandish week in the degenerate garden of Saint Luke's!

With that image fixed in his mind's eye, Dickens left St. Luke's. He concluded his essay with a hope for future Christmases at the asylum:

To lighten the affliction of insanity by all human means, is not to restore the greatest of the Divine gifts; and those who devote themselves to the task do not pretend that it is. They find their sustainment and reward in the substitution of humanity for brutality, kindness for maltreatment, peace for raging fury; in the acquisition of love instead of hatred; and in the knowledge that, from such treatment improvement, and hope of final restoration will come, if such hope be possible. It may be little to have abolished from mad-houses all that is abolished, and to have substituted all that is substituted. Nevertheless, reader, if you can do a little in any good direction—do it. It will be much, some day.

For Dickens the ultimate goal of the asylum is the "restoration" of its inmates to human society, a "restoration" accomplished only through "love."

The Present Moment

To understand the immediate, conscious effect of Dickens's essay on the reader of the late 1850s, one must know that this period saw the conclusion of the debate, in England, concerning the reform of the asylum. While various actions had been undertaken on the continent, culminating in Pinel's reform of Bicêtre during the French Revolution, it was only well into the nineteenth century that a broad, popular interest arose in England concerning the treatment of the insane. Initiated at the very beginning of the century through the activities of the Quakers, the "non-restraint" movement won its major battle with the activities of John Conolly at Hanwell Asylum. "Non-restraint," a term that came to encompass all humane treatment of the insane, was introduced by Conolly into Hanwell in the 1840s.

Conolly, a friend of Dickens, became the spokesman for the new manner of treating the insane.[4] This new manner of treatment implied a new model of viewing the insane. Vieda Skultans, in her study of nineteenth-century ideas on insanity, emphasizes that while the methods of earlier treatment were abandoned, "nineteenth century physicians were not abandoning their role as guardians of the moral order and agents of social control. Physical restraint, coercion and exile are replaced by a philosophy of the self which emphasizes the dual nature of man, the power of the will to prevent and control insanity and which elaborated the arts of self-government."[5]

The control of antisocial behavior is the center of this new system. Its primary goal is the restitution of self-control. "Non-restraint" becomes for Dickens the reform necessary in order to change the image of the mad from the asocial being, existing licentiously beyond the pale of society, to that of a being able to be and desirous of being returned to society. In order to accomplish the creation of this image within the bounds of his essay Dickens begins with an image of insanity acceptable to his readers. Dickens's fiction presents numerous mad characters, ranging from the author of "The Madman's Manuscript" in *The Pickwick Papers* to the schizophrenic John Jasper in *Edwin Drood*. All of Dickens's mad figures have one common feature—their insanity makes them sympathetic rather than horrifying. They are figures who, rather than repelling readers, make them feel superior. The figure of Mr. Dick, the lunatic in *David Copperfield*, can serve as a prime example of Dickens's craftsmanship in shaping the sympathetic image of the mad. The initial draft of Mr. Dick's first appearance in the novel reads as follows:

> I lifted up my eyes to the window above it, where I saw a florid, pleasant-looking gentleman, with a grey head, putting his tongue out against the glass, and carrying it across the pane and back again; who, when his eye caught mine, squinted at me in a manner most terrible, laughed, and went away.[6]

Seen through the eyes of the young David Copperfield, this first meeting with Mr. Dick would have been a terrifying experience. In correcting the proofs, Dickens altered the passage to present a different first impression of the lunatic:

> I lifted up my eyes to the window above it, where I saw a florid, pleasant-looking gentleman, with a grey head, who shut up one eye in a grotesque manner, nodded his head at me several times, shook it at me as often, laughed and went away.

The restructuring of this passage aims at a modification of the horrifying grotesqueness of the madman's squint and laugh. It becomes the not quite comprehensible action of "a pleasant-looking gentleman."

Because the substitution of one model of insanity for another, which Dickens experienced in his own lifetime and which is reflected in his essay on St. Luke's, focused on the introduction of "non-restraint," Dickens deemphasizes the hopelessly insane in his essays and ignores the more grotesque or horrifying aspects of insanity's symptoms, replacing them with comical or endearing ones. The first inmate described in any detail in the essay sits, "sewing a mad sort of seam, and scolding some imaginary person." What disturbs Dickens is the absence of meaningful activity ("work"): "No domestic articles to occupy, to interest, or to entice the mind away from its malady. Utter vacuity." While he sees progress made in "the large amount of cures effected in the hospital, (upwards of sixty-nine per cent during the past year)," he argues that if "the system of finding the inmates employment . . . were introduced into St. Luke's, the proportion of cures would be much greater." A productive restructuring of the insane is Dickens's goal, and for that purpose the insane must be viewed as very close to sanity: "In strictness, we are all mad when we give way to passion, to prejudice, to vice, to vanity; but if all the passionate, prejudiced, vicious and vain people in this world are to be locked up as lunatics, who is to keep the key of the asylum? As was very fairly observed, however, by a learned Baron of the Exchequer, when he was pressed by this argument, if we are all mad, being all madmen, we must do the best we can under such untoward circumstances."[7] So said the *Times* on 22 July 1853. If the sane are indeed so closely related to the insane, then our rejection of the image of insanity is indeed a repression of our inner fear for our own stability.

In a later essay, also written jointly with W. H. Wills, Dickens describes the Asylum for Idiots (Park House, Highgate, London). Here too he turns to his imagined audience and addresses it:

> Madam you are a lady of very fine feelings, you are very easily shocked, you "can't bear" a great deal that a higher wisdom than you would seem to have contemplated your bearing when your little place was allotted to you on this ball. This idiot child of thirteen, sitting in its little chair before the fire—as to its bodily growth, a child of six; as to its mental development, nothing—is an odious sight to you. This idiot old man of eight, with the extraordinarily small head, the paralytic gestures, and the half-palsied forefinger, eternally shaking before his hatchet face as he chatters and chatters, disturbs you very much. But, madam, it were worth while to enquire while the brazen head is yet saying unto you "Time is!" how much of the putting away of these unfortunates in past years, and how much of the putting away of many kinds of unfortunates at any time, may be attributable to that same refinement which cannot endure to be told about them. And, madam, if I may make so bold, I will venture to submit whether such delicate persons as your ladyship may not be laying up a rather considerable stock of responsibility; and you will excuse my saying that I would not have so sensitive a heart in my bosom for the dignity of the whole corporation.[8]

Dickens's goal is to mitigate the horror of insanity and idiocy so that his ideal reader (female, middle-class) can reflect on her social responsibility without being totally overwhelmed by her own inner fears.

The Hidden Moment

Yet another contemporary model of insanity is present in the background to Dickens's essay. It is one that the French critic Hippolyte Taine sensed in his 1858 essay on Dickens, whom he described as follows: "He is a painter, an English painter. Never before, I believe, has the human spirit conceived all of the parts and colors of a picture in greater detail and with more power."[9] For Taine this depictive ability is especially evident in Dickens's portraits of madmen:

> Dickens has painted three or four portraits of the insane, which are quite amusing on first glance, but so true that they are actually quite horrible.

One needs an imagination like his—free of all rules, possessing the potential for excessive, fixed ideas, in order to place the mentally ill into focus. Two figures are especially humorous and horrifying: Augustus, the manic-depressive who is about to marry Miss Pecksniff, and poor Mr. Dick, half-idiot, half-monomaniac, who lives with Miss Trotwood. To understand the sudden bursts of enthusiasm, the unexpected phases of sadness, the unbelievable disconnectedness of a perverted sensibility, to reproduce the retention of thought, the rupture of a course of thought once begun, the interruption by a word, also the same one, which destroys the half-begun sentence and traps the emerging thought; to see the stupid smile, the blank stare, the dwarflike, restless physiognomy of these haggard old children, who painfully make their way from idea to idea, and stumble at every step toward the threshold of truth, a threshold which they cannot cross—to capture all of this one needs the ability which only E. T. A. Hoffmann has to the same degree as Dickens. The play of such fragmented minds is like the squeaking of a door off its hinges: it is painful to hear. One finds there, if one wishes so to label it, an outburst of laughter in dissonance, but even more one registers a moaning and a wailing, and one is horrified, if one tries to measure the clarity, the bizarreness, the excessive enthusiasm and the virulence of the imagination, of the one who has produced such figures, who has carried and supported them to their end without weakening and who found himself in his true medium when he empathized with and created their madness.[10]

It is the visual aspect of the insane, the model of the physiognomy of insanity, which Taine saw in Dickens's "portraits" of the insane. On 27 June 1851, Dickens wrote to P. W. Bankes, "suggesting that, as a painter, he might like to accompany him on a visit he is making to a lunatic asylum."[11]

As was examined earlier, the view that the artist could best capture the essence of insanity had its roots in the theories of physiognomy developed in the late eighteenth century. It was left to John Conolly, in a series of essays in 1858, to work out the most comprehensive theory of this model of madness. Conolly based his essays on a series of photographs taken by a colleague at Surrey Asylum, Hugh W. Diamond. Using these photographs, Conolly presented the strictures for distinguishing between "the ordinary expression of the passions and emotions" and "its exaggeration in those whose reason is beginning to remit its control, and whose wits are just beginning to wander away from the truthful recognition of things."[12] The goal is to draw the fine line between the normal and the abnormal so that a more effective restoration to normality can be achieved.

Dickens, throughout his fictional work as well as the essay under study, had recourse to this manner of distinguishing between the sane and the mad. But, as with the description of Mr. Dick, he tended to limit his descriptions to that fine area just along the borderline between sanity and madness. One sentence from Dickens's essay amply illustrates this procedure through the presentation of four rapid visual images: "There was the brisk, vain, pippin-faced little old lady, in a fantastic cap—proud of her foot and ankle; there was the old-young woman, with the dishevelled long light hair, spare figure, and weird gentility; there was the vacantly laughing girl, requiring now and then a warning finger to admonish her; there was the quiet young woman, almost well, and soon going out."

These four cases are presented in such a manner that the reader observes them in a specific order. The first case is an example of "chronic mania," which Conolly describes in the following manner: "Comical as this picture of an old woman appears at the first view, it tells a somewhat lamentable tale of long mental vexation. . . . The apparently careless air, the reversed bonnet, and a sort of drollery lurking in the cheeks and chin, are largely mixed with traces both of former agitation and excitement, and also with some shadows of lost hope and joy."[13]

The "old-young woman" is an example of "religious melancholy," while the last two cases represent "melancholia passing on to mania" and the final restored state. Here the visualization of the insane enables Dickens to make certain judgments. Insanity is curable and is definable in terms of medical description. It is also the exaggeration of normal states of behavior. In stringing these four descriptions together, however, he is also presenting the evolution of cases from the hopeless (but comical, i.e., acceptable) to the cured. The movement is from abandonment of propriety to quiet acceptance of one's social obligation. When Dickens returned to St. Luke's in January 1858 his purpose, according to his letter to Wilkie Collins, was to see "some distinctly and remarkably developed types of insanity."[14] These types are the visual categories of insanity which Dickens applied when he himself described the insane.

At the very beginning of his essay, Dickens provides an aesthetic structure for observing the insane. This puzzling passage is one of his extremely rare observations of the nature of the visual arts, here using the metaphor of the theater:

How came I, it may be asked, on the day after Christmas Day, of all days in the year, to be hovering outside Saint Luke's, after dark, when I might have betaken myself to that jocund world of Pantomime, where there is no affliction or calamity that leaves the least impression; where a man may tumble into the broken ice, or dive into the kitchen fire, and only be the droller for the accident; where babies may be knocked about and sat upon, or choked with gravy spoons, in the process of feeding, and yet no Coroner be wanted or anybody made uncomfortable; where workmen may fall from the top of a house to the bottom, or even from the bottom of a house to the top, and sustain no injury to the brain, need no hospital, leave no young children; where everyone, in short, is so superior to all the accidents of life, though encountering them at every turn, that I suspect this to be the secret (though many persons may not present it to themselves) of the general enjoyment which an audience of vulnerable spectators, liable to pain and sorrow, find in this class of entertainment.

For Dickens's hypothetical audience the world played out on the stage is a reduction of ordinary, unpredictable life to a shadow-world in which even the most horrifying events have no permanent results. The individual remains untouched by the chance nature of the world. Dickens sees a sense of distance between reality and the observer as a necessary feature of the world. Parallel to this view of the theater is Dickens's own description of St. Luke's. The realities of madness are played out before the observer. He is untouched because of his role as an observer and is able to pattern that which he sees so as to present a world in which cure is a certainty. As part of this procedure, insanity becomes solely a part of an external world. One result of so constructing insanity is to place it outside of the perceiver, to distance it, and, therefore, to lessen its immediacy.

The Historical Moment

In addition to the models of "non-restraint" and physiognomy, both of which the nineteenth century would have recognized as permissible parameters for insanity, there is a third. Even though this model has more complex folkloric overtones than the other two, it is so deeply ingrained in Western images of insanity as not to be immediately apparent. Why does Dickens go to St. Luke's? The major reason he gives in the essay is the festive occasion, the Christmas tree and the dance which "would take place before the distribution of the gifts upon the tree." It is the dance, the ultimate social act of the polite society of his time, which entices Dickens to the asylum on this particular day.

Dances were indeed held in Victorian asylums. Edgar Sheppard, at Colney Hatch Asylum, "had dramatic and musical talent, organized concerts, readings, lectures, 'theatrical representations' and fortnightly balls and formed the asylum band."[15] In a lithograph by Katharine Drake done in 1848 a "lunatic's ball" is portrayed with Dickens's cast of characters already present (Plate 18). They dance to a band playing to the rear of the gallery while over the portal the word "HARMONY" shines.[16]

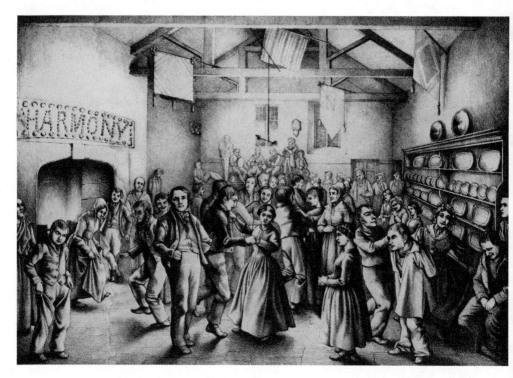

18. Katharine Drake, *Lunatic's Ball* (1848) (Royal College of Psychiatrists, London).

The Victorian "dance of the insane" is but one stage in a long tradition. A seventeenth-century illustration of an "Academy of Fools" shows us "everything which true mania can invent in a bizarre brain of the comic" (Plate 19).[17] The fools, "disguised in masks, exert themselves, spring about. They turn and bend their grotesque bodies in a thousand fantastic figures." The dance of the insane is the total release of the mad from any strictures of society, indeed when Logic wishes to enter the portal it is threatened by one of the fools: "they could be beaten by that fool who is mocking them." This French illustration is closely related to Pieter Breughel the Elder's copperplate engraving of 1559 entitled *The Feast of Fools*.[18] Here too musicians play for the dancing fools, who tumble and gyrate around the stage on which the band is perched.

The close relationship between the world of the fool and that of the insane, at least in terms of sixteenth-century thought, can also be found in Breughel's work. In a series of plates portraying the pilgrimage of epileptics to the shrine at Molenbeek, the illustrations of the pilgrims are preceded by two plates showing the antics of fools.[19] Here too the musical and dancing fool makes an appearance. The popular mind associated

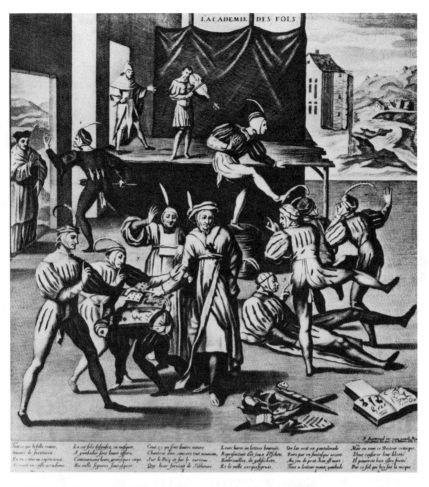

19. *The Academy of Fools* (seventeenth century) (Rene Fülöp-Miller, *Kampf gegen Schmerz und Tod* [Berlin: Süd-Ost, 1938]).

the uncontrolled spasms of chorea with the equally uncontrolled actions of hyperactive mental diseases. They were viewed as dances of the fools or the possessed. Closely related to this development during the late Middle Ages was the appearance of mass hysterical dancing, given the popular names of St. John's or St. Vitus's Dance, still later, Tarantism.[20]

One other strand that runs through the image of the dancing madman should be mentioned. One of the amusements at the court of Charles VI of France was the dance of the wild men, of the *wodwoses*. The wild men were originally the Viking berserkers (the followers of Wodan = Odin), but became the image of the madman as wild man. Their mad dance was a source of entertainment at the court, a fact recorded only by virtue of Charles's narrow escape from being burned alive when, in 1392, the hairy costume of a *wodwos* that he was wearing ignited.[21]

The model upon which all of these images of the mad dancers was based is the late Dionysiac rite of the Corybantes. The Dionysiac ritual, with its possessed dancers and its human sacrifices, became domesticated as it was adapted into Greek tradition from its Eastern origins.[22] But the associations with the harmless Greek festivity surrounding the wine god became inexorably linked with the mindless passion of the Dionysiac ritual.

For Aristotle this madness was a direct result of the "Phrygian mode which inspires enthusiasm."[23] The sound of the flute playing in this mode possessed the listeners and forced them to dance. Their dance is the result of the total suppression of all their logical faculties and their surrender to the power of music. If this were the total evolution of the model of madness which culminates in Dickens's essay, there would be little profit won by following the topos of the dance of the insane back to its origin. For mad dancers are ubiquitous in Western culture. There is, however, one further aspect of the model of the Dionysiac ritual which, through a series of complicated developments, reappears in Dickens's essay. This is the curative nature of the dance of the insane.

Plato, in the *Laws*, describes how mothers, when they wish "to put fractious babies to sleep" employ "not stillness, but its very opposite, movement" as well as a melody of some kind:

> In fact they, so to say, put a spell on their babies just as the priestess does on the distracted in the Dionysiac treatment, by this combination of the movements of dance and song.
> *Clinias:* And pray, sir, what explanation are we to give of these facts?
> *Athenian:* Why, the explanation is not far to seek.
> *Clinias:* But what is it?
> *Athenian:* Both disturbances are forms of fright, and fright is due to some morbid condition of the soul. Hence, when such disorders are treated by rocking movement the external motion thus exhibited dominates the internal, which is the source of the fright or frenzy. By its domination it produces a mental sense of calm and relief from the preceding distressing agitation of the heart, and thus effects a welcome result in both cases, the induction of sleep in the one; in the other—that of patients who are made to dance to the flute in the ritual of the deities to whom sacrifice is done on these occasions—the substitution of sanity for their temporary state of distraction.[24]

Thus dance is not only a sign of madness, it is also its cure. So too with the other forms of the mad dancers or fools. Felix Plater in his *Praxeos medicae opus* of 1656 chronicles how the authorities of Basel hired several strong young men to dance with a girl who had "the dancing mania," to dance with her until she was cured. Clearly Breughel's dancing fools are present on the pilgrimage to serve as a counterforce to the epileptics, helping to cure or at least distract them with their music and antics. So too is Katharine Drake's Victorian ball a manner of restoring sanity to the insane through music and dance. Here, however, we have passed from the miraculous powers of dance to the power of dance as a social force. For, in Drake's lithograph and in Dickens's essay, the restoration of the insane to a recognizable social role is undertaken through the dance.

The construction of madness and its cure which Dickens employs is explicitly described for the reader in the opening of the essay. He criticizes the "good old" manner of treatment, in which madness was treated by torture: "These practitioners of old, would seem to have been, without knowing it, early homeopathists; their motto must have been, *Similia similibus curantur;* they believed that the most violent and certain means of driving a man mad, were the only hopeful means of restoring him to reason." Samuel Hahnemann's homeopathy was well received in Victorian London as well as on the continent. The idea of a treatment which re-created the same symptoms as the disease had already entered, like the physiognomy of insanity, into the popular consciousness.

But Dickens was not arguing that insanity was caused by music in the Phrygian mode and could only be cured by music, according to Aristotle, in the Dorian mode. Dickens sees society itself as one of the prime causes of insanity. Indeed one of the reasons for his trip to St. Luke's was his concern with the unsafe conditions in the Smithfield cattle-market:

Not long before the Christmas Night in question, I had been told of a patient in Saint Luke's, a woman of great strength and energy, who had been driven mad by an infuriated ox in the streets—an inconvenience not in itself worth mentioning, for which the inhabitants of London are frequently indebted to their inestimable Corporation. She seized the creature literally by the horns, and so, as long as limb and life were in peril, vigorously held him; but, the danger over, she lost her senses, and became one of the most ungovernable of the inmates of the asylum.

But it is not just Smithfield market and environs that are the cause of insanity. The entire world through which Dickens passes on his way to St. Luke's is itself unbalanced:

There was a line of hackney cabriolets by the dead wall; some of the drivers, asleep; some, vigilant; some, with their legs not inexpressive of

"Boxing," sticking out of the open doors of their vehicles, while their bodies were reposing on the straw within. There were flaming gas-lights, oranges, oysters, paper lanterns, butchers and grocers, bakers and public-houses, over the way; there were omnibuses rattling by; there were bal-lad-singers, street cries, street passengers, street beggars, and street music.

This is the world of post-Christmas drunkenness, of Boxing Day excess. It is Victorian London's Saturnalia, the Feast of Fools, the world turned into a madhouse.[25]

How narrow is the line between the sane and the mad; how close the external world to the world of the asylum. And the reverse is true. The "Curious Dance" is itself a monument to how close insanity can be brought to sanity through the liberating moment of carnival, a festivity felt to be within the bounds of Victorian propriety.

Dickens Revivified

Some twenty years after the publication (and subsequent republica-tion) of "A Curious Dance round a Curious Tree," after the essay had generally faded from memory, an article appeared in the *London Daily Telegraph* under the title "A Lunatic Ball." The author, a Church of England clergyman, Charles Maurice Davies, had contributed a series of columns to the *Telegraph* on unusual religious practices in London.[26] Here he deviated from his normal practice and went behind the wall of Hanwell Asylum, disguised in the manner of the hard-working London newspaperman, like James Greenwood, to get his story.

"A Lunatic Ball" is distanced enough in time from Dickens's essay to give a sense of the development of the three constructs of insanity pre-sent in the earlier essay. The lunatic ball at Hanwell, John Conolly's first reformed asylum, was also held at Christmastime, during the ancient Roman Saturnalia. It is on a "damp, muggy January evening" during which the author crosses "the Dantesque portal of the institution" dis-guised as a member of a German band. While the location is Hanwell rather than St. Luke's, the atmosphere is identical. The author (and his reader) walk through the galleries, observing that these wards were "very like living in a passage."

Here too we encounter "one old lady, who claimed to be a scion of royalty" in her "resplendent mob-cap." In Davies's essay also the visual vignette plays an important role in determining the borderline between sanity and madness. He sees "one or two, whose countenances really seemed to justify their incarceration." The festivities are less inhibited than in St. Luke's:

In the centre of the room all was gravity and decorum, but the merriest dances went on in corners. An Irish quadrille was played, and an unmistakable Paddy regaled himself with a most beautiful jig. He got on by himself for a figure or two, when, remembering, no doubt, that "happiness was born a twin," he dived into the throng, selected a white-headed old friend of some sixty years, and impressed him with the idea of a *pas de deux*. There they kept it up in a corner for the whole of the quadrille, twirling imaginary shillelaghs, and encouraging one another with that expressive Irish interjection which it is so impossible to put down on paper. For an hour all went merry as the proverbial marriage ball, and then there was an adjournment of the male portion of the company to supper.

The similarities between Dickens's visit and that of Davies are evident. What has changed is the image of the asylum in the implied model of insanity. Davies, along with others who subscribed to the theory of the reform of the insane, "moral management," left his essay open as he pondered:

One question would keep recurring to my mind. It has been said that if you stop your ears in a ballroom, and then look at the people—reputed sane—skipping about in the new valse or the last galop, you will imagine they must be all lunatics. I did not stop my ears that night, but I opened my eyes and saw hundreds of my fellow-creatures, all with some strange delusions, many with ferocious and vicious propensities, yet all kept in order by a few warders, a handful of girls, and all behaving as decorously as in a real ballroom. And the question which *would* haunt me all the way home was, which are the sane people, and which the lunatics?

For the writer the line between sanity and insanity seemed fine. For the inmates, on the other hand, the distinction was clear: "The prevailing opinion inside the walls was that the majority of madmen lay outside, and that the most hopelessly insane people in all the world were the officers immediately concerned in the management of the establishment itself." The distance between sanity and insanity is great, especially if seen from within the asylum.

For the asylum, with its "Dantesque portal" is indeed a place whose motto is "Lasciate ogni speranza voi ch'entrate [Abandon hope, all ye who enter here]!" Release is through "the little dead-house and the quiet cemetery lying out in the moonlight . . . waiting for them when, as poor maddened Edgar Allan Poe wrote, the 'fever called living,' should be 'over at last.'" For Davies the reform of the asylum lies hidden in the past. His historical consciousness is reduced to a single mention of lunatics "being chained and treated as wild beasts." For him the wall of the asylum is indeed the dividing line between the world that calls itself sane and the world of the mad. For the festivities at Hanwell are not a bridge upon which the insane may re-enter the world of the sane. They are the activities of and for the asylum. The asylum has become "a small town in itself, and to a large extent self-dependent and self-governed." But at the same time it is a closed world that senses its own distance from the world of the sane. The madhouse has ceased being an asylum, a refuge from the world, and has become an institution, a structure harboring the insane. From the former there was the promise of a return to the outside world; from the latter, this promise was lacking.

Tracing Madness

In Dickens's essay "A Curious Dance round a Curious Tree" three constructs of insanity exist simultaneously. The model of "moral management," rooted in the contemporary reform of the asylum, is on the most conscious of these levels. Also present in Dickens's essay as well as in psychiatric practice of the period is the model of the physiognomy of insanity. This model, while only an undercurrent in the essay, supports the general thesis of the nature (and therefore the treatment) of the insane.

The primary model postulates sanity and insanity as single moments on a continuum. Affecting only one aspect of the individual's personality, the disability of madness is an exaggeration of some normal state. Once this exaggeration is corrected, the individual can be returned to society. Indeed, the relationship between sanity and insanity is so close that only the practiced eye can really distinguish between the sane and the insane. Once trained, however, this eye can judge those asocial members of a community and institutionalize them to be cured and returned as productive members to that selfsame society. The process of resocialization is present in the third strand in Dickens's essay. The therapeutic nature of the dance for the insane is a pattern of treatment recurring throughout Western thought. The motto of the curative dance is like cured by like. Madness induced by music is cured by music. Here Dickens varies his theme slightly. It is society itself which contains the seeds of potential madness hidden in its institutions. But it is through other institutions, such as the dance, that mental balance can be returned.

When Davies's essay is examined, written as it was some twenty years after the publication of Dickens's work, certain alterations in levels of consciousness can be seen. First, the historical contrast of old and new manners of treatment is no longer bright and vivid in Davies's mind's eye. The reform of the asylum lies in the past. The model implied by this reform, resocialization, has been shown to be in practice idealistic. The asylum had become solely the place where the insane were kept away from society. Here the tradition of moral insanity, the belief in the total and overwhelming nature of madness, begins to replace the concept of moral management. Davies is on the path to this view. For him the physiognomy of insanity is but further proof of the easily recognizable distinction between sanity and madness. His asylum is the inferno—with no exit.

This exercise in the analysis of the historical constructions of insanity in specific literary texts illustrates how complex, hidden, and often contradictory the stereotypes of insanity can be. For the text mirrors one moment in an understanding of the nature of a specific time. It contains all the confusions and contradictions present in any given moment of time concerning the nature of difference.

Dickens's need to place the insane, the Other, in a world that was sympathetic, in which difference was not a stigma that excluded the outsider from the human race, was his own personal reading of the image of the insane. As can be seen in Davies's essay, much the same reality can be represented in a quite contradictory manner. It is the processing of these dyadic images which points to the underlying structure of the stereotype as well as to its protean surface nature.

CHAPTER SIX

The Insane See the Insane:
Richard Dadd

Art by the Insane

The collection of the artistic production of the insane assembled by Hans Prinzhorn of the University of Heidelberg during the first decades of the twentieth century has been and remains a major source of our information about the modes of representation of reality by those labeled as "insane."[1] A recent German catalogue of an exhibition drawn from the collection, which toured various galleries in the Federal Republic in 1980, managed to convey the impression that the works of art, especially those that were selected to represent various "themes" in the Prinzhorn collection, provided a mimetic reflection of the horrors inherent in the patients' environment rather than a representation of the patients' structuring of reality.[2] It begins with a long section entitled "the asylum," which purports to describe life in the various German, Austrian, and Swiss hospitals that housed the patients at the turn of the century. Accompanying pages of text on "admissions," on the "closed ward," on "life in the asylum," and so forth lend strength to this impression.

The level of naiveté which such an approach to art reveals is also reflected by the polemical intent of the 1980 exhibition from the Prinzhorn collection. In line with the influence of the antipsychiatric movement's image of the schizophrenic as seer and artist, the producers of the German exhibition wished to illustrate the axiom that the patient alone possesses true insight into his or her illness and truly understands the implications of his or her treatment.[3] This insight is denied to the "sane," who are, rather, responsible for the illness of those in the asylums, either by labeling the patients as "crazy" or by creating a world so mad that their insanity can be understood as their only reasonable response.

The private worlds created by the insane in their anguish are quite real. They are the expressions of the myths they cast about the world and the fears they project into it, just as those who see themselves as "sane" use images to control their world. These myths shape our understanding of the daily realities that all of us experience, whether our perception of the world is at the end of the spectrum which we label "normal" or at that radically different end, which we label "pathological."[4] That such a spectrum exists autonomously of societal labeling is accepted as long as we remain in the realm of somatic illness. Who among us would doubt that our self-representation is altered when we are physically ill? But it is unimportant if the source of this altered sense of self is psychological or somatic. For mental illness is marked by the same quality of suffering as organic illness. Mental illness alters our self-perception in a manner that indeed may be even more marked than the alterations of somatic illness. The mentally ill, in the view of the antipsychiatric movement in the United States as well as in the Federal Republic of Germany, are denied the status of suffering which accompanies illness. Part of human suffering is represented in an altered image of the world. When their representation of their suffering is seen as "exalted" or "fabricated," the mentally ill are set apart and perceived as "different." This is, of course, a false image of difference, a difference that creates the abyss between the reality of the observer and that projected onto the mentally ill. By accepting the mundane existence of mental illness, we can gain a more valid understanding of the perception of "difference" held by the mentally ill. It is a perception of the "difference" that exists, however, on a spectrum on which we too have our place.

My thesis in this chapter is simple: when you look at the images of the asylum or other images of madness in the artistic work of the mentally ill, you are looking at highly symbolic representations of internal states for which a structure of expression has been found in the representation of the idea of madness. And that representation is not merely a mimetic reflection of the daily world of the insane, but rather is also tied to the long Western tradition of representing psychopathological states. Not only is madness, to paraphrase Oscar Wilde slightly, represented in art but art shapes our conceptualization of madness. It is a long and intricate tradition of the symbolic function of images of insanity. Taken from folk belief, high and low literature, and art, these constructions of disease (through the image of the diseased) provide at least the external matrix for the representation of the insane by the insane. This generally accepted tradition of representing difference is then put to private use within the individual symbolic systems of those within the asylum (and without).

Images of Madness

In this discussion of some of these borrowed constructions from the artistic traditions of portraying madness, I will begin by a further exploration of the implications of melancholy. The female image of melancholy, as portrayed by Dürer, presented among other topoi the exaggeration of emotional states. (See the discussion in Chapter 2.) Indeed, when male characters in the late medieval epics were portrayed as melancholic, they were often given passive, "feminine" attributes. Often the source of their madness was labeled as "love sickness," a direct result of their pathological feminization. Not all forms of madness are represented by the figure of melancholy, but only that form which is within the stereotyped perception of the nature of woman—for melancholia is passive madness.

It is important to remember that most medieval texts of the early Middle Ages comment that the male, very specifically the nobleman, is primarily at risk in contracting love madness.[5] "Love madness" is a sign of a higher sensibility. Thus the prescription, proposed by Avicenna (and following him a number of medieval physicians), that the best cure for love sickness is the purchase of a prostitute's favors. By the Renaissance, it is the woman who becomes the exemplary sufferer from love sickness. The shift can be observed already in the thirteenth century in the work of Peter of Spain, later Pope John XXI, who, in a series of commentaries, observed that the origin of the love sickness was not in the mind (the highest sense) but merely a reflex of the genitalia. As sexual physiology came to be seen as the source of love sickness (in analogy to physical illnesses such as gonorrhea), the social status of "love sickness" shifts, from the nobleman to the woman, from the top of the social ladder to its bottom. If the roots of the disease are corporeal, it must most directly influence the female, the epitome of the physical. Feminine gender was also accorded to the physical attributes of the deadly sins, such as slothfulness, most frequently represented by the female. The perception of madness in the Middle Ages was structured on the level of activity ascribed to the insane, and activity was equated with the domination of the humors over the mind or over the body. The other three major categories of insanity—mania, epilepsy, and frenzy—were all perceived as highly agitated states of mind and were most often represented by male figures. But as the shift in status of love illness occurs, from that of a disease of noble males and their more noble sentiments to that of mere biological reflex of woman, the other forms of madness are forced into the background. They are diseases of the mind, as influenced by the humors or the temperaments. Their higher levels of activity signify them as "male," in contrast to the marked passivity of the melancholic. The melancholic becomes the essential image of psychopathology for an age that understands madness as a physical (and therefore a feminine) disease. Madness is feminine and the feminine is passive.

We can turn again to Hogarth's picture of the asylum for the classic example of a world of madness in which both aggressive and passive images are juxtaposed. In the final plate of *The Rake's Progress*, Hogarth's protagonist, Rakewell, is portrayed in exactly the same position as the statue of "raving" madness in chains, carved by Caius Gabriel Cibber in 1680, which adorned the portal of Bedlam (Plate 20; cf. Plate 5). Opposite "raving" madness, Cibber placed "melancholy," with his hands hidden from view. In Hogarth's portrait of the asylum, the melancholic figure is also present, hands clenched, with a dog, that most sensitive of beasts in the medieval bestiary, barking at him. He is "love mad," as much the victim of the feminization of his world as Rakewell is the victim of the financial corruption of inherited rather than earned wealth.

The idea of the insane as the object of "humane treatment" slowly began to dominate the popular as well as the medical characterization of the image of madness, first among the Quakers in Great Britain, and then was institutionalized by Philippe Pinel after the French Revolution. Vincenzo Chiarugi's 1794 drawing of the "British straight-waistcoat" (which seems to be the first medical illustration of insanity, though not in a textbook) is a positive image, since it replaced the popular notion of the mad in chains, an image that associated insanity with criminality as well as with uncontrolled actions (Plate 21). In Chiarugi's picture, the violent, aggressive image of madness dominates the idea of passive madness. And therefore the figure used to model the appliance is male. The specificity of the "straight-jacket" as an instrument of medical treatment, rather than merely of restraint, turned this instrument into the icon of the new treatment of the insane. But it was a highly ambiguous one. To understand the ramifications of this paradigmatic shift in the perception of the insane we shall turn to a mid-nineteenth-century witness who captured the altered sense of the asylum against the still remembered images of Hogarth's Bedlam.

Richard Dadd's Madness

In turning to an image from the world of the reformed asylum, one can judge how such fantasies function even in psychopathic systems. The paradigm of "non-restraint" and its juxtaposition to older visual icons of madness present, for example, in Charles Davies's portrait of Hanwell Asylum, are representative of the general perception of the reformed asylum in Great Britain in the mid-nineteenth century. (See the discussion in Chapter 5.) From the reformed asylum I have taken a single image

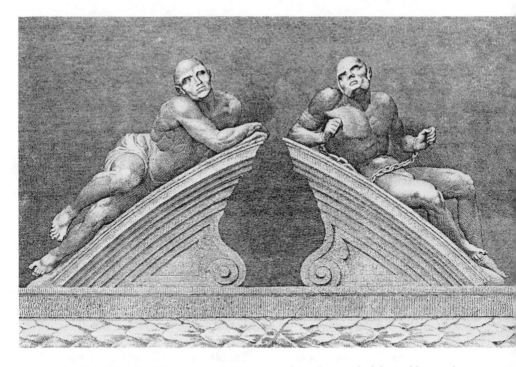

20. Caius Gabriel Cibber's statues of madness, from the portal of the Bethlem asylum (Thomas Bowen, *An Historical Account of the Origin, Progress, and Present State of Bethlem Hospital* [London: n.p., 1783]).

produced in the asylum by a patient and attempted to reconstruct the perception of madness that the patient incorporated into his own private symbolic world. The patient is Richard Dadd, whose reputation as an artist has grown considerably in the past few decades.[6] Dadd is certainly best known as the artist of "The Fairy Feller's Master-Stroke," which has hung in the Tate Gallery since 1963, when it was presented by Sir Siegfried Sassoon, in whose wife's family the painting had been since it was painted in Bethlem asylum in 1864.

Born in 1817 in Chatham, Richard Dadd was one of seven children of an apothecary in Brompton, four of whom were to die insane. Educated at The King's School in Rochester, he began to draw seriously when he left school at about thirteen. In 1834 the Dadd family moved to London, where Robert Dadd, Richard's father, took up practice as a carver and gilder. In 1837, after a period of self-study, Richard was admitted to the Academy School, where he studied under Henry Howard. He became closely allied with two other young painters, John Phillip and William Powell Frith, and they formed a group which they called "The Clique."

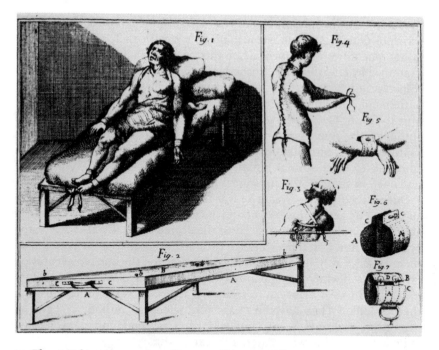

21. The straight-waistcoat, from Vincenzo Chiarugi, *Della pazzia ingenere* (1794) (Oskar Diethelm Historical Library, Cornell Medical College, New York).

These young painters were clearly the stars of the Academy. Dadd won numerous prizes and had commissions for his work from various publishers.

In 1842 Dadd and Phillip undertook an extensive trip that was to take them through Europe into Asia Minor and eventually as far as Egypt. In Egypt Dadd experienced his first attack of madness. He writes to Frith of having often "lain down at night with my imagination so full of wild vagaries that I have really and truly doubted of my own sanity."[7] Upon returning home to England, it was clear to his family and friends that he had slipped into insanity. He became violent, heard voices, and saw things that did not exist. He began to preach of his mission to free the world from the devil, believing himself to be persecuted for this mission by the devil's minions. He later wrote of this period: "On my return from travel, I was aroused to a consideration of subjects which I had previously never dreamed of, or thought about, connected with self; and I had such ideas that, had I spoken of them openly, I must, if answered in the world's fashion, have been told I was unreasonable. I concealed of course, these secret admonitions. I knew not whence they came, although I could not question their propriety, nor could I separate myself from what appeared my fate."[8] During the summer of 1843 he continued to work, producing a series of drawings of his friends, all shown with their throats cut. His father was quite concerned about this turn of events and had his son examined by Dr. Alexander Sutherland, who held Richard to be no longer responsible for his actions. A few days after the consultation with Dr. Sutherland, Richard Dadd lured his father into Cobham Park and stabbed him to death. Dadd believed his father to be the devil incarnate, "the author of the ruin of my race." Richard fled to France, where he was captured and eventually returned to England. On 22 August 1844 he was admitted to the criminal lunatic department of Bethlem Hospital. He remained in mental hospitals until his death on 8 January 1886.

During the forty-two years he was in mental hospitals Dadd produced an unceasing series of works of art (and poetry). His reputation remained alive outside the asylum, indeed to the degree that officials had to stop permitting him to sell his works to the outside because of the pressure on them to serve as his agents. I shall concentrate on the one representation of "madness" which Dadd painted during his many years in the asylum (Plate 22). In 1854 he began to produce a series of "sketches to illustrate the passions." They covered "passions" such as "brutality," "pride," "ambition," "drunkenness," and so forth. One represented "agony-raving madness." This watercolor is an extraordinary image.

Remember Charles Dickens's image of the modern asylum juxtaposed against the pentimento of remembered visual fragments from the past. The Bethlem Royal Hospital, into which Dadd was admitted in 1844 and where he found himself in 1854 as he painted "agony-raving madness," was a modern asylum like Davies's Hanwell, in which chained patients were to be found only in fantasy. Indeed, the kennellike environment in which Dadd's chained patient is found, his half-nakedness, his animallike nails, his tousled hair, his vacant glance all speak not to the mimetic representation of the reality in which Dadd found himself, but to a highly symbolic fantasy of madness. We have seen what the context of this image is, but Dadd's picture relates to one further tradition, a tradition that can be reconstructed out of the various strands of the portrayal of the insane.

Dadd's Reading of Bell

Richard Dadd was a trained artist. One of his textbooks would certainly have been Sir Charles Bell's 1806 *Essays on the Anatomy of Expression*. As I have discussed in Chapter 2, Bell provided a specific image of the madman (see Plate 8) which incorporated the traditional notion of the bestial nature of madness. Bell's image of "madness" summarized,

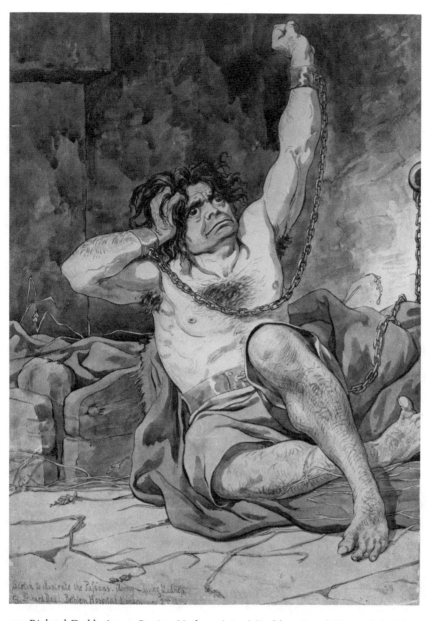

22. Richard Dadd, *Agony-Raving Madness* (1854) (Bethlem Royal Hospital Archives and Museum, London).

within the new science of physiognomy, a traditional British manner of representing insanity as an atavistic state. But this tradition was understood by Bell and his readers as an artistic tradition, much like the representation of the passions within the *Encyclopedia* or Camper's analysis of the differences of facial angle among the various races. But, as in these examples, the line between art as the representation of a perceived reality and the reality itself was blurred. There was still a strong ideological message to be delivered in the iconographic representation of the "difference" of the insane. In analyzing Richard Dadd's refunctioning of Bell's image of "madness," we can use the ideological matrix in which this icon is embedded to help us understand the function of Dadd's image of "agony-raving madness" within his paranoid system.

To place Dadd's image side by side with Bell's reveals a series of continuities in the overt structure. These, combined with the refunctioning of Bell's image in the historical context of the reformed asylum of the mid-nineteenth century, can provide us with some clues to the meaning of madness in Dadd's world view. What strikes the eye initially is that the figure portrayed by Bell is passive—"watchful," to use Bell's term. Like the chained animal, the madman sits drawn together, eyes averted, and hands clasped under his arms. The visual impression is that of a topos of the representation of madness, that of the "hidden or clenched hands," which, as we have seen, has been part of the standard topos of insanity since the Middle Ages. Playing on the biblical motif of Proverbs 19:24 ("A slothful man hideth his hand in his bosom. / And will not so much as bring it to his mouth again."), this motif is present in numerous images of "madness." The ineffectuality of the insane, their inability to function in the world of work, is echoed by this image. Like the animal, the madman has no place in a world dominated by the Protestant ethic with its strong emphasis on the role and value of work.

Dadd's image is not of passive madness, but of the passions of agony and raving madness. His madman's hands are not hidden but raised in a gesture of aggressive (and, therefore, masculine) insanity. One hand, raised above his head, is thrown out with the clenched fist, signifying a madness restrained by the chains. In Bell's image these chains seem to lack any function, as the madman is portrayed as passive (even though potentially aggressive). The other hand is clasped to the head in a traditional representation of grief or pensiveness, as in Dürer's image of melancholy. But even here the gesture turns into a meaningful sign of madness, since it is visually associated with the tearing of hair, a sign indeed of grief, but grief out of normal bounds (as represented in Hogarth's Rakewell). Even the feet of Dadd's "raving" madman, like those of Blake's *Nebuchadnezzar* (see Plate 9), reveal his madness through their bestiality, a factor also present in the unruliness of his hair. Dadd stresses, with his iconographic references, that this is an exemplum of

"agony" as well as "raving madness." The passivity of Bell's image, with
its threatening potential, is the model for the actively distraught nature
of Dadd's madman. And yet the faces of the two figures are quite different. Bell's image is that of the potential of aggressiveness present in
madness; Dadd's of its actual presence. The madman in Dadd's portrait is
acting, struggling, but against what?

Bell's image of the madman would have been his own internalized
representation of the concept of "difference" as formulated in 1806. Following John Haslam's dismissal from Bethlem in the next decade, there
was a marked improvement in the status of the insane. A further reform
came in 1853 when the Commissioners in Lunacy again examined the
status of the mental hospitals in Great Britain and suggested the appoint-
ment of a resident physician superintendent for Bethlem. The appoint-
ment of William Charles Hood, who took great interest in his prize
patient, Richard Dadd, was the result. Under Hood Dadd began to paint
his cycle of the "passions" while confined to the "criminal wing" of the
asylum. Even the "criminal wing" of the hospital, with its prisonlike
features of iron bars and the lack of any organized activity, was not the
older, unreformed asylum, even though it was quite primitive. It had
cages that, in a contemporary view, were "more like those which enclose
the fierce carnivora at the Zoological Garden than anything we have
elsewhere seen employed for the detention of afflicted humanity."[9] Dadd
may well be making a reference to the older, unreformed perception of
the asylum in his visual quotation of Bell's image, contrasting the daily
reality of the other patients in Bethlem with the world of the "criminal
wing" which he would have experienced. To do so he employed the
artistic representation of an older reality, in which the patients were
perceived not merely as being hospitalized but (from the perspective of
mid-century) as being punished.

The eyes of Bell's figure are cast toward the ground; Dadd's figure gazes
upward. Indeed, the entire thrust of Dadd's portrait, following the line of
the upraised arm, is skyward. This very raising of the perspective of the
madman places him within the tradition of religious art, with the eyes of
the martyr raised to the presence of the divine, unseen by the observer
but impressed upon the imagination of the madman as martyr. So Dadd's
madman, represented as such, also relates in some way to the divine. But
to what divinity?

Delusional Structures and Representations: Dadd and Schreber

At this point let us make the leap from simply describing the history of
the representation of insanity and the structure of these two images to an
interpretation of Dadd's picture given the historical context in which it is

found. Here speculation must replace information, but we shall see that the representation may well function in the world that lies between an understanding of self and the delusional structure Dadd employed to give form to his anxieties.

First, the picture of "agony-raving madness" points to a conventional (even archaic) understanding of the image of the madman, not that unlike the other conventional images Dadd employs for the other "passions." With these conventional icons he distances the representation of the passions, but especially that of "madness," from his own life and world. These images belong to the world of art, a world necessarily perceived as separate and distinct from the mundane realities of daily life. Yet, unlike the other representations of the "passions" which Dadd uses, that of madness reflects the stereotypes of the world in which he found himself. And he ties his idea of madness to this archaic image, in which madness is linked with punishment.

Dadd was aware during his hospitalization, indeed as early as the late 1840s, of his own instability. This instability was structured into a delusional system that revolved about the Egyptian gods, especially Osiris. This obsession with the world of Egypt was a continuation of the actual fascination with Egypt present in Europe during the first half of the nineteenth century, a fascination that took Dadd to Egypt on the journey during which his breakdown occurred.[10] He described his belief system to William Charles Hood:

> My religious opinions varied and do vary from the vulgar; I was inclined to fall in with the views of the ancients, and to regard the substitution of modern ideas thereon as not for the better. These and the like, coupled with the idea of a descent from the Egyptian god Osiris, induced me to put a period to the existence of him whom I had always regarded as a parent, but whom the secret admonishings I had, counselled me was the author of the ruin of my race. I inveigled him, by false pretences, into Cobham Park, and slew him with a knife, with which I stabbed him, after having vainly endeavoured to cut his throat.[11]

Osiris is Dadd's true father. And Osiris is the god of the underworld, of death. This delusional structure reappeared in slightly altered form when he was taken prisoner in France. There he spent his time in the asylum at Claremont gazing at the sun "which he calls his father," according to the French authorities.[12] Thus the raised eyes of the madman point to the divine nature of his calling, which, as understood by Dadd, is both mad and meaningful. The raised arm—the "raving," that is, active rather than passive, image of madness—also reflects on the act of parricide, the stabbing of the father.

But the father is an all-encompassing concept of the forces of control. Dadd was captured in France on his way to kill the emperor of Austria, yet another powerful father-figure to be executed by Dadd in his role as the envoy of Osiris. We cannot help but make the leap from this image of the sun as father to that other document of late nineteenth-century madness, the autobiography of the German jurist Daniel Paul Schreber, written a half century after Dadd's image was created and the subject of Sigmund Freud's most extensive investigation of a paranoid system.[13] For Schreber too, the godhead as father is central to the system; similarly, the sun serves as an icon of the father to be both honored and destroyed. But we do not wish to fall into Freud's trap of simply accepting Jung's theory that the symbolism of the paranoid schizophrenic is an atavistic throwback to the images implanted on the world soul at some more primitive stage of our evolution, a stage captured in the symbolic systems of the madman. Dadd and Schreber seem to recast universals such as light and darkness, sun and shadow, into a system which helps them explain to themselves their real or imagined act of parricide.[14] And both systems see the punishment for the act of parricide in the madness of the son. Both systems, in their act of creating aesthetic objects (texts or images) that represent the structure of madness, enable the creator of the object to stand, at least for the moment, outside of the system. This existence outside of the paranoid system represented in the structure of the aesthetic object is itself a projection of the patient's wish to stand apart from and observe his madness.

But in the creation of such distancing devices there is a need to call upon patterns for the organization of reality which exist in the world. As in all art, the source for these patterns is found in earlier works of art which are in some way related to the basic pattern the artists require. Dadd draws on Bell for the outward images of madness, divinity, and punishment. But even a further level of representation links Dadd's image with Schreber's autobiography. There is a common symbolic ground for Schreber's ability to look at the sun without being dazzled and the sun-father present in Dadd's Egyptian mythology. Both are structured by a literary image, the image that gives shape to the discourse about madness which is present in Schreber's language as well as in Dadd's picture.

This source is the language and imagery of Byron's *Manfred* (1817). Dadd had selected this poetic drama as the subject of one of his first major commissions, the decoration of 26 Grosvenor Square for Lord Foley in 1841–42. But it was also one of the favorite subjects for a number of early nineteenth-century British artists. Schreber quotes from the play (which was influenced by Goethe's *Faust* and after it was one of the most popular Romantic dramas in Germany during the nineteenth century). Indeed, Schreber borrows the central vocabulary for his pantheon of the gods directly from Byron's work. The plot of Byron's play, with its fury-driven hero whose incestuous relationship has driven him insane, haunts the image of the madman present in both Schreber and Dadd. The "agony" of Manfred, whose tortured death closes the drama, is incorporated in the image of "raving madness," with its solitary figure of the madman. Thus the focus of the single figure of the madman, which Dadd adapts from Bell's portrait, has a hidden significance, the solitary and insane end of Byron's title figure. Madness becomes externalized through the image of Manfred's furies, which are present in the delusional system of Dadd as the Egyptian gods, and in Schreber's image of madness as the spheres of Ahriman and Ormuzd, the two segments of the godhead. The projection of the internalized guilt, with its sexual references, onto the external world is thus perceived in an aesthetic mode and can become the material for art. It is thus doubly projected—first, outside of the self onto the world and second, onto the world within the clear artifice of the work of art.

Here we must limit our speculation about Dadd's delusional system, but we can now see that the image of the madman, raving and in agony, is a symbolic representation of part of that system. It is the isolated and condemned madman as the adept of Osiris, in chains because of his aggressive, dangerous insanity, which relates to his role as the violent murderer of authority, of the father, and the needed sense of punishment for that act. But the image also stresses the masculinity of the madman. This masculinity can only be proved in the denial of the power of the father, a power that is perceived to be so overwhelming that to deny it is itself an "insane" act. And this act is represented in the active (rather than the passive) madman. Yet in differentiating his image from Bell's, Dadd stresses the difference between the feminine and the masculine to such an extent that the very act of differentiation becomes a sign of their parallel implication.

The killing of the father is the act of establishing oneself as the masculine force that replaces the threatening masculinity of the father. This act defines the source of dread and localizes it outside of the self. However, it employs a vocabulary of images to do so which labels the self as mad. Dadd's paranoia was coupled with his awareness of the reality of his life in Bedlam. He translated these two factors into an image of madness which drew on an artistic precedent—Bell's picture, with its references to the passivity and animallike condition of the insane—and reversed many of that earlier image's implications. The perceived "agony" felt by the patient may be tied to his perception of the control now imposed upon him by the structure of the asylum. But it may also relate to the limitations placed on his role as a follower of Osiris. "Raving madness" is the label the asylum doctors have placed upon the patient, much as

Dadd places his label upon the watercolor. Dadd can thus displace his sense of rupture with the "real" world onto an aesthetic object (his watercolor), which itself has a primarily aesthetic reference (Bell's picture). Since Bell's image is that of a world quite different from his own, one that existed but no longer exists except in the mythic iconography of art, it relates as much to the world of art as to the world of madness. Dadd's image is tied as much to his transcendental delusional system as it is to the representation of reality within the asylum.

Images and Realities

Dadd's image, like the images of madness in the Prinzhorn collection, represents complex systems of structuring psychotic delusions. We can begin to explore them, given enough information about the systems and their context (for no delusional system is independent of the realities of the cultural context experienced by the patient), but we can probably never completely reconstruct them without knowing the patient's interpretation of the system. For an archeological recreation of the system is of little use: what is vital is understanding how the patient dynamically perceived the functioning of the system. Thus the objects collected by Prinzhorn, like the lists of tales or proverbs collected by nineteenth-century ethnologists, may provide texts, but they do not provide the ground necessary to understand not what the texts said but what they meant. When we observe the works in the Prinzhorn collection, we must therefore keep the individuals who created them firmly in mind, each quite different from his or her neighbor, each rendering commonly held systems of symbolic representation into personal code. Without the voice of the patient, without an understanding of the patient's anguish and pain, such works remain mute, open to our comprehension, but quite incomplete. This lacuna must be kept in mind when the fascination of these works spins its web around us.

CHAPTER SEVEN

The Insane See the Insane:
Vincent Van Gogh

By the end of the nineteenth century the construction of the image of the mentally ill in medicine and the fine arts had achieved an amazing complexity. Strands of meaning from earlier representations of various psychopathological conditions had become so intertwined and submerged in popular thought that their antecedents were no longer apparent at first glance. Examples of such difficulties of interpretation can be found in the late work of Vincent Van Gogh.[1]

As early as the beginning of the 1880s, Van Gogh's work reflected a fascination with the restructuring of some of the classical images of aberrant mental and emotional states. In 1881 and 1882 he drew a series of seated and weeping figures. Sketches of a weeping female, her head covered by her arms, drawn in black pencil, exist from his stay in The Hague (F 1060, 1069), and there are at least four different views of an old man weeping from the same period (F 863, 864, 997, 998).[2] These seated, weeping figures culminate in two major works, the nude female figure in *Sorrow* (F 929, 929 bis, 1655; Plate 23), in its three versions, and the seated weeping male figure in *At Eternity's Gate* (F 702, 1662; Plate 24), in its two states. Iconographically, all of these works stand in the tradition of the Renaissance representation of the figure of melancholy, typified in nineteenth-century popular thought by Albrecht Dürer's etching *Melancolia I* (see Plate 1). Van Gogh altered the implications of these figures in a manner that reflects both his personal views of depression and the altered attitude toward mental illness in the late nineteenth century.

The background to Van Gogh's lithograph *Sorrow* illuminates the artist's evolving view of the classic model of melancholy. Van Gogh's earlier

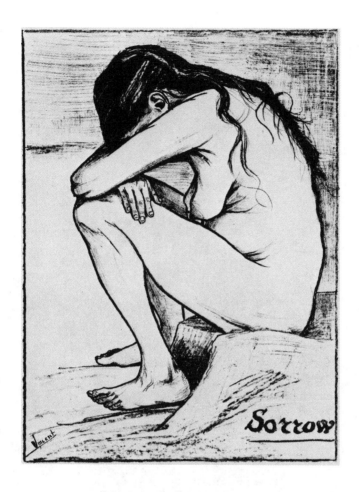

23. Van Gogh, *Sorrow* (1882) (Stedelijk Museum, Amsterdam).

studies of seated, weeping peasant women give way to an angular representation of the emaciated, pregnant figure of *Sorrow*. Like the earlier studies, it was based on firsthand observation of working-class models. Van Gogh's relationship to the model for *Sorrow*, the woman he calls "Sien," is detailed in his letters to his brother Theo in 1882. Perhaps even more striking is his description of the aesthetics of his model in a letter to his friend Rappard in the spring of that year: "I never had such a good

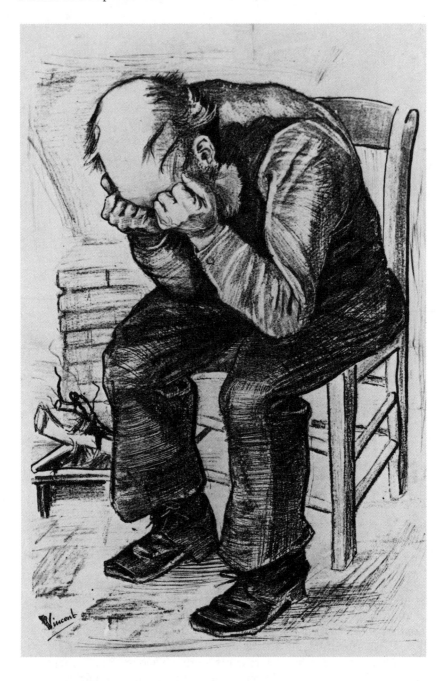

24. Van Gogh, *At Eternity's Gate* (1882) (Stedelijk Museum, Amsterdam).

assistant as this ugly, faded woman. In my eyes she is beautiful, and I find in her exactly what I want; her life has been rough, and sorrow and adversity have put their marks upon her—now I can do something with her."[3] Since this effect is so successfully captured in the drawing that the model's individuality vanishes, it is evident that the lithograph reflects those qualities he sought to capture—a figure weighed down by the world.

In the Renaissance, melancholy was regarded as an inherent attribute of the individual, reflecting the dominance of certain internal biological forces under the more general influence of the cosmos. But Van Gogh's figures in *Sorrow* and *At Eternity's Gate* are individuals driven to the brink by society's inhumanity. They are isolated from society since they can no longer function in it. Both the old man, his time of useful work behind him, and the cast-off, pregnant woman are pariahs in the ordered world of society since they have no economic benefits to offer. Their biological state is but an aspect of their exploitation by society. They have no way out of their dilemma and thus depression becomes a realistic reaction to their position in life.

Van Gogh has also filtered his impression of Sien through yet another paradigm, because his caption for the drawing of *Sorrow* (F 929 bis) is a quotation from Jules Michelet's *La Femme* (which he had read as early as 1874): "How is it that on earth there can be a lonely, forsaken woman?" Jean Seznec comments that "according to Michelet, the nineteenth century was the century of woman's misery, abandonment, and despair; man's mission was to liberate her, to free her from all the servitudes that oppress her."[4] Indeed, Van Gogh's *Sorrow*, even though it stands in the tradition of the Renaissance figure of melancholy, is a substantial extension of that philosophic concept of affective disorder.

These figures of depression represent not merely social comment, however; they are also representative of the potential for change, a major alteration in the nineteenth-century attitude toward mental illness.[5] They evoke the sense of meaninglessness reflected in Van Gogh's quotation from Michelet: how can such waste be permitted? Van Gogh evidently felt that the figure was sufficient to carry this message, since he did not place the quotation from Michelet below the lithograph of *Sorrow*.

The reworking of the classic theme of melancholy in the light of Van Gogh's strong social conscience presents a paradigm for the understanding of two late paintings. These works, *Men's Ward at Arles* (F 646) (Plate 25) and *Head of a Patient* (F 703) (see Plate 30), exist in a similar continuum of the representation of mental and emotional disorders, having their roots in the late eighteenth century. But they are not such explicit descendants of an iconographic tradition as are the figures of the melan-

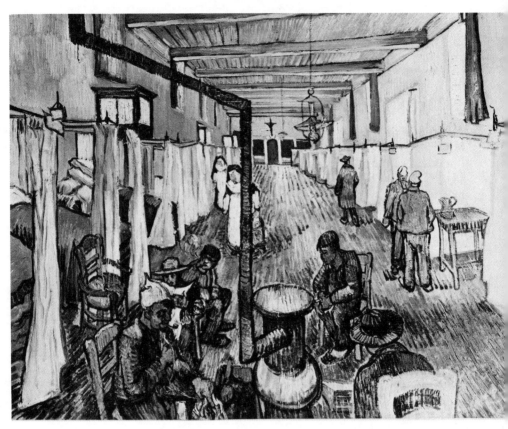

25. Van Gogh, *Men's Ward at Arles* (1889) (Oskar Reinhart Collection, Winterthur).

cholic since their historical context is much less well known. *Men's Ward at Arles* stands in a tradition of the asylum scene whose first and best-known representative is the final plate from William Hogarth's *Rake's Progress* (see Plate 5). The final decades of the eighteenth century saw the Hogarthian model of the madhouse scene continued by Goya in two paintings of the madhouse at Saragossa (Plate 26). As in Hogarth's picture, the types of the inmates are clearly recognizable—from the madman as king at the right to a crouching maniac in his "casa de locos" at the left—as defective inhabitants of a walled world. Unlike Hogarth, Goya freezes single moments in his paintings. The sequence of images in *The Rake's Progress* provided a context for the final image of Rakewell in Bedlam. In Goya's work this context must be supplied by the observer.

The tradition was continued by Wilhelm von Kaulbach, whose *Narrenhaus* (1835) provided a radically delineated set of visual topologies

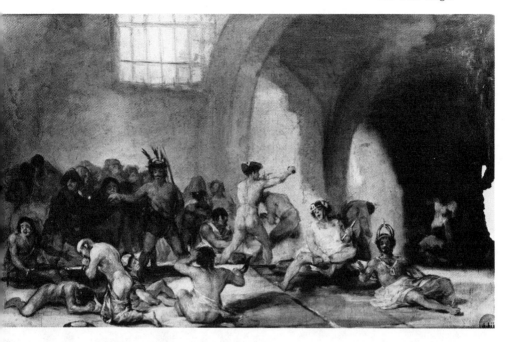

26. Francisco Goya, *The Madhouse at Saragossa* (1794) (Royal Academy of San Fernando, Madrid, Spain).

(Plate 27). The sense of action present in Goya has been eliminated and the observer is presented with a set of frozen figures. This etching was so popular that it spawned a series of psychological interpretations based on Kaulbach's visual classifications of the physiognomy of insanity. The madman as warrior, as scholar, and as ruler are figures who would have been at home in Hogarth's Bedlam.

In the early 1850s Paul Gachet, a young doctor at the Salpêtrière, introduced his friend the painter Amand Gautier into the world of the famed Paris asylum. The intention was to provide the painter with models representing the various types of insanity. Out of Gautier's studies came *Les folles de la Salpêtrière* in 1855, continuing the earlier tradition of the madhouse scene (Plate 28). Gautier attempted to catalogue the insane not so much according to their physiognomy (as Kaulbach did) but in terms of specific categories of illness ranging from hebephrenia to mania. One further continental representation of the madhouse in the late nineteenth century should be mentioned. Daniel Urrabieta y Vierge's illustration of Charenton is similar in structure to Gautier's view of the Salpêtrière (Plate 29). As with all the asylum images, the space is differentiated by the walls of the institution. But the figures, as

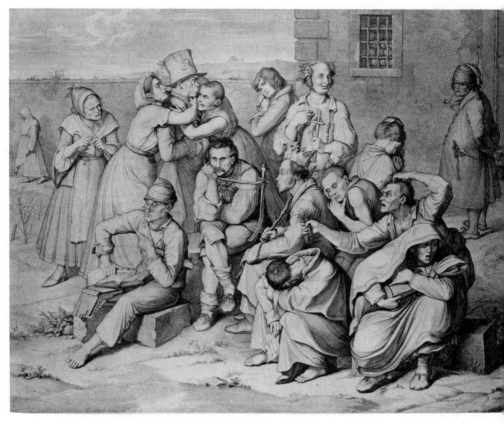

27. Wilhelm von Kaulbach, *Das Narrenhaus* (1835) (Pennsylvania Academy of Fine Arts, Philadelphia).

in Gautier's work, are specific representations of psychopathologies, from the fixed gesture of the figure at the lower left to the depressed seated figure at the right foreground. Of some interest is the miniscule dancing figure at the rear of the scene. In an earlier asylum scene, Katharine Drake's *Lunatic's Ball* of 1848 (see Plate 18), the eventual return of the insane to the world outside is indicated through the motif of the dance as a social convention. Some knowledge of the complexities of the iconology of the madhouse scene in art during the eighteenth and nineteenth centuries is vital to an understanding of Van Gogh's *Men's Ward at Arles.*

Van Gogh described his completion of the canvas in a letter to his sister written from the sanatorium at Saint-Rémy-de-Provence in October 1890.

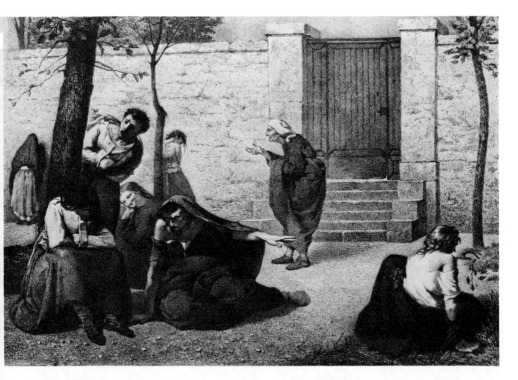

28. Amand Gautier, *Les folles de la Salpêtrière* (1857) (Clements C. Fry Collection, Yale Medical Historical Library, New Haven, Conn.).

I am now working on a ward in the hospital. In the foreground a big black stove surrounded by a number of gray and black figures of patients, behind this a very long room with a red tile floor, with two rows of white beds, the walls white, but a white which is lilac or green, and the windows with pink and green curtains, and in the background the figures of two sisters in black and white. The ceiling is violet with big beams. I had read an article about Dostoevski, who wrote a book *Souvenirs de la maison des morts*, and this induced me to resume a large study I had begun in the fever ward at Arles. But it is annoying to paint figures without models. [3:461]

The roots of Van Gogh's painting lie in his experiences in the hospital at Arles after his self-mutilation at the end of 1888, and again in February of the following year, when he was admitted suffering from a delusion of persecution. In spring 1889 he voluntarily admitted himself to the private sanatorium of Saint-Paul-de-Mausole, which lay on the outskirts of Saint-Rémy-de-Provence. He remained there a year, during which he

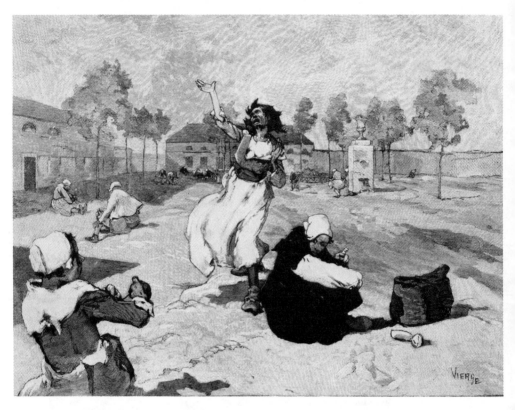

29. Daniel Urrabieta y Vierge, *Yard of an Asylum* (Clements C. Fry Collection, Yale Medical Historical Library, New Haven, Conn.).

painted numerous studies of the physical surroundings of the asylum, but *Men's Ward at Arles* is unique in its presentation of a hospital scene with patients. If anything, his painting is closest in spirit to the copies from Daumier he made during his hospitalization, which represented closed spaces with figures.

Van Gogh's letter to his sister illuminates his image of the hospital. First, the picture is a composite. Begun at Arles in the "fever ward," it was completed while he was at the asylum at Saint-Rémy; his complaint about the lack of models for the figures implies that he was reconstructing the closed world of the ward while in another hospital. Thus the image of the hospital at Arles is filtered through the experience of Saint-Rémy. It becomes an abstraction of the world of the living dead, of the madmen with whom Van Gogh lived and with whom he identified. Dostoevski's work, known to him only through its title, *Notes from the House of the Dead*, served as the motto for this work, much as the quotation from Michelet served to provide a broader social context for the drawing of *Sorrow*. In a letter to his brother he wrote: "Some days ago I was reading in the *Figaro* the story of a Russian writer who suffered all his life from a nervous disease which he finally died of, and which brought on terrible attacks from time to time. And what's to be done? There is no cure, or if there is one, it is working zealously" (3:204). Van Gogh identified with Dostoevski's purported epilepsy as the illness from which he himself suffered. And their illness was made manageable, or at least acceptable, through created work.

Van Gogh's understanding of the suffering of the mind underwent a radical shift after his voluntary admission to Saint-Rémy. The earlier representations of mental or emotional disorders were part of his understanding of man's total suffering in this world. In Saint-Rémy he was confronted with the specific reality of mental illness as the totality of the world in which he found himself. On 9 May 1889, almost immediately after his arrival, he writes: "Though here there are some patients very seriously ill, the fear and horror of madness that I used to have has already lessened a great deal. And although here you continually hear terrible cries and howls like beasts in a menagerie, in spite of that people get to know each other very well and help each other when their attacks come on" (3:170). Just as depression came to be expressed in Van Gogh's art through his personal experiences as well as his reading, his understanding of the insane became colored by his firsthand experiences.[6]

Van Gogh was afraid of madness when he arrived at the asylum. "But all joking aside, the fear of madness is leaving me to a great extent, as I see at close quarters those who are affected by it in the same way as I may very easily be in the future" (3:174). His sympathy with the plight of the other patients is reflected in his identification with them. He writes that "formerly I felt an aversion to these creatures, and it was a harrowing thought to me to reflect that so many of our profession . . . had ended like this. I could not even bring myself to picture them in that condition" (ibid.). Among the artists Van Gogh suspected were in madhouses was the illustrator Vierge, the creator of the famed madhouse scene (3:243).

The structure of Van Gogh's painting of the hospital ward reflects the tradition of the madhouse scene. The clearly limited space of the hospital with its inhabitants marks the universe of the asylum. The seated figure holding a cigarette is a version of the melancholic old man of *At Eternity's Gate*. Indeed, a sketch (F 1601 verso) that Van Gogh most probably used for this figure is even more evidently a representation of chronic depression.

Van Gogh's hospital ward, however, is different from the earlier hospital scenes.[7] The manic figures present in the earlier works are missing, and there were indeed none in Saint-Rémy (3:174). But a more significant difference lies in the fact that Van Gogh's figures, rather than represent-ing specific types or classifications of mental illness, reflect the daily existence of the inmates in the hospital. These are the quintessential inmates of the house of the dead, made dead because of forced inactivity. They smoke, sit, read newspapers, talk, but have no constructive roles, like that which Van Gogh ascribed to his activity as a painter. He writes in September: "The treatment of patients in this hospital is certainly easy, one could follow it even while traveling, for they do absolutely *nothing;* they leave them to vegetate in idleness" (3:213).

For the nineteenth-century observer the house of the dead was the house of idleness. Charles Dickens, Van Gogh's favorite writer, con-demned the absence of any meaningful activity in the English asylums, arguing that if "the system of finding the inmates employment . . . were introduced . . . the proportion of cures would be much greater."[8] It is this absence of work, or meaningful activity, which is portrayed in the canvas begun at Arles and finished at Saint-Rémy. Van Gogh's fear of pur-poseless existence, of vegetating in the asylum, is triggered by the mere mention of the title of Dostoevski's novel. The picture is Van Gogh's own note from the house of the dead, the asylum.

After Van Gogh was released from Saint-Rémy he was placed in the care of a physician who was himself a patron of the arts. Paul Gachet, Gautier's friend, had earlier established himself in Auvers-sur-Oise and offered to supervise Van Gogh. During his stay in Auvers, Van Gogh turned out a remarkable series of portraits and landscapes. One of the works evidently completed in Auvers, though it may have been begun earlier in Saint-Rémy, is his *Head of a Patient* (Plate 30). This portrait of an anonymous patient descends from another tradition of depicting the madman.

Van Gogh had earlier been fascinated by Eugène Delacroix's portrait *Tasso in the Asylum* and requested while still living at Arles that his brother send him a lithograph of the work (3:109) (Plate 31). He referred to this portrait as "representing a *real* man. Ah! portraiture, portraiture with the thoughts, the soul of the model in it, that is what I think must come" (3:25). However, Delacroix's image of the sixteenth-century Ital-ian writer in the madhouse recalls the structure of Hogarth's Bedlam, with other inmates and gawking visitors watching the melancholic Tasso.

For the prism through which to depict the inmate at Saint-Rémy, Van Gogh turned instead to Théodore Géricault, an artist whom he placed parallel to Delacroix in his own collection of prints. His portrait of the inmate at Saint-Rémy contains a visual echo of Géricault's *Monomanie du vol*, painted at the Salpêtrière between 1821 and 1824 (see Plate 10). The position of the head, the coat and scarf, the lidded eyes, all reflect Géricault's work. Van Gogh thus makes use of a classic portrayal of the

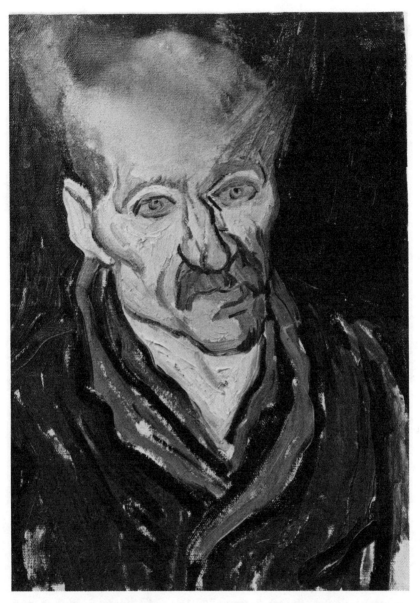

30. Van Gogh, *Head of a Patient* (1890) (Rijksmuseum Van Gogh, Amsterdam).

insane to underline the banality of madness. For the subject's abnormality is apparent only if one knows that the portrait was painted in an asylum. The line between madness and sanity in these portraits is invisibly fine.

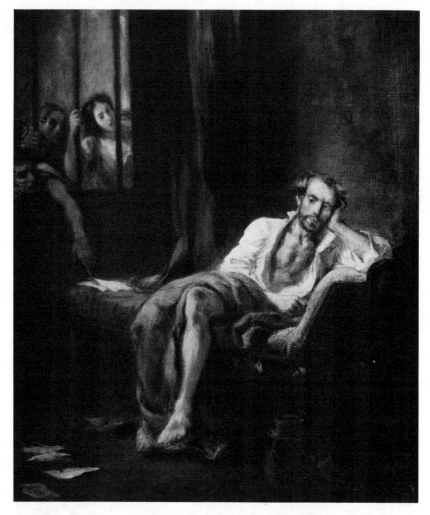

31. Eugène Delacroix, *Tasso in the Asylum* (1839) (Oskar Reinhart Collection, Winterthur).

One can contrast such an artistic approach with that of the attempts of medical illustrators at the close of the nineteenth century to capture psychopathologies. Byrom Bramwell's *Atlas of Clinical Medicine*, published in 1892, brought out portrait studies of remarkable diagnostic accuracy, such as a study of chronic insanity (Plate 32).[9] But the distinction between the tradition of Géricault and Van Gogh and that of Alexander Morison and Bramwell is the former's emphasis on passive rather than active states of madness.[10]

In the asylum scene painted by Van Gogh there is a surface appearance of normal activity, and the same is true in his portrait of the inmate. Van Gogh, however, makes reference to the greater historical context of these works through his adaptation of earlier structures of depicting the insane.

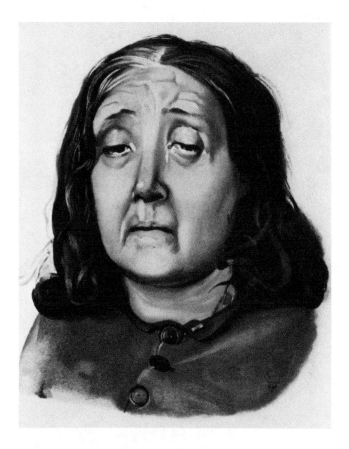

32. Byrom Bramwell's chromolithograph of chronic insanity, from his *Atlas of Clinical Medicine* (Edinburgh: Constable, 1892) (private collection, Ithaca, N.Y.).

The importance of the two paintings of the mentally ill in Van Gogh's work lies partly in their uniqueness. When one examines Van Gogh's production during the final two years, years spent in institutions and under the threat of imminent mental collapse, there are few direct references to mental illness. Landscapes, portraits, and copies make up the bulk of his work. When he copies Delacroix, his model is not *Tasso in the Asylum*, but rather *The Good Samaritan*. His attempt to repress his fear of madness, a fear echoed in most of the letters following his self-mutilation, finds few direct outlets in his work, and these are encased in iconographic structures that stand in a long tradition of classifying the insane as inhabitants of another world, isolated from the observing eye of the artist.

CHAPTER EIGHT

The Science of Visualizing
the Insane: Charles Darwin

Browne and Psychiatric Photography

In the epilogue to the major collection of essays on Charles Darwin's contributions to the theory of facial expression, Paul Ekman comments on the "hundreds of photographs which Darwin had collected in preparing the expression book. Most are of mental patients, are rather gloomy to inspect, and are not very informative about more than the clothing of that time."[1] What Ekman misses in his "reading" of Darwin's photographic collection (which included extensive ethnographic materials gathered from major contemporary investigators of expression such as Paolo Mantegazza) is the development of Darwin's understanding of the function of such images, including those of disease, in Darwin's construction of his theories. Darwin's fascination with and extensive use of photographic material in his pendant to *The Descent of Man*, his *Expression of the Emotions in Man and Animals*, are evident upon examination of the illustrations in the volume itself.[2] Darwin's construction of the image of the mentally ill reveals itself as well upon a careful reading of the book. That these two interests were closely interrelated is not, however, evident from the printed page. Darwin's interest in the mentally ill and his reliance on photographs of their expressions illustrate a changing attitude toward the nature of empirical evidence for behavioral studies. This change relates to technological developments in both neurology and photography and their reflection in the nineteenth-century understanding of visual documentation. These confluent factors are most clearly revealed in Darwin's unpublished correspondence with Sir James Crichton Browne and his incorporation of material written by Browne in his monograph on expression.

James Crichton Browne (1840–1938), the son of William Browne (co-founder of *Brain* in 1878), was one of the most distinguished psychiatrists of the late nineteenth century.[3] Not only Darwin but other behaviorists such as Henry Maudsley consulted him concerning the most modern research on neurology and psychiatry. Trained in Edinburgh under Lister, Syme, Laycock, and Goodsir, Browne became associated with the West Riding Asylum (Wakefield) in 1866 as medical director. There he founded the first pathology department in a British asylum as well as a house journal, the annual West Riding Lunatic Asylum Medical Reports. These volumes, the first of their kind in Great Britain, combined psychiatric and neurological case studies with theoretical essays.

Browne was also an amateur photographer. In the 1850s this same happy combination had led Hugh W. Diamond (see Chapter 2) to evolve his theory of the use of the photograph in the treatment of the insane. As late as 1874 four of Diamond's photographs were used by J. Thompson Dickson to illustrate his *Science and Practice of Medicine in Relationship to the Mind*.[4] The relationship between the application of photography and the evolving understanding of mental illness was established in Great Britain by the time Browne began photographing his patients in the late 1860s.

The rationale behind the introduction of the photograph in studies of physiognomy and affect is clear. Eighteenth- and early nineteenth-century students of the physiognomy of the insane relied on various forms of artistic reproduction as the basis of their interpretations (see Chapter 2). Not the individual but the artist's interpretation of the individual stood as the basis for their studies. The more sensitive among the early nineteenth-century psychiatrists, such as Etienne Jean Georget, were aware of this problem and confronted it directly, by insisting that primary direct observation of the patient could lead to more meaningful results. Still, most theorists dealing with the expression of the insane, such as Morison and Esquirol, commissioned artists to represent the insane as accurately as possible. But it was only with the introduction of the photograph that an objective portrait seemed to be accessible.

Arthur Schopenhauer, at mid-century, opened his essay on physiognomy with the comment:

That the outer man is a graphic reproduction of the inner and the face the expression and revelation of his whole nature, is an assumption whose *a priori* nature and hence certainty are shown by the universal desire, plainly evident on every occasion, to see a man who distinguished himself in something good or bad; or, failing this, at least to learn from others what he looks like. Therefore, on the one hand, people rush to the places where they think he is; on the other, newspapers, especially the English, endeavor to give minute and striking descriptions of him. Thereafter, painters and engravers give us a graphic representation of him and finally Daguerre's invention, so highly valued on that account, affords the most complete satisfaction of that need.[5]

Schopenhauer's ironic scale of reproduction places the "realism" of the photograph at the pinnacle of accuracy. So too was it perceived by psychiatrists fascinated by the appearance of their patients. A caveat, however, must be added. Though the introduction of photographs into the daily life of the asylum during the 1860s became commonplace, reproduction of such material for general scholarly consumption was difficult. John Conolly used lithographs based on photographs to illustrate his studies of insanity, as discussed in Chapter 2. A similar means of reproduction was used to illustrate the standard textbook of the period.[6] Though photographs in books were directly reproduced as early as 1851, the procedure was cumbersome and expensive.[7] It was only with the popularization of the paper negative in the 1860s that photographs of all types could be inexpensively incorporated in popular as well as scientific studies.

When Darwin approached Browne to obtain photographs of the insane as well as some aid in understanding the nature of their mode of expression, he became involved in an ongoing debate as to the relationship between the means of perceiving the insane and the validity of interpreting what was seen. It was generally understood that definable categories of expression, if not physiognomy, existed for the various types of mental illness. Using models such as cretinism and paresis, nineteenth-century psychiatrists believed themselves able to recognize the varieties of expression in the various forms of insanity and to employ these categories for diagnostic purposes. The contemporary research into localization of brain function gave promise that such alternations in expression would be concomitant to specific brain diseases.[8] These diseases were understood as the ultimate etiologies for all mental illness. Here too, Browne functioned as Darwin's expert on the most recent findings on brain structure. He also altered the idea of illustrating mental states through his combined interests in both areas.

The Image of the Insane in *The Expression of the Emotions*

In the introduction to *The Expression of the Emotions in Man and Animals*, Darwin documented sources of evidence for his view that there is a continuum of modes of expression throughout the animal kingdom.[9] He notes that "in the first place" he observed infants, his own children, recording the development of their emotions in a manner similar to

Piaget but predating him by more than fifty years. "In the second place, it occurred to me that the insane ought to be studied, as they are liable to the strongest passions, and give uncontrolled vent to them."[10] Darwin relied on material supplied primarily by Browne for his observations. In the book there are nine specific references to the correspondence with Browne, whom Darwin described in his introduction as "an excellent observer" who "with unwearied kindness sent me copious notes and descriptions."[11]

Darwin first discusses the insane in his chapter on weeping, citing cases of depression: "One melancholic girl wept for a whole day, and afterwards confessed to Dr. Browne, that it was because she remembered that she once shaved off her eyebrows to promote their growth." Such a vignette lends authenticity to Darwin's discussion of grief. Later, Darwin again cites Browne concerning the expression of grief among the insane:

> Dr. Browne carefully observed for me during a considerable period three cases of hypochondria, in which the grief-muscles were persistently contracted. In one of these, a widow, aged 51, fancied that she had lost all her viscera, and that her whole body was empty. She wore an expression of great distress, and beat her semi-closed hands rhythmically together for hours. The grief-muscles were permanently contracted, and the upper eyelids arched.[12]

Here one aspect of the visage is singled out for comment as if it were indicative of the entire physiognomy. Darwin implies a relationship between the delusional state and the radically delineated expression of the patient. He sees in this relationship a proof of the existence of exaggerated expression in the insane.

A parallel observation is made in regard to the expression of an idiot, who "complained to Dr. Browne, by the aid of signs, that another boy in the asylum had given him a black eye; and this was accompanied by 'explosions of laughter' and with his face covered with 'the broadest smiles.'"[13] Inappropriate affect is also the topic of Darwin's sole reference to Browne's scholarly work. Browne, who had long had a special interest in the problem of the general paralysis of the insane, contributed an extensive discussion of Robert Boyd's paper on the topic in the *Journal of Mental Sciences.*[14] He paraphrased a section of it for Darwin, who used Browne's paraphrase in his volume. This passage concerned the "optimistic" visage of the paretic and Browne's emphasis on the physiognomy of expression in general paralysis as a primary means of diagnosis.[15]

Darwin's chapter on anger, the classic sign of mania, draws upon Browne's comment on the "angry scowl" of an epileptic idiot, whose contracted lips expose a "prominent row of hideous fangs."[16] In this context Darwin cites Henry Maudsley's *Body and Mind* to the effect that the idiot is the arrested form of a human at an earlier (and more primitive) stage of development.[17] Darwin's views on insanity seem greatly influenced by Maudsley's formulation. While it is never clear that Darwin subscribed to Maudsley's general view that all insanity is a form of genetic reversion, this idea was certainly consistent with his understanding of the expression of emotions among the insane. This loss of control would be the absence of civilized standards of behavior and a return to earlier modes of uncontrolled expression.

Pride is the first emotion among the mentally ill actually "seen" by Darwin. Darwin directly comments on photographs supplied to him by Browne:

> In some photographs of patients affected by a monomania of pride, sent to me by Dr. Crichton Browne, the head and the body were held erect, and the mouth firmly closed. This later action, expressive of decision, follows, I presume, from the proud man feeling perfect self-confidence in himself. The whole expression of pride stands in direct antithesis to that of humility.[18]

This is the first attempt in his study to extrapolate the relationship between the state of mind and the mode of expression of the insane based on visual material. Darwin does not supply the reader with the photographs. His comments are unqualified and relate to his own interpretation of the nature of the medium as well as to Browne's clinical notes. Darwin would have been aware that the exposure time of such photographs was so long as to record the fixed visage over a length of time: he knew that he was not dealing with an instantaneous freezing of an emotion. Nevertheless, he believed himself able to extrapolate one feature (the function of the lower lip) from the complexity of frozen structures. Further, he sought out exactly those photographs of the insane which supported his view by presenting an unwarranted and exaggerated aspect of pride. A parallel procedure exists in Darwin's discussion of "fear."[19]

In what is perhaps the most difficult chapter in his work, Darwin cites the expression of the insane in his discussion of the "erection of the hair in man and animals." Browne had supplied him with multiple cases of the insane who manifested this symptom.[20] But Browne's patients were probably suffering from myxedema, a variety of hypothyroidism, which can have mania as an auxiliary symptom. It is in this context, however, that Darwin presents the sole illustration of a mentally ill patient in his book (Plates 33, 34). Darwin had this photograph reproduced as an engraving, and he noted the gulf between the original and the copy: "I have had one of these photographs copied, and the engraving gives, if viewed

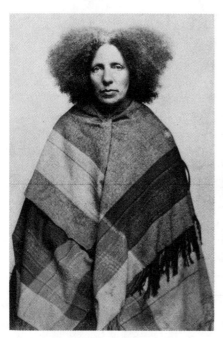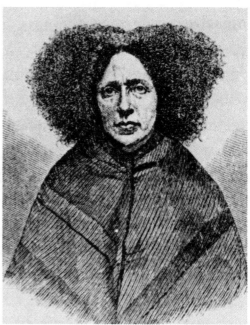

33, 34. James Crichton Browne's photograph and the engraving made from it, used by Charles Darwin in his *Expression of the Emotions in Man and Animals* (London: Murray, 1872) (private collection, Ithaca, N.Y.).

from a little distance, a faithful representation of the original, with the exception that the hair appears rather too coarse and too much curled."[21] The erection of the hair in the photograph does appear quite different from that in the engraving. Here, for the first time in the book, Darwin notes the difficulties that the medium of reproduction presents. But in no way does he call into question his own ability to interpret the visual material presented to him, even when drawing a totally false analogy between erection of the hair in animals and the insane. Darwin's final reference to Browne is in the chapter on blushing, where he refers to the total incapacity of idiots to blush. Here he had to rely on Browne's written information, which differentiated between a blush (a "civilized" reaction) and a flush (a "primitive" reaction), since no photograph of the period could capture the distinction.

The Unpublished Correspondence between Darwin and Browne

The material concerning the insane in Darwin's study of expression was culled primarily from his exchange of letters with Browne.[22] On 19

May 1869 Browne wrote to Henry Maudsley, sending him "some notes on expression for Mr. Darwin." Darwin had approached Browne through Maudsley, and Browne found himself confused by Darwin's request. Though Maudsley's initial letter is lost, it is evident from Browne's reply that Darwin wished to have some specific information concerning the expressions of the insane. Browne was not clear as to the form his answer should take: "To tell you the truth I have been greatly puzzled to know how to reply to the two queries. I do not exactly understand what sort of information Mr. Darwin wishes—whether statistics, cases, or generalizations founded upon experience. I have thought it safer to stick to facts" (19 May 1869). By facts, Browne meant case studies with relatively detailed comments. The six-page manuscript appended to the letter discusses at some length the state of hair, the "obtrusive display of teeth or 'girn' as the Scotch have it," and the action of the platysma myoides, the muscles of the neck, in the expression of the insane.

Browne also supplied two photographs to accompany his case notes. The first was of a female patient whose hair bristled whenever morphium was administered to her. (Darwin incorporated this case in his discussion of the "erection of the hair.") The second photograph was

> of a man who died of "horror" and in whom the bristling of the hair was only present to a very trifling extent. He believed that he not only brought ruin upon himself but upon all with whom he was brought in contact—that *"an awful doom"* (awful because of its very vagueness) awaited him. He was perpetually endeavoring to "fly into the arms of death to avoid the terrors of his countenance" and attempted suicide by hanging, by scratching the veins of his arm, by drowning, by beating his head upon the wall and by throwing himself before a loaded wagon. When he died no organic disease was found in his body. Only emaciation and redness of the grey matter of the brain.

This case study is typical of Browne's discussions, but this and the other case noted above are of special interest because of the accompanying photographs. Darwin, who collected illustrative material from many sources, must have been particularly fascinated by this approach. Not only was he presented with a relatively detailed case study but he could also evaluate at least some aspects of it which might be of interest to him (for example, the bristling hair) in a semi-direct manner. Darwin made at least two specific references to Browne's first manuscript in the final study, so he must have found it of help in understanding the expression of the insane. Browne's efforts, however, only tempted Darwin to make further, direct requests. On 22 May 1869 he thanked Browne for his notes, commenting that "they contain exactly and fully the information which I wanted; and besides being of the greatest use to me, are most interesting and graphic as to be almost painful." He requested further information concerning the problem of the bristling hair and the action of the platysma myoides in cases of extreme fear or anxiety. In this regard he inquired whether Browne had seen Duchenne de Boulogne's volume of photographs illustrating the effect of electric stimulation on the muscles of the face.[23] Duchenne's photographs are, however, themselves quite problematic. He referred to posed photographs of an actor miming various expressions and then used electric stimulation on the patients to recreate the mimed expression. Although Duchenne was in most cases able to document what muscles (or grouping of muscles) caused each expression, there was no attempt to verify the universality of the expressions. Rather, the theatrical expressions of the French stage were taken as an accurate reflection of the scale of all human expression.

On 1 June 1869 Browne replied to Darwin that he would be very interested in seeing Duchenne's photographs and that he had already reciprocated by sending him "another packet of photographs. . . . Let me know if there are any you would like to possess. I must ask you to return these as they are out of my album, but of most of them I believe that I can procure copies. They are all patients of my own." Browne also enclosed extensive notes on the subjects earlier mentioned by Darwin, in part illustrated with further photographs:

> Along with it (the manuscript) I will send five photographs of an idiot girl under my care who has many singular ways of expressing her emotions. When pleased she flaps her hands in front like little wings and when displeased throws the head back in the most extraordinary manner (shown in photograph 5), so that the occiput rest upon the dorsal vertebra between the scapulae. It is an anatomical puzzle to me how this is accomplished.

Darwin's interest in the physiognomy of insanity was heightened by Browne's two manuscripts. He wrote to Browne on 8 June 1869 concerning the psychiatrist's remarks on the "grief muscles" in the insane. Darwin doubted their specificity as an expression of sorrow, but his interest in Browne's photographs echoes throughout the letter: "Sometime ago I went into several shops in London to try to buy photographs of the insane, but failed; so you may believe with how much interest I have carefully looked at your excellent ones, and made some notes."

After an extended exchange, Browne returned Darwin's copy of Duchenne with detailed notes. He accompanied them with "a photograph of a female patient in the Southern Counties Asylum (Dumfries) under the care of Dr. Gilchrist in whom the bristling of the hair was well seen. The woman was in a tranquil mood when the portrait was taken. When she was agitated—the ascendant emotion being horror—the hair stood out like *wire*" (6 June 1870). He also observed that "we are beginning to take large photographs here the size of Duchenne's and will, I think, secure some interesting observations. I shall send you some. Is there any point connected with expression that you would particularly wish to have illustrated?" The manuscript comments on Duchenne are ten pages of foolscap. They are highly impressionistic but follow Darwin's intent in having Browne comment on the plates: "In order to test Duchenne's plates I have shown the most characteristic (hiding any indication of what they were meant to express) to between 20 and 30 persons of all kinds, and have recorded their answers: when nearly all agree in their answer, I trust him" (8 June 1870). By requesting numerous interpretations, Darwin was able to see whether a consensus of opinion could be found as to the emotion expressed. Darwin ignored the evident ethnocentricity of such interpretations as well as the difficulty of interpreting fleeting emotions based on static representations. Browne's comments are very much in the direction Darwin requested. As always, however, he cites numerous parallel cases in his comments, many of them of psychopathologies. In thanking Browne for his comments, Darwin emphasized that Browne "always tell[s] me exactly the things which I am anxious to hear" (8 June 1870).

Darwin then returns to his desire to observe (even indirectly) the cases he wishes to study:

> You propose to send me a photograph of a case of "general paralysis of the insane," and I should be very glad to see it: I have been trying to get a London photographer to make one of a young baby screaming or crying badly; but I fear he will not succeed. I much want a woodcut of a baby in this state. I presume it will be hopeless, from constant movement, to get an insane person photographed, whilst crying bitterly. [8 June 1870]

Darwin understood the technological difficulty of his request; he needed a photograph that would stop a fleeting emotion at one point during its expression so that the totality of that emotion could be extrapolated from that one instant. This was beyond the technical capability of photography in the early 1870s. Indeed, it was only in the 1890s that Eadweard Muybridge used high-speed photography to register the movements in a case of locomotor ataxia, a neurological disease.[24]

On 8 February 1871 Darwin wrote to Browne with more inquiries concerning the weeping of the severely depressed and the laughing of idiots. He inquired whether the bristled hair in the photographs Browne sent to him had ever been or would ever again become smooth. And again he took up the question of Browne's photographs:

Are the large photographs of the insane you lent me, and others which you said were to be made, to be purchased in London? Or could I purchase them through you at the asylum? I should like to get one or two with the corners of the mouth depressed, in order to be engraved or woodcut. Possibly others might be of service to me for the same end, if I could see them. Lastly, you told me that photographs had been taken of patients suffering from "general paralysis of the insane," in which a smiling benevolent expression occurs.

In the course of the month Browne sent Darwin yet another manuscript, fragments of which were preserved. It is concerned with the relationship between capillary circulation and mental state and reflects many of the latest scientific views concerning brain localization. On 20 February 1870 Darwin replied, thanking Browne for his efforts and requesting even more photographs: "After I have seen all you can send, I will then ask whether I could have some (supposing any suit my purpose which is of course a chance) copied: there would however be the risk of the copiers dirtying the photograph. I go to London for a week on Thursday, and intend to enquire about the new plans for engraving direct from photographs." Although Darwin did have a selection of the illustrative material for his study of expression engraved for inclusion in the forthcoming volume, he also learned that he would be able to incorporate direct reproductions of photographs in the volume. He included none of the insane. On 3 April 1871 Browne sent Darwin the photograph of the paretic he had requested:

They are I regret to say most unsuccessful and only indicate very imperfectly the labial tremor which I have described to you. The difficulty of photographing such shaky subjects is however immense and the artist a novice. . . . In all those whose photographs are now forwarded to you, the exalted extravagant profusive ideas have been well marked. They have given away millions daily.

Darwin's reply on 7 April 1871 records his successful discovery of a source for usable photographs to illustrate his book:

I have received the photographs and am greatly obliged for all your never-ceasing kindness. They are not expressive enough for my purpose. I am, however, now rich in photographs for I have found a photographer in London, Rejlander, who for years has had a passion for photographing all sorts of chance expressions exhibited on various occasions, especially by children, and taken instantaneously. One of the insane women with

bristling hair has been copied by photography on wood, and a most skill-
ful man is now cutting it on wood and is convinced that he will succeed.

Darwin's "discovery" of Oscar Rejlander, perhaps London's most popular photographer, added a new dimension to his study. In his book
Darwin reproduced twenty-eight of Rejlander's photographs. But Darwin
was not using "instantaneous" photographs. Because of the limitations
of the silver collodion process, Rejlander posed his subjects and directed
them to react on cue. His photographs are conscious works of art, not
unlike the carefully posed "assemblages" for which Rejlander was justly
famous.[25] Several of the photographs reproduced by Darwin are of Rejlander himself in a series of posed expressions. Although such a procedure has an ancestry in Duchenne's use of posed photographs, the
empirical value of such material is slight. Indeed, the public saw that
Rejlander's photographs had more aesthetic appeal than scholarly value;
sixty thousand copies of the image of "mental distress" were purchased
within a short time after it was offered for sale.

During 1871 Darwin turned to writing his study of expression. On 26
March 1871 he requested from Browne official permission to use the
photograph of the woman with the bristling hair in the book. Darwin also
requested further information on the blushing of the insane, its physiology and context. On 16 April 1871 Browne sent Darwin his notes on
blushing among the insane and idiotic. Browne saw a direct relationship
between the diminution of the circulation of blood in the brain and the
absence of blushing among the severely impaired. On 28 February 1873
Browne received a copy of the finished book with a note thanking him for
his aid. In response Browne broke an extended silence on 2 March 1877 to
acknowledge receipt of the book and to thank Darwin profusely for his
kind words.

By 1873, after the publication of his study of expression, Darwin's
views on the use of visual materials as empirical proof of the nature of
expression had undergone a substantial change. On 16 April 1873 Browne
sent Darwin fifteen photographs of his wife, who had "voluntarily assumed the expressions which she believed to be indicative of certain
emotions and frames of mind of which I had given her a list." Darwin's
reply is extremely polite: "The photographs are very curious and show
great power of acting; but still I think I should have known that the
expressions were acted, if I had not read your letter first" (17 April 1873).
Here Darwin is not only polite but cautious, a circumspection missing
from his own earlier search for photographic material.

How careful Darwin had become in evaluating the photograph as proof
in behavioral studies can be judged in his final exchange with Browne.
On 27 December 1873 Browne wrote to Darwin requesting that he con-

tribute to a volume on the pathology and treatment of general paralysis covering every aspect of the disease.

> Now it occurred to me that you might immensely aid us in our work if you would consent to give us a few remarks on the Physiognomy of the Disease. I could submit to you a series of photographs illustrating its various stages, and a very few words of yours would I am certain embody the true significance of the whole.

In effect Browne was asking Darwin to give them something similar to his earlier interpretations of the expressions of the insane which he had based on Browne's photographs. Darwin answered Browne promptly, declining participation:

> But I really think it will be impossible for me to write even a short essay on the subject. I have a good deal of experience, and am convinced that the utmost that I can do is to give you the impression which each produces on my mind; and I doubt whether any one could safely do more. Though photographs are incomparably better for exhibiting expression than any drawing, yet I believe it is quite necessary to study the previous appearance of the countenance, its changes, however small, and the living eyes, in order to form any safe judgement. I suspect moreover that our judgement is in most cases largely influenced by accessory circumstances. From your being able to study the living patients, and more especially from your various letters to me, I am fully convinced that you could do *well* that which I could effect only in the most imperfect manner. Nevertheless I shall be very glad to give you the impression a careful inspection of any photographs which you may send me produces on my mind.

Darwin never wrote his interpretation, and the scholarly correspondence concluded on this note except for an exchange of publications and pleasantries.

The Darwin-Browne correspondence reveals some of the working techniques employed by Darwin in his construction of an understanding of human expression and his use of visual sources in his undertaking. Of the masses of material solicited from Browne concerning the expressions of the insane, Darwin wrote to him: "I have been making immense use almost every day of your ms. The book ought to be called by Darwin and Browne?" (26 March 1871). Indeed, Browne's contributions form an important subtext to Darwin's own work.

Darwin's Eye

In examining Darwin's understanding of the insane and the means through which this understanding was achieved, it becomes evident that Darwin's position in the history of observing the insane was a pivotal one. On the one hand, he was indebted to the older physiognomic tradition (Lavater) as well as the older theories on expression (Bell); on the other, he was able to postulate expression as a physiological rather than a purely cultural phenomenon. How he achieved these ends is of interest. Darwin's reliance on data provided by others is certainly known, but his extensive use of visual material to buttress his arguments has been little understood. This research device becomes extremely important when the question of Darwin's perception of insanity is involved. What was Darwin looking for in the photographs of the insane? What did he see? What he sought was proof that raw, uncontrolled emotions in humans exist and that they parallel other forms of expression in the higher mammals. The insane, for Darwin, were those individuals who, through their illness, lost the protective structure by which civilized humans control their expressions of emotion. In a way the insane and idiotic form a "missing link" to our emotional past. It is not surprising that Darwin found what he sought in Browne's photographs. The idea that the photograph supplied an objective source from which observations could be made, the underlying concept of scientific photography in the nineteenth century, had been transferred from microphotography to psychiatric photography.

Darwin, once his initial enthusiasm waned, began to see the innate subjectivity of such photographs. For even a purely phenomenological description of the action of the various muscles in the expression of certain emotions presupposes that the emotions can be elicited and registered in an uncontaminated manner. Darwin avoided this problem (as did Duchenne) by employing posed photographs of emotions, through which a common denominator could be used to delineate the various expressions of emotion. Such an ethnocentric procedure could have little or no scientific value. Darwin became aware of this during the course of his work and expressed it in the final letters to Browne. Darwin's self-conscious awareness of his construction of the image of the insane out of visual evidence that he believed to be suspect (i.e., non-scientific in the sense of a positivistic definition of science) illustrates the complexities of our social construction of icons of disease. Darwin became aware that while he needed this visual material to buttress his evolutionary theory, it was material that reflected a clear cultural bias, and his subsequent distancing of his work from Browne's later investigations into the expression of the paretic is an indicator of this consciousness.

CHAPTER NINE

Medical Colonialism and Disease: Lam Qua and the Creation of a Westernized Medical Iconography in Nineteenth-Century China

Chinese Medicine and Western History

The relationship between Chinese models of science and those in the West has been the topic of one of the most striking scholarly undertakings of the last thirty years, Joseph Needham's multivolume history of science and technology in China.[1] The central theme of Needham's study is the autonomy of Chinese science and its central role in the development of an "Oriental" scientific world-view, which is of equal stature to that of "Occidental" science. The myth that Needham succeeds in destroying is that the Chinese, although able to evolve rather sophisticated technologies, remained on a relatively primitive level of technical sophistication, especially in comparison with the parallel rate of scientific and technological progress in the West. Needham counters this by showing the complexity as well as the autonomy of Chinese scientific thought and by stressing its progress within a model of Chinese science.

As of yet only peripherally covered in Needham's monumental undertaking is the development of the theories and technologies of Chinese medicine.[2] This area, however, more than most others, has been the subject of Western fascination since the earliest contacts between East and West.[3] For Chinese medicine, in all of its aspects, postulates a concept of human nature and anatomy so different from Western presuppositions (to all appearances) that it immediately captured at least the antiquarian interests of those fascinated by the "difference" of the Chinese. As more and more is known, it becomes clear that Western and Eastern medical theories share a stratum of preconceptions. And that what strikes the Western eye as "different" is the recapitulation of the familiar in a context in which the "different" is expected.

Medicine, more than any other area of science, served as one of the earliest and most important touchstones for marking the difference between the "aggressive and young" civilization of the West (in its own estimation) and the "corrupt and ancient" civilization of the East. For while concepts of difference evolved within traditional Chinese culture which gave special value to Chinese art or music or drama in contrast to the art or music or drama of the West, in the sphere of science it was only Chinese medicine (*chung-i*) that was consistently contrasted with Western medicine (*hsi-i*). There was no sense that it was necessary (or perhaps possible) to defend Taoist alchemy against Western chemistry.[4] The need to validate the difference between "Oriental" and "Occidental" spheres of culture within the realm of science was in general limited to the world of medicine. And the need for this distinction arose specifically during the course of the nineteenth century.[5] There was an implied association at this time between aesthetics and science or technology. The world of indigenous medicine, like that of art and music, needed to be defended against the intrusion of Western concepts and perceptions that made it appear inferior or at least "different."

This defensiveness was especially necessary after the 1820s, when the Western contempt for all things Chinese began to manifest itself in Europe and the Americas. Until this point most things Chinese seemed to have higher value because of their origin. No clearer example can be found than that of Chinese porcelain. Once the secret of manufacturing porcelain was uncovered in Europe in the late eighteenth century, the value of porcelain as an aesthetic object produced by an alien but higher culture was diminished. With the decline of the porcelain trade, the association of Chinese art and science in the West became a negative one, especially given the evident decline of Chinese political and economic power during the same period. The link between science/technology and aesthetics was heightened through this negative association. Now that Western technology had conquered the manufacture of Chinese aesthetic artifacts and Western political powers had begun to perceive China as a goal for colonialist expansion, the positive image of the ancient civilization with its higher forms of science and art was reversed. Chinese science became of purely antiquarian interest or became the target of Western mockery, as a sign of the stagnation of Chinese civilization.

This conflict between the Chinese and the Western traditions in medicine reveals a deep-seated reassessment of the nature of the understanding of the self. Medicine provides the historian of ideas with an extremely forceful set of mental images about the self in the form of the qualities and structures ascribed to the bearer of pathology as the antithesis of the implied health of the observer. And nowhere in the history of medicine can these fantasies be better examined than in the history of medical illustration. The history of Chinese medical illustration is yet to be written in detail, even though Needham began to address it in his study of acupuncture. This chapter, however, will focus on a problem that haunts Needham's greater study of Chinese science and which is central to any understanding of the presumed autonomy of any semiotic system: the interference that may well exist from competing systems of representation—especially the interference from systems that are understood to be more powerful than the traditional codification present within any given institutional framework. Thus, for example, Renaissance anatomical illustration in the West, with its complex (and historically discontinuous) iconography, simply drove out (or absorbed) the conventions of medieval medical illustration to such an extent that such representations were perceived by contemporaries as "old-fashioned" or "wrong." (See the discussion in Chapter 3.)

There is a traditional manner of understanding Chinese medical illustration which stresses its autonomy. It sees Chinese medical illustration as an ancient tradition primarily representing modes of treatment (rather than pathologies) which are clearly tied to systems of treatment as portrayed in herbal treatises and studies of acupuncture and moxa. The representations are overtly abstract (and thus parallel to the medieval European anatomical representations) or highly symbolic (and thus parallel to Renaissance anatomical illustration). Especially the manuals on acupuncture provide the reader (and student) with images that are either schematic or keyed by overt symbols (e.g., objects held by the figures) to external symbolic systems of reference (Plates 35, 36). Such images clearly conform to an "Oriental" mode of representing the ill.[6] For in no case is the pathology the focus of the representation, but rather the underlying structures that permit treatment. The individual patient vanishes (as Hegel's view of the Orient would have led us to expect). What remain are the generalized structures of the healthy body which permit treatment for a host of ailments.

The problem with this rather simple view of the nature of Chinese medical illustration is that it denies any shared representation with the more "sophisticated" images of pathology which were developed within Western systems of medicine. Yet we know that such interference did occur. Without a doubt the best example is a late seventeenth- or early eighteenth-century Chinese medical manuscript held by the National Library of Denmark. In his introduction to the facsimile of this manuscript, J. W. S. Johnsson documented the source of the illustrations as the anatomical illustrations of the Danish anatomist Thomas Bartholin and his school.[7] Just as schematic as the images of the patient in handbooks

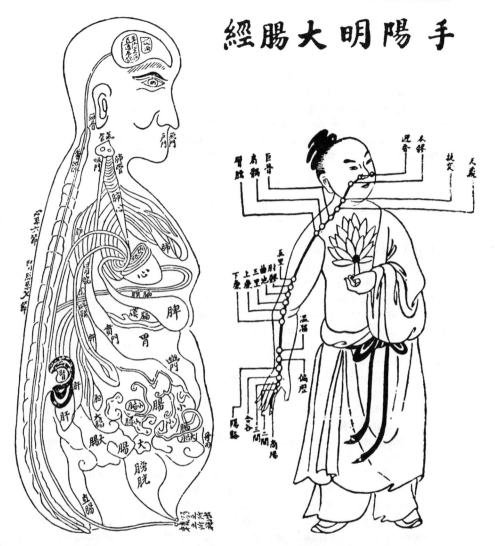

經腸大明陽手

35, 36. Two traditional images of the body in Chinese anatomy, one schematic and one symbolic, from William R. Morse, *Chinese Medicine* (New York: Hoeber, 1938).

on acupuncture, these images reflect the new iconography of the Renaissance masters of anatomy. That such influence exists elsewhere in the history of Chinese medical illustration, at least during the past three centuries, is without doubt.

Western models have been available at least for the past three hundred years to Chinese medical illustrators. Shih Fen, in what remains the best study of Western influences on Chinese medicine, documented many other areas of such influence.[8] The Copenhagen manuscript provides a classic example of the direct borrowing of representations from an external system. What would be of real interest is how (or if) such codes, isolated from their complex iconographic references, were absorbed, altered, and became part of the dominant mode of Chinese medical iconography during the eighteenth century. While such documentation is not presented by Johnsson, we do have an extraordinary example of the Chinese restructuring of conventions in medical representation in an extended corpus of mid-nineteenth-century illustrations.

Lam Qua and Medical Illustration in Canton

Lam Qua's series of at least 115 oil portraits of pathological conditions forms one of the major resources for any reconsideration of the representation of pathology in nineteenth-century China.[9] Trained by George Chinnery—the exponent in China of the "English Grand Style"—in Western artistic techniques during the 1820s, Lam Qua is the best known of the many indigenous artists who accepted the Western mode of representation.[10] This system, together with Western political power, appeared to the mid-nineteenth-century Chinese as more powerful than, and therefore preferable to, their own.

While perspective was known to Chinese artists as early as the sixteenth century, it was only in the nineteenth that it was associated with the power of Western cultural politics and thus became the preferable mode of representation. The difference between the two systems of aesthetic representation was thus endowed with ideological significance— one system was seen as weaker and less valid than the other. Indeed, tradition has it (at least a tradition within the Fearon family) that Lam Qua had been a houseboy in the Fearon home in Macao when Chinnery arrived in China.[11] The houseboy became entranced by the skills of the Western artist while watching him paint in Christopher Fearon's garden. Here, too, the parallel between the domination of Western political power (the position of the Fearon trading family in Macao) and the aesthetics associated with this power in the form of Chinnery's portraiture places the "house boy" in the position of Robinson Crusoe's "Friday," trained in the outward manifestations of Western society in order to be permitted to share in the power of his master's technology.

Lam Qua was important enough among his contemporaries in Canton (Guangzhou) that when a French traveler, M. La Vollé, visited the artists of that city, it was to Lam Qua's studio that he was first taken.[12] Above the door was a sign that pointed to the double focus of Lam Qua's art: "Lam Qua, English and Chinese Painter." William Fane de Salis, who visited Lam Qua, commented on the distinctions between these two styles and their value. A painting in "English" style was worth £10 and was "fashioned with good drawing and perspective"; a "Chinese" painting was only worth £8 because it was "out of all drawing proportion and perspective."[13] The indigenous art of China (like its medicine) was of less value because it was competing with a system that was assumed by the Western viewer to be more sophisticated.

Lam Qua, who employed as many as ten to twenty artists in this studio, was clearly the most prolific of the local painters as well as the most renowned. He had most probably begun his career by copying portraits as a member of a similar studio. By the 1840s he had become the best-known Chinese artist in Canton and began to sign his canvases "The Sir Thomas Lawrence of China," certainly calling more on Lawrence's status as a portraitist and as the head of the Royal Academy than on any claim to Lawrence's facile style. Lam Qua's portraits of Chinese merchant-princes, such as Sam Qua (now at the Peabody Museum in Salem, Massachusetts), were shown at the Boston Athenaeum in 1851. These portraits were both part of and symbolic of the China trade. Commissioned by the Ipswich, Massachusetts, merchant Augustine Heard, they represented his trading partners in Canton. They are portraits in the general style of the British academic painters of the period, such as Chinnery, Lawrence, or Sir William Beechey, but unlike the smooth, precious nature of these artists' works Lam Qua's portraits strove to capture the individuality of the sitter. They in no way sought to glorify the sitter, but rather used conventions of portraiture to capture the illusion of each individual's uniqueness.

Osmond Tiffany, Jr., visited Lam Qua's studio in 1844 and commented: "He takes portraits in the European style, and his coloring is admirable. His facility in catching a likeness is unrivalled, but wo [sic] betide if you are ugly, for Lam Qua is no flatterer. I might repeat a dozen stories of his bluntness, but they have probably found their way into print."[14] This attitude toward the aesthetics of portraiture has a fundamental influence on Lam Qua's medical illustration, as will be discussed. The power of Lam Qua's academic portraits, with their juxtaposition of a familiar style with an "exotic" subject matter as well as an "exotic" creator, can be judged by the fact that Lam Qua's "Head of an Old Man" was exhibited at the Royal Academy in London (1835). Likewise, Lam Qua was the first Chinese artist working in a Western tradition whose work was exhibited in America (*Portrait of Moushang, Tea Merchant, Canton, China* in 1841 at the Apollo Club in New York City).

Peter Parker and the Medical Missionaries

Lam Qua painted his series of portraits of patients (or at least had this series of portraits painted in his studio) within a very specific historical context. Peter Parker, the first Protestant American medical missionary in China (who had taken his medical degree at Yale in 1834), commissioned Lam Qua, beginning in the 1830s, to capture the likeness of a number of the most interesting cases in his hospital in Canton. (The case notes for many of these are preserved at Yale.) Lam Qua first sketched these images on rice-paper and then transferred them (or had them transferred) into a series of Western-style portraits in oil on canvas. One series of these portraits was prepared before Parker's return (because of the unrest during the Opium Wars) to the United States in 1840. Another series was undertaken (because of the success of the first) upon his return to Canton in 1842. The first portraits were used by Parker on his trip to England and in the United States to illustrate his presentation of his case studies to such groups as the Boston Medical Society in order to raise funds for his missionary work by showing the success of his medical practice in China.

Peter Parker was the first foreign doctor to undertake the training of Chinese paramedicals. Senior among these Chinese students was Kwan A-to, Lam Qua's nephew, who was trained in basic ophthalmological and surgical procedures. There is a portrait of Peter Parker by Lam Qua reproduced in Edward Gulick's monograph on Parker, in which Kwan A-to appears in the act of examining a patient's eye.[15] There the master is seated in a prominent position in the right foreground holding a Chinese manuscript, while the student undertakes the actions he has been trained to perform, in the left background. The patient, the least "Westernized" figure in the portrait, has his back to the viewer so that his primary attribute is his "pig-tail," the sign of servility. Parker's commission to Lam Qua documents an attitude toward the representation of somatic illness which is inherently Western and—given the relationship between the "master" and the "houseboy," between the Westerner and the Chinese—dominant.

What is most striking is that Lam Qua's painting is clearly a version of George Chinnery's 1835 portrait of Thomas R. Colledge, surgeon of the East India Company, in terms of the position of the two Chinese. In Chinnery's portrait, however, the pig-tailed figure is not the patient but, much more traditionally, the Chinese paramedic. It is Colledge who is actively examining the patient's eyes. Lam Qua has marginally subverted the original portrait, putting the apprentice Kwan A-to in the active role of Western healer, but has maintained the boundaries of power in placing Parker in the foreground role of teacher. Parker's greater size, a reflex of the use of Western perspective, gives him the dominant role in the portrait, assuring the retention of power within the Western model of representation in science.

It is the refunctioning of the Western model for the representation of pathology within the world of nineteenth-century China which forms the context for any understanding of Lam Qua's undertaking. Lam Qua's relationship to *his* master, Chinnery, parallels Kwan A-to's relationship to Parker. Each must learn to see the world through new models of reality perceived as much more powerful than those in traditional Chinese art or science.

Lam Qua and the New Science of Medical Representation

Lam Qua represents this new reality in his portraits of his patients and brings to these portraits, either consciously or unconsciously, some of the ideological implications of nineteenth-century European medical illustration as well as certain specific ideological needs that he, as a Chinese artist in Canton, perceived as inherent in his representation of pathology.

The image of the identifiable patient as the bearer of a specific pathology arose in European medical illustration as an outgrowth of the medical philosophy of the Idéologues, who believed that only single cases could be validly examined and could serve as the basis of any general medical nosology.[16] (See Chapter 2 for a more detailed discussion of this movement.) For scientists such as Helvétius, Condorcet, and Pinel held to a radical empiricism that demanded that specific patients and their phenomenologies be the focus of the medical gaze. As a result, Pinel produced the first illustrated textbook of psychiatry (see Plate 7). It was from this textbook rather than from the observation of patients that students of medicine in revolutionary France were taught about the insane. Pinel offered visual representations of specific cases as his substitution for the empirical reality of specific patients. This substitution was possible for Pinel and his students only because a theory of the pathognomonic nature of the appearance of the insane had evolved during the eighteenth century which provided specific external signs for madness in the physiognomy of the patient.

But it was Jean-Louis Alibert in the 1810s who began—with his twelve-volume atlas of skin diseases—a tradition of illustrating medical studies with images that were perceived as mimetic rather than schematic. Extraordinarily well illustrated (and costing more than the annual salary of a surgical assistant), Alibert's work stressed the visual representation of the external manifestations of dermatological diseases in a series of case studies. It is evident that the illusion of mimesis which Alibert's images had for his contemporaries resided to no little extent in his use of the engraved portrait technique of the early nineteenth century coupled with the application of color. Much of the perceived improvement of Alibert's illustrations over those of Pinel, for example, lay in this adoption of the technology of "high" art. This type of "realistic" medical illustration broke with what in retrospect was seen as the highly schematic images of seventeenth- and eighteenth-century physiognomic representation.

Alibert continued the tradition of Pinel in yet another way—both presented aspects of disease which were understood to have a specific external structure. Medical illustration followed the idea of science as classification which dominated the early nineteenth century. Skin disease, like madness, had specific external signs, all of which were pathognomonic. The external, pathognomonic sign is the definition of disease, and therefore the line between the patient and the observer.

When Lam Qua went to Peter Parker to paint the 80 patients represented in the 115 portraits, he was confronted with a conflict. Parker wanted his most appalling cases documented so that he would have a way of proving his value in China. It was therefore necessary to document those cases where the external manifestation of the disease labeled the individual as overtly diseased and therefore dependent on the new medicine from the West. Tumors were the most evident sign of such illness. The ability easily to remove large benign tumors (some as large as thirty-five kilograms) with relatively narrow pedicles was a sure sign of the superiority of Western medicine (since Chinese medicine did not undertake surgery, as it disfigured the body and thus violated Confucian dogma)—as valid a sign in the West, as documented through Lam Qua's paintings, as it was in China. It is important to understand that Parker's medical practice had an ideological purpose. He was a medical missionary and, as a missionary, interested not only in the spread of Protestant Christianity but also in the Westernization of China. Indeed, his activities were so successful that he was seen to have "opened the gates of China with a lancet when Western cannon could not heave a single bar."[17] Parker's view was that Western medicine was proof of the superiority of all things Western. An anecdote is told of him that when he found himself in Guy's Hospital, where a series of the patient portraits were on display, he boastfully corrected his guide, who commented that nothing could have been done for these poor fellows, by retorting that he had operated on all of them![18] The extraordinary appearance of Parker's patients, even to the European eye, shows the special role that the Western medical practitioner had in China, curing the seemingly incurable. This notion is parallel to the missionaries' view of the conversion of the Chinese to Christianity. For the Chinese, so different in culture (and race) from the European, can become Christians, just as Parker's patients can become healthy.

But Lam Qua was evidently also given some visual guidance in preparing his drawings and paintings. He did not simply paint portraits of the patients in the manner of Lawrence, for his images follow the general traditions of the post-Alibert illustrations of pathologies. Indeed, one can compare them with a slightly later text, Rudolf Virchow's 1863 lectures on tumors, in order to judge their similarity.[19] The patient is represented in isolation, as a single figure; the focus of the observer is on the pathology of the patient. And the pathology, the tumor, is the overt sign of the role of the observed as the proposed object of treatment. Indeed, in the illustrations to Virchow's lectures the representation of the patient with a tumor, found as the frontispiece to the first volume, is gradually replaced with the image of the tumor itself, in keeping with Virchow's own stress on cellular pathology. The patient quite literally vanishes in the course of Virchow's lectures, to be replaced by the emblem of the disease, the tumor. In Lam Qua's paintings the patient becomes an extension of the pathology, representative of the pathology much as the English country gentlemen in Lawrence's paintings become representative of a class or an attitude toward life. In Lam Qua's paintings the patient "vanishes" since the patient becomes the perceived object shared between the physician-missionary, Peter Parker, who is lecturing about them, and his Western audience. The audience, whether of physicians or of Christian missionaries, has its belief system concerning the nature of the Chinese reified in the establishment of its sense of superiority to the patient. The patient bears a double stigma—first, the sign of pathology, and second, the sign of barbarism, his or her Chinese identity. Each patient must still appear to be unique in order for the scientific value of the illustration to dominate. There is no attempt to present a schematisized image of the pathology independent of the image of the patient. But the power of this scientific mode of representing difference establishes the boundary between the viewer and the patient. The Western audience was provided with this sense of their own superiority to this Chinese inferiority through the use of Lam Qua's paintings (Plate 37).

Parker brought a series of early nineteenth-century textbooks with him to China which would have provided similar images to those found a decade or so later in Virchow's work (or, indeed, in almost any medical handbook from the 1820s on). Lam Qua was given models (much as Chinnery had supplied him with portraits to copy when Lam Qua was his apprentice) in order to establish the correct, acceptable image of the patient for the Western (not the Chinese) observer. For Parker and his medical associates in the West were the implied viewers of Lam Qua's canvases. What Lam Qua provided, however, may well have transcended

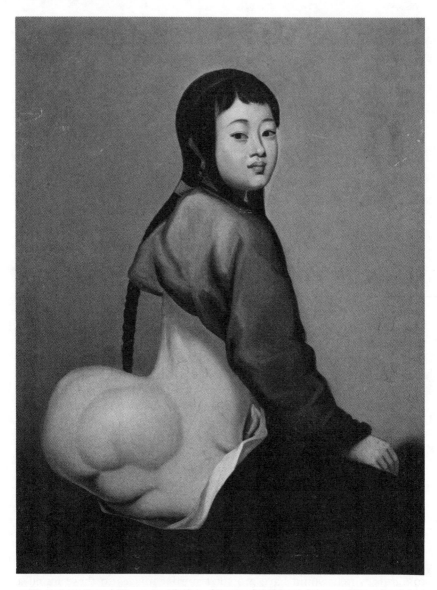

37. Lam Qua, *Young Woman with Spinal Tumor* (Herbert F. Johnson Museum of Art, Cornell University; Gift of Dr. and Mrs. Ronald M. Lawrence).

the merely mechanical reproduction of pathologies represented through the conventions of Western medical illustration. His images illustrate what happens when systems of representation meet and one is dominant over the other that is perceived by all involved to be weaker.

Reading Lam Qua's Portraits

Lam Qua presents his patients so as to stress their pathology. The visual impact of the tumors and other gross pathologies would have been striking (especially for the Western eye of the mid-nineteenth century), though certainly not unfamiliar. Thus the association of the image of the untreated pathology with the perceived weakness of indigenous medicine in China, as opposed to the newly introduced medicine from the West, would have provided one possible level of interpretation but not the only one. The portraitlike quality of the reproductions (again as seen by the Western observer) seems to stress the individuality of the patients. But for the indigenous Chinese observer the "English" portrait was an alienating manner of portraying reality. Just as William Fane de Salis commented on the "good drawing" of Lam Qua's "English" portraits and the crudity of the traditional "Chinese" images "out of all . . . proportion," so too must the "English" portraits have struck the mid-nineteenth-century Chinese viewer as deformed. But this quality would have been associated with the obvious political power controlled by the West. It was given a positive quality (and thus had a greater value in the marketplace).

Yet in spite of this "portraitlike" quality, the dominance of the pathology still served as the focus of the representation. The analogy to Lam Qua's painting of Peter Parker and Kwan A-to is striking. For there the qualities ascribed to the figures are highly symbolic: Parker sits holding (and therefore controlling) a Chinese manuscript, showing his domination over the world he has entered; Kwan A-to is the proof and instrument of this domination as he undertakes a Western medical technique with Western ophthalmological tools; and the faceless, anonymous patient is characterized by his subservience to both, placed in such a way as to allow the viewer to see only the sign of his position in the subordinate culture. Here Lam Qua provides us with a mode of reading his representations of illness. He is the observer—Parker is not the only one—and in stressing the centrality of the new vision of humanity, that of Western medicine and Christianity, he shares in the power that makes the patient vanish.

The pathological sign has an ideological message, placing the Western observer in a dominant position over the indigenous patient. By producing medical illustrations that were not overtly schematic or symbolic (as in the traditional mode of Chinese medical illustrations), Lam Qua allies himself ("The Sir Thomas Lawrence of China") with the power of the new mode of seeing the patient and thus shares the separation that Parker senses between his perception of the patient and that of native medicine. The portraitlike quality of Lam Qua's paintings is the sign of his role as an "English" observer. The open hostility to him on the part of such English painters as Chinnery, because of his command of their style, is not unexpected. Furthermore, Lam Qua's use of models taken from the new medicine (*hsi-i*) shows that he is part of a new elite, the Chinese who have command over Western tools, no matter what their area. Western art and science have replaced Chinese art and science as representations of power. Those Chinese who control these tools are exercising a power denied to them under most circumstances. Thus Lam Qua is able to use those facilities employed by the Westerner to stress the inferiority of the Chinese to show that the Chinese can assume control of power.

Lam Qua's hidden agenda is manifest in the fact that the very signs of difference which for Alibert were the indicators of specific disease entities come to have a symbolic function. The diseased Chinese, artfully painted in the manner of Western portraiture and posed in the most up-to-date Western scientific manner, secretly signifies the power of the new order over the old, not just over Chinese medicine (*chung-i*) but over all of the older and therefore weaker means of organizing and controlling reality.

Lam Qua and the Westernized Illustrated Book

The images of disease which Lam Qua records are also images of the diseases of the Chinese past (as understood by the medical missionary), of the weakness and corrupt practice inherent in indigenous modes of representation. Lam Qua, however, was a master of both styles, the new English and the now debased Chinese. It is clear that for Peter Parker's gallery of the gross pathologies of Imperial Canton only the new style would do. With this action Lam Qua created the necessary association between the new medicine and the new art, an association that placed the new Western modes of representation in a dominant position in late nineteenth- and early twentieth-century China. In handbooks of Western medicine produced in China this association was simply assumed, even though it provided for the Chinese an alienating set of images for anyone who equated the traditional aesthetics of China with the "correct" self-image of the Chinese. It is no surprise that when the British physician Benjamin Hobson, who arrived in China in 1839, sought out illustrators for these first texts, produced in the 1850s, which were to teach Western medical knowledge to the Chinese, he turned to the Cantonese artists.[20] The illustrations, while primitive, are clearly in the tradition of nineteenth-century European anatomical illustration. There is no place in the transmission of European knowledge, with all of its ideological implications, for Chinese medical illustration. This tradition continued to develop through the publication of the central text that still defines Western medical knowledge (in the popular mind) in terms of a system of representation, *Gray's Anatomy,* in Osgood and Whitney's translation of 1880.

The domination of Western medical representation between 1834 to 1851, from Peter Parker's arrival in China to the publication of Benjamin Hobson's first medical textbook, can be understood as part of the general competition of Western and indigenous systems of visual representation in China. For the domination of Western medical representations can be paralleled to the domination of yet another system of representation, that of Western religious art, during the same period. In 1851 the "Association of God Worshipers" (*Taiping tianguo*), preaching a unique form of Evangelical Christianity, appeared in southern China. The rebellion that they fomented employed much of the imagery of Evangelical Christianity, including biblical imagery, but most specifically that of John Bunyan's *Pilgrim's Progress,* which was translated with illustrations in 1851. Rudolf Wagner has shown, in an insightful study, that the iconography and imagery of the central text of the Taiping Rebellion, the vision of its leader Hung Hsiu-ch'uan, were rooted in the conventions of Evangelical Christianity read as a program for action in terms of Chinese canons of rationality.[21] What is striking is that the illustrations to Hung Hsiu-ch'uan's vision, reprinted by Wagner, are simply reworkings of the representations taken from Muirhead's translation of Bunyan, the standard Western vocabulary of Evangelical religious images.

These images are, however, given a quite different level of importance, for they are not understood merely as allegorical representations but as the actions that are necessary for a successful act of political rebellion. The Protestant missionaries, such as Parker and Hobson, initially welcomed the Taiping Rebellion as a sign that Christianity had taken root in China. They had, of course, associated the externals of the Taiping vision, cast in the well-known images taken from Bunyan and the Bible, with traditional Christianity as they understood it. Only when it became clear that the Chinese were repeating the action of the British during the Opium Wars, that they were attempting to undermine the existing state for political reasons (rather than religious ones), did they reject the Taiping revolutionaries. For the Western system of representation initially controlled the actions of the missionaries, who first saw only the external signs of Evangelical Christianity in the iconography employed in the revolt. It also controlled the actions of the revolutionaries, who accepted the meaning of the texts and their illustrations quite literally, and who ceased advancing once the limited goals described in the vision had been accomplished. Each group saw in the iconography of Evangelical Christianity quite different meanings and acted upon them. Something quite similar had already happened, but on a much more limited scale, with the adoption of Western medical illustration. The Western-trained artists accepted the power given them by the new system of representation but used the power for their own purposes, not those of the missionary-doctors. They achieved status for themselves, placing themselves in the role of the masters of the new science. From the perception of the medical missionaries they were, like the patients they painted, invisible. They were merely technical extensions of Western modes of perception. But they were able to subvert this invisibility to achieve a new status as part of the new world of power invested in Western modes of perception. And, unlike the Taiping revolutionaries', their refunctioning of a Western symbolic system was never exposed.

Western medicine came to stand for the dominance of the West in China. Indeed, the appearance of traditional Chinese medical practitioners in 1925 at the deathbed of Sun Yat-Sen, the representative of modern China and a Westernized medical practitioner, symbolized the central role that medicine came to hold in distinguishing between the imposed Western tradition and Chinese tradition. With the rise of the new nationalism in the early twentieth century, traditional medicine became an icon for Chinese national aspirations. And this was a reaction to the general decline in reputation it had experienced in the generations following Lam Qua, when the aesthetics of power had been introduced into the world of medicine in China.

CHAPTER TEN

Opera, Homosexuality, and Models of Disease: Richard Strauss's *Salome* in the Context of Images of Disease in the Fin de Siècle

Disease and Culture

To document the construction of popular as well as medical images of the diseased, I have asked a series of questions about the social context of an opera libretto, about an author's intention in selecting a theme for an opera, about the cultural significance of selecting any given text to be set to music. My object is one of the most popular operas of the twentieth century, Richard Strauss's *Salome*, first performed in the Dresden Opera on 9 December 1905. My contention is that in selecting a libretto composers take into consideration much more than aesthetic appropriateness. They are aware of the cultural implications, including images of disease, and of the force that cultural presuppositions will have in shaping the audience and drawing it both into the work, as well as, perhaps even more important than, into the theater.

With Richard Strauss the problem of the libretto seems on first glance to be rather trivial, for did he not simply, to quote his own words, "purge the piece [i.e., Oscar Wilde's French drama of 1892] of purple passages to such an extent that it became quite a good libretto"?[1] Would it not, therefore, be sufficient to read the play, to understand the drama's admittedly complex genesis, in order to comprehend Strauss's libretto? As we have seen, it is the culturally determined reading of any text or image in its historical (and, indeed, national) context which determines its particular meaning; and one basic aspect of this culturally determined reading of a text is the image of disease which dominates any given culture. There is a "text in this opera," to paraphrase Stanley Fish, but it is a text constructed through the demands of the interpretative community in which the text is understood to function.[2] It is clear that I will be able to illuminate only a very small corner of the context generated by the interpretative community in which Richard Strauss's reading of Oscar Wilde took place, but I hope that this example will suffice to indicate the extraordinary complexity of reading a libretto in its full cultural, intellectual, and political matrix.

I shall be examining three major contexts for the interpretation of Strauss's libretto. First, I sketch the history of Oscar Wilde's image as the homosexual writer par excellence in the German-speaking lands during the period of Strauss's concern with Wilde's text; second, I explain how the basic associations within the German reception of Oscar Wilde are reflected in Strauss's presentation of the characters of the opera as stage Jews with all of their intimation of disease; third, I give a rationale for Strauss's selection (and defense) of Wilde's *Salome* in light of these two factors. I do not wish to present an exhaustive reading of the libretto. What I offer is an attempt to reconstruct a set of cultural presuppositions about disease and difference which existed in Germany and Austria at the turn of the century and an inquiry into how these presuppositions shaped the choice of the libretto and its contemporary interpretation. These models of disease and pathology play themselves out in Strauss's reading (and our re-reading) of Oscar Wilde's text in an intricate but illuminating manner.[3]

The Pervert: Wilde in Germany

Oscar Wilde was dead only three years when the Viennese poet Anton Lindner approached Richard Strauss with the libretto of an opera he had begun, which he had based on Wilde's play *Salome*.[4] (Lindner was the author of the text for Strauss's "Hochzeitlich Lied" [opus 37], which Strauss had set in 1889.) While Strauss was taken with the theme at the time, he did not think enough of Lindner's idea to view it as any more than potentially a minor pendant to his recently completed opera *Feuersnot* (produced at the Viennese Court Opera on 29 January 1902). Eventually he rejected Lindner's libretto. Strauss's first two operas, *Guntram* (1894) and *Feuersnot*, were settings of mock-Wagnerian themes. *Guntram* was, as George Marek observes, "a farrago of Wagnerian ideas," pseudomedieval plot and all. *Feuersnot*, according to Marek, is the librettist Ernst von Wolzogen's version of *Die Meistersinger*.[5] With the choice of *Salome*, Strauss clearly broke with his early attempt to write mock-Wagnerian operas, or at least music to mock-Wagnerian texts, and rethought his views on the nature of opera. Here he associated himself with the musical as well as cultural avant-garde, adapting the model of Claude Debussy's 1902 setting of Maeterlinck's *Pelléas et Méli-sande*, without a doubt the first important opera of the post-Wagnerian avant-garde. Strauss had already begun to identify himself with the "moderns," but only in his selection of the programs for his symphonic tone poems. As with the shift from the "folkloric" theme of his tone poem *Till Eulenspiegel's Merry Pranks* (1895) and his "Nietzschean" *Thus Spake Zarathustra* (1896), with *Salome* Strauss discovered the avant-garde opera and was in turn discovered by the avant-garde.

The theme of Salome as the virginal dancer erotically attracted to John the Baptist was reintroduced in European culture during the 1830s and 1840s in the work of Jacob Grimm and Heinrich Heine.[6] There were at least two widely read prose treatments by famous (if not notorious) members of the intellectual avant-garde by the closing decades of the nineteenth century, Gustave Flaubert's last published work, "Herodias," and J. K. Huysmans's quintessential novel of self-conscious decadence, *A Rebours*. In the visual arts *Salome* was a major theme of high (and not so high) art during the fin de siècle, from Wilde's inspiration, the gore-dripping image painted by Wilde's contemporary Gustav Moreau, to the cool and distanced lithograph of Salome by Strauss's contemporary Edvard Munch. But it had not yet been the subject of a musical setting (with the exception of Pierné's incidental music to the French production of Wilde's play). In 1903 Strauss saw Max Reinhardt's production of the play in the "Kleines Theater" in Berlin (with the young and brilliant actress Gertrud Eysoldt in the lead). Reinhardt had chosen the best of the four competing German translations, that of Hedwig Lachmann, for his production. After his visit to the theater, a friend (the cellist Heinrich Grünfeld) suggested to Strauss that the play could provide real material for an opera.[7] Strauss immediately answered that he was already at work, having been inspired by Lindner's earlier mention of the theme.

The point of setting Wilde's play, according to the composer some four decades later, was his belief that "Oriental and Jewish operas lacked true Oriental color and scorching sun."[8] It is important to note the hyphenated phrase, "Orient- und Judenoper." Strauss, writing as late as 1942, acknowledges that he was writing a "Jewish" opera. Other works in this genre, biblical operas such as Verdi's *Nabucco* (1842) and Saint-Saën's *Samson et Dalila* (1877), or post-biblical representations of the Jews such as Halévy's *La Juive* (1835), lacked the "Orientalism" that Strauss understood as necessary for a "Jewish" topic. Strauss's words also reflect the concept of the Jew held by both anti-Semites and some Jews in the German-speaking world by 1905. The anti-Semite's charge (to be found in works as far removed from one another as Friedrich Ratzel's geographic studies and Houston Stewart Chamberlain's anti-Semitic diatribes) that Jews were merely Orientals who would always be outsiders in the

West was internalized by at least one radical fringe of European Jewry. Early Zionist writers such as Theodor Herzl and Martin Buber accepted the charge that they would always remain outsiders, remain Orientals in a world of Occidentals, and they acted upon this belief: Herzl, by seeking a national homeland for the Jews outside of Europe; Buber, by finding the true wellsprings of Jewish culture in the world of the Eastern European Jew.[9] Strauss's acceptance of this form of projection, with all its ambiguities, is a clear reflection of the reception of *Salome* in Germany and Austria. And Strauss's association of the Jew with the cultural avant-garde influenced his selection of the *Salome* libretto in a most complicated manner. There was a strong popular image of Jewry as the bastion of the cultural avant-garde, an image shared by some Jews as well as promulgated by much of the German anti-Semitic literature of the period.[10] Even the initial impetus, to set Oscar Wilde's play rather than a rewritten version that would not have borne Wilde's name, came from its production by a Jew leading the dramatic avant-garde, Max Reinhardt, and a suggestion from another Jew, Heinrich Grünfeld, that Wilde's play (not a watered-down libretto written by a third party) could provide material for a new opera.[11] It is the link between Wilde, the homosexual poet, and the Jews as representative of the avant-garde which will continue to appear in our unraveling of Strauss's libretto.

Oscar Wilde's play, written in French in 1891 and 1892 for Sarah Bernhardt, had been performed only in 1896 in Paris (without the Divine Sarah). In London the Lord Chamberlain forbade any production of the play, because of its representation of biblical figures, until 1931. Wilde, who died in Paris in 1900, had an extraordinary popularity in Germany during the early twentieth century. Between 1900 and 1934 there were more than 250 publications of Wilde's work (more than any other British author except Shakespeare), and during the 1903–4 season alone, 248 performances of his dramas were seen on the German stage, including 111 performances of *Salome*.[12] While Reinhardt's production of *Salome* was not the German premiere (this took place in the winter of 1901 at the "Freie literarische Vereinigung" in Breslau), it was by far the most famous of the period and served to link the names of Reinhardt and Wilde in the public imagination.[13] Indeed, Wilde's popularity grew in Germany almost in inverse proportion to its decline in Britain following his trials (and conviction) in 1895–96 on charges of sodomy.

The trials, held in London, were reported in detail in Germany. A long, factual report ran in the liberal newspaper *Die Zeit*, and two extraordinary essays were published in the socialist magazine *Die neue Zeit* by the exiled politician Eduard Bernstein.[14] In the first of these essays, Bernstein stressed the popular British image of Wilde as the effete aesthete. He revealed how the British public condemned the "unnatural" aspect of a behavior that had existed in society since the Greeks and Romans. Bernstein's thesis concerning the nature of homosexuality is, however, most clearly presented in the second essay, which counters Friedrich Engels's "Origin of the Family." Bernstein argues that it is only in the more complex societies that homosexuality is viewed as deviant. Indeed, he observes that it is a "commonplace" in the popular British attack on Wilde, "that with increased wealth and luxury sexual excesses increase" (p. 230). This popular equation, against which Bernstein argues, formed the basis for the German conservative attack on Wilde as a typical product of British capitalism. The Socialists had in general supported the cause of homosexual emancipation in Germany.[15] Wilde thus became part of the litmus test between the right, which condemned him as representative of the decay of the British, and the left, which saw the persecution of homosexuality as a sign of the inherent hypocrisy of German society.

Bernstein was clearly arguing against such writers as the conservative commentator Moeller van den Bruck, who in an essay on Wilde uses Wilde's homosexuality as a means of condemning British imperialism.[16] For van den Bruck it is the specter of "brutal or ignorant" British colonialism which gives rise to writers like Wilde. Wilde is his prime example of British degeneration, an unnatural reaction to the materialism that dominates the British soul. Wilde's is an example of "sexual insanity" (and van den Bruck uses the English words as if to stress the particularly British nature of this disease). Wilde is quintessentially British, typical of the ideology of colonialism: "Morally this people does not know what else to do. It seeks a replacement for morals in eccentricity. The proverbial British brutalization of the masses is nothing more than misdirected sexuality in a society deeply embedded in the perversions of all quarters of the earth" (p. 251). The British are perverted because they have internalized in their wanderings all of the perversions of the world. In response to such "Brit-bashing," Bernstein stressed the parallels between the persecution of Wilde and the potential for similar public persecution of homosexuals under German Imperial law.

But he does not recognize the insidious racist subtext of the conservative's argument. (Indeed, given the Socialist view that anti-Semitism was a reflex of the latter stages of capitalism, he could not recognize this feature, even though his own reference to the degeneracy of increased luxury is a phrase borrowed from the anti-Semitic literature of the period.) For the British are merely substitutes for the Jews. This apposition can be seen in van den Bruck's image of the homosexual's discourse: it is the "dissipation of thoughts in sophistry," a term long used to represent the discourse of the Jews (p. 250). The British are seen as the most degenerate nation in Europe; they become, by association, the new Jews of

Europe. This link was made even more overt with the general mid-nine-teenth-century European understanding that in the *Realpolitik* of the Middle East the "Jews [were] a possible *avant-garde* of England's imperialism," to quote Barbara Tuchman.[17] Nietzsche, in *The Antichrist[ian]*, had already denounced this view of the Jews as true decadents: "The Jews are the antithesis of all decadents: they have had to *represent* decadents to the point of illusion; with a *non plus ultra* of histrionic genius they have known how to place themselves at the head of all movements of decadence (as the Christianity of Paul), in order to create something out of them which is stronger than any *Yes-saying* party of life."[18] But within German conservatism this association remained. Wilde's sexual deviancy is thus nothing more than further proof that materialism (read: Judaism) leads to perversion, a thesis long applied to the Jews of Europe. For the Christian focus on the Jews had centered on their sexual difference, a difference seen in Jewish ritual practices, such as circumcision, and fantasies about Jewish sexuality, such as the myth about Jewish male menstruation. In the late nineteenth and early twentieth centuries, much of the fantasy concerned the special case of Jews and incest, a factor that plays a large role in shaping the contemporary reading of Strauss's libretto.

In 1896 Oscar Sero wrote a detailed, almost day-by-day account of Wilde's trials in a monograph published in Leipzig by Max Spohr, who served as the major outlet for popular as well as scholarly works on homosexuality during the years following the Wilde trials.[19] Sero appends to his account of the trials a long "dialogue" on the treatment of and attitude toward homoerotic activity in Germany. This repeated much of Bernstein's theme of the parallel rather than difference between British and German society. The trials of Oscar Wilde had a major impact in shifting the attitude of German homosexuals toward the importance of repealing the law against homosexual activity (section 175 of the Imperial Criminal Code) which had been in force since 1872 (continuing the older laws in the Prussian Criminal Code). In other words, it was the Wilde trial, the trial of art and the artist by the materialistic and anti-intellectual British (according to German perspective), which thus crystallized the homosexual emancipation movement in Germany. Indeed, the appearance of Adolf Brand's homophile periodical *Der Eigene* in 1896, as well as the founding of the first homosexual emancipation organization on 15 May 1897, the *Wissenschaftlich–humanitäres Komitee* (by Max Spohr, the sexologist Magnus Hirschfeld, and the civil servant Erich Oberg), was to no little degree stimulated by the trials of Wilde. The homosexual emancipation movement, even though initially it was broadly based politically (and included some members of the anti-Semitic right), quickly became identified with the avant-garde (and therefore

Jewish) left. It is significant that the image of the Wilde trials in Germany was shaped by individuals who were seen as liberals—but also very clearly understood as Jews (especially Eduard Bernstein and Magnus Hirschfeld). It was this link, rather than any other, which remained in the popular mind.

Wilde, after his trials, became as much the image of the persecuted artist as he had been the representative dandy of the 1880s. He became the symbolic artist persecuted by the forces of aesthetic conservatism, represented in the writing of avant-garde Germany by the metaphor of Victorian (read: Wilhelmian) prudery. In an obituary of Wilde, published in Magnus Hirschfeld's *Jahrbuch für sexuelle Zwischenstufen* in 1901, "Numa Prätorius" (the pseudonym of lawyer Eugen Wilhelm) centers his account of Wilde's life on the trials and discusses their impact in Germany. For him, the use of paid informants and blackmailers on the part of the prosecution was "for Germans" incomprehensible.[20] Wilde remains the persecuted artist, persecuted by the state for his sexual orientation but also for his status as a member of the intellectual avant-garde.

By 1905 the merger of artist and works is complete. Hugo von Hofmannsthal, in an essay written in that year, sees Wilde as the essential symbolist poet, whose life and art are inseparable.[21] Wilde takes on this role not merely because of the nature of his work, but because his life too was created from a series of symbolic masks, including the final one, the mask of degradation, Sebastian Melmoth (Wilde's pseudonym after his release from prison and his escape to the continent). Here Hofmannsthal follows Wilde's own suggestion, made in his essay "The Truth of Masks," in reading nature, even the nature of the poet, through the work of art. For Hofmannsthal, "Wilde's essence and his fate were one and the same. He approached a catastrophe with steps like Oedipus, the seeing-blind" (p. 89). The reference to Oedipus, the essential symbolic actor in the fantasy of the fin de siècle, the actor representing sexual perversion, incest, and divine punishment, is significant. It is this world of sexual pathology, represented not by homosexuality but by incest, which Hofmannsthal focuses on and which is reflected in Wilde's *Salome*.

The view of Wilde's life as the apogee (or nadir) of self-reflexive creation is present as early as 1896 (under the impact of the trials) in a letter from Richard Beer-Hofmann to Hofmannsthal. Beer-Hofmann praises Socrates's defense in which "death did not seem to be too high a price for the joy of having had so many beautiful talks with young and old. There is a remarkable relationship between Wilde and Socrates. Of course in Wilde everything is distorting, debased."[22] For Hofmannsthal, Wilde's life is representative of the magnificent failure of living out the desire of the avant-garde, the desire to create a series of masks through which to exist. The marginality of such a life is stressed by Erich Mühsam, who writes of the Bohemians' "brutally representative exaggeration of their difference."[23] It was the public representation of Wilde's sexual difference, the trials that Wilde initiated, which fascinated Hofmannsthal. Wilde becomes for Hofmannsthal (understood by his opponents as just another avant-garde Jew) a touchstone for understanding his own internalization of his homoerotic feelings and society's view of the perverted sexuality of both homosexual and Jew.

Karl Kraus's *Salome*

Without a doubt this image of the persecuted artist had its most elaborate presentation in a long series of essays (beginning in 1903) by Karl Kraus, published in his influential periodical *Die Fackel*.[24] In December 1903 (or roughly when Strauss began to be seriously concerned with the Salome theme), Kraus opened his discussion of Wilde with a polemic against a German book on the sexual life in Britain: "The uncomplicated German can only gaze upward jealously at the British nation, which is so far above the continent in the culture of sexual perversion and the development of sexual hypocrisy, which, as well as murder, can bring forth the genius of Oscar Wilde, and which has flagellation-bordellos and laws that can threaten the nuances of sexual activity with a ten-year jail sentence."[25] The importance of this review is not merely that Kraus (like Bernstein before him) points out the parallels between British sexual attitudes and those in contemporary Viennese society, at least in terms of the barbarity of the public executions and their popularity in England. (He represents such executions as parallel to the Wilde trials.) Kraus also introduces that term which is central in any understanding of the complex link between Wilde, Strauss, the Jews, and the avant-garde: *Perversität*. Kraus's manner of indirect citation shows here (as elsewhere in *Die Fackel*) that he is using a term from the general contemporary discourse of difference. It is the category of the "perverted," not merely the unnatural but the anti-natural, which provides the link that can help us understand the power of reading Wilde in the opening decade of the twentieth century.

At the close of that issue of *Die Fackel*, Kraus reports two items of gossip back to back: the anti-Semitic attacks abetted by the official city government (with its publicly anti-Semitic mayor, Karl Lueger) to limit the promotion of Jewish civil servants; and the permission granted to perform Wilde's *Salome* in Vienna (but only "if the head of John the Baptist, which Salome brings in, is covered with a cloth. Too dumb!" Kraus retorts.)[26] This seemingly random juxtaposition makes one aware of how closely Kraus—Jew, cripple, aesthete—links such varied categories of difference as Semitism and homosexuality, the Jews and Oscar Wilde.

In the Christmas issue of 1903, Kraus devotes the first fourteen pages to a detailed review (and review of the reviews) of this production of *Salome*.[27] It was performed in the Deutsches Volkstheater (the Viennese parallel to Reinhardt's Kleines Theater), a theater that, by inviting German guest productions, was able to produce European avant-garde plays otherwise banned in Austria by the censor. On 12 December 1903 Adele Hartwig brought her version of *Salome* from the Neues Theater in Berlin; it was a *succès de scandale*. Kraus begins his review (as was his usual practice) with an attack on a text, here Friedrich Schütz's review of the play in the *Neue freie Presse*, the paper edited by Kraus's bête noire, Moriz Benedikt. It is important to read Kraus's opening of this review in light of the rhetoric to which he is responding and in which he clothes his understanding of the play:

> "When critics disagree the artist is in accord with himself," wrote Wilde in the wonderful introduction to his *The Picture of Dorian Gray*. In the arena of his noble culture of the spirit, the argument of proletarian idea-mongers can only be heard as the Yiddish-accented German [*Gemauschel*] of the Pharisees, moderated by the excellent direction of *Salome*. I do not have the pleasure of enjoying works of art as an observer. A fatal sharpness of hearing forces me to listen to the voices that come from the depths and I cannot pray before I curse the sacrilege. Like the *Gemauschel* of the Pharisees in *Salome* [when they cry out]: "One sees, that he is not the Elias!" One cries who has forced himself gesticulating into the foremost row and whose name is Friedrich Schütz. [p. 1]

While Kraus uses this review to defend Wilde and his drama (with the parodied cry echoing the closing of the play: "Kill that critic!" ["Man erschlage diesen Kritiker"], p. 2), it is his attempt to decouple homosexuality and the Jews which makes up the greater part of his long and detailed examination of Schütz's review. He observes that "Mr. Friedrich Schütz is not a pederast" (p. 2), the unspoken theme of Schütz's review, according to Kraus's reading, being, If in a review of a work by a known homosexual such as Oscar Wilde, I, as a reviewer, do not attack homosexuality, then am I not "one of them"? Kraus's defense of Wilde is linked to his opposition to the prosecution of homosexuality and his libertarian view that sexuality has no business being under the control of the state. But the central thrust of the first paragraph has little to do with this question, and Kraus himself drops this theme after a long paragraph.

His main concern, the center of his review, is also the central theme of the opening paragraph. It is his focus on the role of the Jews, represented for Kraus (but not for Schütz) by their discourse, by the language of the "Pharisees" in the debates before Herod about the divinity of Christ and the mission of John the Baptist. For Schütz, Wilde is merely an anti-Semite, a "Briten-Goi" who attacks Jews in the basest manner. (Here, the attack on Britain as the source of all evil is redirected into an attack on the victim, Wilde, for being merely one of them, an anti-Semite.) Kraus quotes Schütz that the Jews are reduced to "'a quintet of tottering Jews represented with ugly gestures, which fulfill the deepest sense of subjugation.' The direction of the Volkstheater does even more and 'lets these Hebrews speak in a Jewish tone [*mauscheln*].' And that has to be inflicted on Mr. Schütz for whom every work of art must have but one law: 'There is no Jewish ill-breeding'" (p. 9). But even Kraus admits that the use of Gemauschel, the Jewish tone fall, on the Viennese stage was tasteless: "Indeed the jargon [*Jargon*] of the group of Pharisees should have been moderated—at least with an eye toward the audience at the premiere" (p. 9). For the use of Gemauschel points, as I have indicated in much more detail elsewhere, to the double-bind of a Jew such as Karl Kraus writing in German.[28]

Kraus, Herzl's most violent early opponent in Vienna, rejects the call for an Orientalization of the European Jews. He sees acculturation, if not assimilation, as the only possible means of overcoming the hostility to the Jews of the world in which he lives. He shares the general assimilationist point of view that the recent political opposition to the Jews, at least in Vienna, is the result of having large numbers of unacculturated Eastern Jews from the provinces of the Austro-Hungarian empire in the capital. With his focus on the Gemauschel of Wilde's Jews, Kraus points to the incompetence of a specific group of Jews—the Eastern, Yiddish-speaking Jews, the Jewish parvenues in Vienna, the object onto whom Viennese Jews projected their anxieties. These anxieties arose because of the charge, heard in the political speeches and read in the pamphlets and scholarly monographs of anti-Semites of all persuasions, that all Jews (not merely the newly arrived) did not, could not, command the discourse of high culture, the discourse of the Germans. It is, of course, in Richard Wagner's "Judaism in Music," that this view had its most often quoted representation.[29] Kraus points to his separation from those specified by this charge with his own "translation" into "Pharisees" of Wilde's designation of these argumentative figures as "Jews." For Kraus, Wilde's stage Jews are but "Pharisees," with all of that term's negative connotations in Christian-German rhetoric. They are not merely "Juden," as the German translation of the text states, for that designation, read as a racial category by a German reader, would also include Karl Kraus.

In Kraus's review of the *Salome* review, he condemns the German (read: Berlin) version as unnecessarily altering Wilde's intent in the drama, but even more so the thin-skinnedness of the critic for that daily paper (understood as "Jewish" by both anti-Semites and Jews such as Kraus) who saw in every representation of the Jews an oblique attack on them. Kraus mockingly asks Schütz to allow some "perverted" views, so that the theater can serve up peacock's tongues as well as peasant dumplings (*Bauernknödel*) (p. 12). "Perversion" becomes a positive label, the label of libertarian aesthetics, of the cultural avant-garde with which Kraus, on one level, identifies himself. He thus closes his review of the review with the acerbic observation that the clerical newspaper *Vaterland*, as well as Benedikt's *Neue freie Presse*, have both condemned the play. Both Catholics and Jews conspire to damn true art, while Kraus represents the defender of the "perverted."

Let us for a moment examine not Kraus's response, which is that of a Viennese "Jew" who is internalizing his own ambivalence about the hidden language attributed to the Jews by the anti-Semites, but rather Friedrich Schütz's original feuilleton.[30] Kraus's reading of Schütz presents a clear case of his projection onto the "Jewish" writer (Schütz as the agent of the "Jewish" newspaper, Moriz Benedikt's *New Free Press*) of his own fears about the nature of Jewish (i.e., "perverted") discourse. Schütz does indeed spend over half of his review recounting the biography of Wilde in a condemnatory manner, contrasting him with Byron and Heine. Kraus reports quite correctly Schütz's condemnation of the poet as homosexual. But his reading of Schütz's discussion of *Salome* as a text and of the visiting Berlin production has a different slant once the original review is examined. Schütz stresses the historical marginality of the court of Herod, does not glorify the history of the Jews under the Romans, and comes only in his penultimate paragraph to condemn "the direction of the Volkstheater" in having "the Hebrews *mauschel*": "if such a concept were correct then one would need to perform [those dramas such as Hebbel's] *Judith* . . . which play on the soil of Judea in Yiddish [*Jargon*]." Kraus places Schütz's condemnation at the very opening of his review since it was the quality of the production (and the language of the review) which spoke most directly to his own sense of identity. He read Schütz's review as an attack on the homosexual poet Wilde from the standpoint of the Jewish press, an attack that set the corrupt discourse of the self-conscious Jew, Schütz, against the forces of pure art, represented by Wilde's representation of the Jews. Schütz's was an attack on the avant-garde from the side of the forces of reaction—but a Jewish reaction, which Kraus labels ironically as no different from the forces of Catholic reaction.

But, of course, the perverted discourse of the Jew, no matter what the ideological identity of the individual, was inexorably linked with the polluted language of the homosexual. Thus Kraus needed to separate his discourse about the avant-garde (a discourse that was not "Jewish" but about Jews) from that of the "bad" Jews, such as Friedrich Schütz.

Kraus's view was no more an unambiguous affirmation of the label of "perverted" for the cultural avant-garde than Nietzsche's aphorism had glorified the "degenerate" as the sole image of the true artist. On 4 January 1904 Kraus followed his review of *Salome* with a further attack on Friedrich Schütz under the title "The Picture of Dorian Gray (Toward a Picture of Friedrich Schütz)," which again begins with a paraphrase of the homophobic rhetoric of the period: "In that rag, the advertising pages of which are open to the offering of every perversion and whose owners in a notorious manner financially benefit from the procuring of pederastic contacts, a certain F. Sch. has fumed about Oscar Wilde in a moral wrath."[31] While Kraus proceeds to quote from Wilde on the corruption of critics in general, as he had at the beginning of the earlier review, he began by condemning the homophobic Schütz for writing for a mere homosexual rag. The Jew, who condemns the homosexual, is not above pandering to (and for) him. The importance of this statement lies in the ambiguity of Kraus's use of the term *perversion*, applying it not only to the homosexual but also to the Jewish press. Jews, such as Moriz Benedikt, are no better than their own image of the homosexual.

The image of Oscar Wilde in the public press of the fin de siècle ties together a string of seemingly unrelated elements: a strong anti-British attitude, a sense of sexual pathology, the image of an author as identical with the image of his work, popular images of the language of deviance. All of these elements are linked through the association of accepted stereotypes of the Jews with characteristics of difference ascribed to the homosexual. And all of this was during a period of growing concern with the homosexual scandals among the nobility and the upper class in Germany and Austria, such as the Krupp scandal of 1902.[32] It was the very awareness of difference—sexual, cultural, racial—which set the stage for the most notable of these scandals, that concerning Wilhelm II and his friend Philipp Eulenberg, which broke in 1906, shortly after the premiere of Strauss's *Salome*. There the association of anti-Semitism, homosexuality, and the discourse of the Jews (in the role of Kraus's German alterego, Maximilian Harden, who brought this scandal to the surface) is illustrated. Strauss was composing during the very period in which Harden's material was appearing and forcing the discussion of homoeroticism into the political arena.

Salome and the Pervert

Having set the stage for our reading of *Salome*, we can now move to the opera itself and see how its contemporary reception was shaped by that representation of difference labeled "perversion." It is precisely this term that had ubiquitously been used to designate not only the author, Wilde, or his world, but the nature of his drama. Strauss was quite aware of the implications of selecting a text by Wilde. In 1948 he remarked upon the publication of Hesketh Pearson's biography of Wilde: "How times have changed!"[33]

The very term *perversion* itself became closely associated with the opera. During the rehearsals for the first performance in Dresden, the producer demanded of the singer who had been cast as Salome that the role be full of " 'perversion and outrage,' " a demand that she, "the wife of a Saxon Burgomaster," of course refused to obey.[34] On 10 December 1905, a review of the dress rehearsal in the *Dresdner Nachrichten* (the very first review of the opera) begins with a reading of Wilde's play: "The raw actions, the exaggeration of everything which Wilde's text demands of normal feelings by its perverted actions, the disgusting nature of the material, all of this is transfigured through the music."[35] Over and over again this theme is sounded: Strauss's great music redeems the perversion of Wilde's text. But the perversion is present. When Gustav Mahler, the head of the Viennese Court Opera, submitted Strauss's opera to Dr. Emil Jettl, the court censor, in order to have it approved for performance, Jettl's rejection mentioned an objection to the representation of biblical characters on the stage; but, even more important, he saw the drama, in the light of the opposition and critical reaction to the 1903 Viennese production of Wilde's play, as a work that represented sexual pathology: "Irrespective that the representation of actions from the New Testament raises considerations for the court theater, the presentation of the perverted sensuality, as incorporated in the figure of Salome, is morally repugnant."[36] The censor objects to the "perversion" of the subject matter, of Salome's character, and to the play, which incorporates into its reading the image of its author as "pervert."

The theme of "perversion" is ubiquitous in the contemporary reading of the opera—whether pro or contra. In the first scholarly reactions to the opera, such as Eugen Schmitz's monograph of 1907 on Strauss, there is a clear defense against the accusation that "Wilde's *Salome* is an artistic representation of perversion."[37] Oscar Bie's monograph of 1906 asks the question, "Is it possible to represent perversion?" And answers: "Childish catchwords—perversion and decadence."[38] In Strauss's correspondence with the French novelist Romain Rolland (whom he had requested to check the French version of the libretto), Rolland launched a series of attacks on Wilde and his text. Wilde's language was "literary jargon." In 1907, after the initial performance of *Salome* in Paris, Rolland wrote Strauss a long and detailed condemnation of the text as "not worthy of you. . . . It has a nauseous and sickly atmosphere about it: it exudes vice and literature. . . . Wilde's *Salome*, and all those who surround her are unwholesome, unclean, hysterical or alcoholic beings, stinking of sophisticated and perfumed corruption. I fear . . . that you have been caught by the mirage of German decadent literature. However talented these poets may be . . . the difference between them and you is the difference between an artist who is great (or famous) at *one* time (a fashion)—and one who is—who should be—great for all time. . . . You are worthy of better things than *Salome.*"[39] The resonance of Bernstein's attack on the stereotypical belief that sexual perversion results from increased sophistication and luxury is unmistakable.

This view echoes many of the contemporary notions about the homosexual found in the popular press during the so-called Eulenburg scandal, but it also reflects much of the popular (and literary) understanding of the nature of Jewish sexual pathology. The connection is made in one of the pamphlets that circulated in 1906 as a result of the premiere of Strauss's opera.[40] H. Ernstmann labels the Wilde play an example of a "medical (gynecological?)" theme in biblical clothing; a play that reveals the inner workings of the author's mind: "The play should be called *Oscar Wilde* rather than *Salome.*" While condemning Wilde's "bigoted fellow countrymen" for their persecution of the poet, he still damns Wilde's immorality and his creation of this "song of perverted love." Concerning the opera, Ernstmann claims that "if you tell me what you set to music, I'll tell you what you are," and he proceeds to link Strauss with one other figure of the avant-garde—Max Liebermann—to illustrate the relationship between the theme of the work of art and its true essence. Liebermann, the dean of German Impressionism and the most visible "Jewish" artist of the avant-garde, is attacked for having stressed (in a 1906 polemic against German regionalism) that art is form and is not dependent on subject matter. Ernstmann's linking of Strauss with the "Jewish" avant-garde labels both as diseased; only "sick artists produce sick art." The author of the play and the composer of the opera are "sick," and their disease is Jewish modernism.

The objections to the play and the total identification (as we have seen) of the play and the author provide a setting for the understanding of the term *perverted,* but it is a setting that must have a wider and more detailed context. For not only are homosexuals perverted, and their advocates, the Jews, perverted, even their characters are perverted. Perversion becomes the label that joins all forms of sexual deviance, linking heterosexuality and homosexuality. For, if Salome is perverted, her perversion certainly has nothing to do with the representation of homosexuality on stage, but rather (in a German reading of 1905) with the representation of a sexual hysteric and the source of her hysteria. The symptom, Salome's sadism—manifested by her desire to possess a fetish, the severed head of a man who has rejected her—had its origin in the trauma of her attempted seduction by her stepfather, Herod. For just as, from the very opening of the opera, Salome desires to possess the eyes, hair, and lips of Jochanaan, so too does Herod have a fetishistic wish to possess the cup from which Salome would drink or the fruit that she would eat. A simple case for the master solver of cases of hysteria, Sigmund Freud.[41] Salome suffers from memories, memories acted out for the audience in Herod's attempts to seduce her. This was certainly not Herod's first attempt, as the text documents. Is Salome then perverted because she is a victim who in turn victimizes? Is she perverted because she is presented as mentally ill, as a hysteric, where the signs, symptoms, and etiology are clearly present for the audience to see? This would clearly be but a superficial reading of the opera's libretto.

Salome is perverted because she serves as the audience's focus for a set of representations of difference, all of which are understood as perverted. They include appropriate signs and symptoms as well as the resultant psychosexual pathology. And, more basically, they reflect on Strauss's sophisticated understanding of his ideal audience and their self-representation. For there is one social group whom Strauss would have desired as his ideal audience, who were understood by fin-de-siècle medicine as being especially at risk for hysteria, with its roots in seduction and incest: the Jews.[42] Jean Martin Charcot, among many others, stressed the "especially marked predisposition of the Jewish race for hysteria."[43] It was a hysteria that had its source in Jewish sexual selectivity, which European medicine understood in terms of late nineteenth-century eugenics as "inbreeding." Jews, both male and female, are hysterics because they indulge in perverted sexuality; the signs and symptoms are clearly marked on their physiognomy. But incest was not merely the source of disease—it was also a crime. There is a complex literature that documents (or refutes) the special nature of Jewish criminal sexuality, the higher incidence of "moral crimes" among Jews.[44] Thus the sexual "perversions" of the Jews have both a medical and a legal dimension and are understood as parallel to the "perversions" of the homosexuals.

Strauss provides for his audience a set of signs and symptoms that enable them to understand the libretto as a "Jew-opera." *Salome* is more than an opera about perverted sexuality—it is a play about Jewish sexuality and criminal incest, a topic that even a contemporary critic such as Friedrich Schütz, who seemed to be attuned to reading the anti-Semitism inherent in Wilde's play as seen in Austria, could not articulate in his review of the first Viennese production of the play. Strauss accepts Schütz's interpretation of the work as a play about perverted Jews, Jews with money. It is a "Jewish" reading of the play, as Karl Kraus is at pains to point out, a reading that reflects the heightened sense of vulnerability felt by many German and Austrian Jews at the turn of the century.

Let us begin with those scenes that Friedrich Schütz understood as the most problematic in Oscar Wilde's play, the presentation of the Jews as speakers of Gemauschel, a "Jewish" discourse. In preparing the play for the stage, Strauss pares down Wilde's text, cutting it almost in half. He removes a number of the peripheral characters such as Tigellius and Salome's slaves, and he reduces the repeated appearances of the Jews to one major scene. However, they are first presented in musical form, as a leitmotif, during the opening scene of the opera. Narraboth, Herod's guard, is observing, "How beautiful is the Princess Salome tonight," when a din breaks out in the banquet hall where Herod is entertaining. One subsidiary motif in their cacophony is labeled by Strauss as "howling [*heulend*]." The Jews arrive onstage as the first soldier turns to the second and asks: "What an uproar! Who are those wild beasts howling?" And the second soldier replies: "The Jews. They are always like that. They are disputing about their religion."[45] (For Strauss, as for Wilde, these are "Jews," not Kraus's "Pharisees.") The animal nature of this music line later resurfaces as one of the motifs that characterize the Jews by pointing to the irrational nature of the Jews' discourse. Thus the Jews' language is depicted as aggressively argumentative, as barbaric, but this quality only reflects the hidden, contaminating nature of their discourse. There was already a nineteenth-century tradition of representing the Jews' discourse on the operatic stage as different. Stendhal, in his *Life of Rossini*, comments on how an acquaintance of the composer remarked to him, while Rossini was working on *Mosè in Egitto:* "Since you intend to have a Chorus of Jews, why not give them a nasal intonation, the sort of thing you hear in a synagogue?"[46] Rossini did not represent the Jews in this manner, but "composed a magnificent chorus, which in fact does open with a most curious harmonic combination strongly reminiscent of the Jewish synagogue." Stendhal evidently sees Rossini's musical quotation as the fulfillment of the suggestion of Rossini's friend, while it was, of course, something quite other, the use of musical intertextuality to create the illusion of the world of the Jews.

Strauss is less subtle in his musical representation of the Jews' discourse. For example, he consistently associates the Jews' leitmotif with one particular instrumental sonority: that of the oboe, an instrument that produces a thin, whining sound and which has a specific contemporary musical reference, as shall be discussed below. He also has the cacophony of the orchestra reach its peak when the first and second soldiers use the words "howling" and "Jews." This motif of the "howling Jews" reappears clearly and on its own to herald the entry of the Jews when they take the stage later in the opera. The quintet of Jews appears to protest Herod's refusal to turn Jochanaan over to them. The quintet consists of four very high tenors and a very low bass, introduced for comic effect. The numerous appearances of the Jews in Wilde's play, with their comic

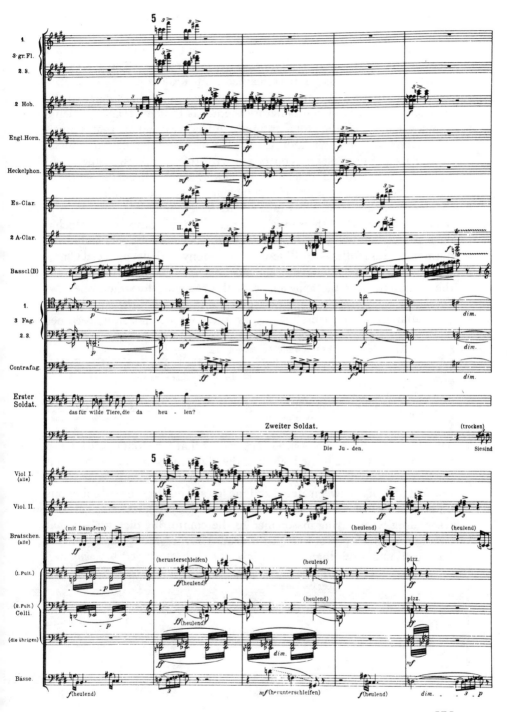

presentation as stage Jews, are now concentrated into this one intense scene. Strauss, as he notes in a letter written in 1935 to Stefan Zweig, is caricaturing the five Jews as well as Herod, but he is doing so within a German, rather than a British, mode of representation.[47] The overt topic of the Jews' debate, as we have learned from Kraus's satire of Schütz's review, is whether or not Jochanaan has seen (or perhaps even is) the Messiah. A quintet of contradictory themes is presented, and in such a manner that the result is total unintelligibility, a cacophony that is musically avant-garde but also indicative of the nature of the Jews' discourse. Their cacophony is clearly contrasted with the opera's two other principal modes of musical discourse, the shimmering, chromatic world of Salome and the firm diatonicism of Jochanaan. Unlike them, Jews argue; they don't make sense. Their music is basically out of key. This point is made incisively when their musical language is set against that of Jochanaan and his followers. Both in the opening scene of the opera and in the quintet, Strauss follows shrill Jewish cacophony with deep-voiced Christian response and diatonicism. The most extreme juxtaposition comes in the argument over the appearance of the Messiah, in which one Jew, described as "screaming," shows complete disregard for the prevailing, "Christian" tonality. Herod, to whom the Jews are appealing, becomes

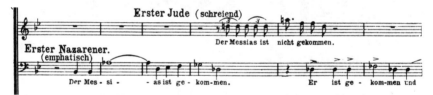

part of this debate, and it is surely significant that, like four of the Jews in the quintet, his voice is the highest of the high tenors. In fact, throughout the Jews' main scene, Strauss makes every effort to forge a sense of musical identity between Herod and the Jews. And after the cacophonous quintet has finished, it is Herod who continues the Jews' musical role, responding with jarring dissonance to the comforting diatonicism that announces Jesus's power to raise the dead. The message is clear: Herod is (musically) no more than another Jew.

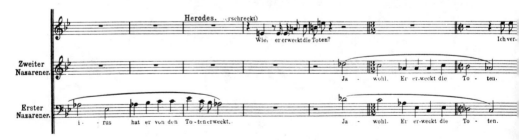

For Strauss's audience, the discourse of the Jews would have been marked not only by their argumentation, by their "howling" and "screaming," but also by the sexualized nature of their voice. Indeed, Strauss introduces a musical joke, playing on their discourse and their sexual identity, halfway through the Jews' quintet. The highest note in that quintet is on the word *beschnitten*, "circumcised." The late nineteenth-

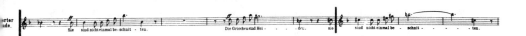

century view associated the act of religious circumcision with the act of castration, the unmanning of the Jew by making him a Jew.[48] And the high-pitched note used by Strauss pointed toward that association as well as the link between the Jews' discourse and that of the homosexual, the feminized male.

This is a theme that, like the potential of the Jews for mental illness, haunts the pseudoscientific literature written against the Jews during the nineteenth century, the literature given the "scientific" label of "anti-Semitism" during that period. By the beginning of the twentieth century the pseudoscientific literature of Jewish race hatred had become a genre in and of itself. Its most representative work was published in German in 1904 and became the topic of wide discussion as Strauss was setting Wilde's text. Otto Weininger's *Sex and Character* is a work, by a self-hating Jew, that attempts to reveal the inner, destructive nature of both Jews and women. Published posthumously after the author's suicide in 1903, *Sex and Character* was seen as a major scientific contribution to the discussion of human psychology. Weininger sought to create parallel categories of difference, showing that all Jews are merely women. Important for Weininger was discourse as a marker for difference, for Jews, like women, express their nature in their language.[49] Women flirt or chatter rather than talk. But most important for Weininger is the quality of the male Jews' song, which reveals their nature: "Just as the acuteness of Jews has nothing to do with true power of differentiating, so his shyness about singing or even about speaking in clear positive tones has nothing to do with real reserve. It is a kind of inverted pride; having no true sense of his own worth, he fears being made ridiculous by his singing or his speech."

Such a view of the nature of the Jews' discourse has its clearest representation in the language spoken by comic Jews on the stage of the fin de siècle; it is a language that is *mauscheln*, unclear, muddy. By the twentieth century, one of the signs of the Jews' language is that "he *mau-*

schelt. His voice often breaks."[50] It is this break that is signified by the musical voices in Strauss's portrait of the Jew. And thus Herod is as much a Jew as are the disputatious quintet, his discourse signifying his incestuous sexuality. Strauss's audience would have heard in the high-pitched, breaking voice of the Jews an audible sign of the Jews' difference, a sign that would have been completely understandable given the "perverted" nature of the Jews' sexuality as represented on the stage.

Strauss's setting of the discourse of the Jew is central to any reading of the opera. It is the key to the figure of incestuous father and child, the Jew as the seducer and object of seduction, the hysteric and her father surrogate. Thomas Mann made this link overt in his tale of mock-Wagnerian passion, "Wälsungenblut" (1905), in which the use of Yiddish (suppressed after the first printing of the story) by the incestuous twins marks them as merely Jews—Jews of the cultural elite, but Jews nonetheless.[51] Mann suppressed the "Yiddish" conclusion to the tale because of the violent objections of his father-in-law, the Jewish educator Alfred Pringsheim, to the racial characterization of the incestuous couple. This was a basic cultural assumption, that the upper class, especially Jews, were perverts, and their perversion took the form of a crime: incest. Incest was but the ultimate form of sexual selectivity. Popular medical knowledge of the period believed that "inbreeding" led to a weakening of the stock, to the appearance of specific illnesses, such as hysteria. This is the subtext of Freud and Breuer's *Studies in Hysteria* (1895), which accounts for why its Jewish authors suppress any mention of the religious identity of their patients in the published version of their cases, while it looms relatively important in their case notes.[52]

The link with the idea of "perversion" incorporated in the figure of Oscar Wilde, both homosexual and criminal, becomes overt once the association of the quality of voice as a signifier of difference is made. For the feminizing "break of the voice," the inability to speak in a masculine manner, is also one of the standard stigmata of degeneration borne by the homosexual for late nineteenth-century medicine and popular culture.[53] Homosexuality, by the close of the nineteenth century in the work of Krafft-Ebing, Tarnowski, Moll, and others, was generally understood as being an innate, biological error, which not only manifested itself in "perverted" acts, but was written on the very body of the homosexual through the appearance of specific, visible signs. And one of the most evident, cited in almost all case reports, is the quality of the voice. With the increased knowledge of the endocrinological system during the latter half of the nineteenth century, the biochemical link between the breaking of the voice and sexual change during puberty became known. The change of voice signaled the masculinization of the male; its absence, the breaking of the voice, the male's inability to assume any but a "perverted" sexual identity. It is, however, also accepted within the fin-de-siècle nosological system describing homosexuality that those who become homosexuals, usually through the act of seduction, have some type of inborn predisposition that may well announce itself through the stigmata of degeneration.

The tension between "nature" and "nurture," between these two models of homosexuality, also had its parallel in attitudes toward race during the same period and with much the same confused response on the part of those stereotyped. It is assumed that the stigmata are "real" signs of perversion, whether present or future, whether endogenous or exogenous. This assumption is internalized by those stereotyped and ofttimes in the most complex manner. One would imagine that the endogenous explanation for difference would have been rejected by those individuals so stigmatized. Not so. Karl Heinrich Ulrichs, the first major advocate of homosexual emancipation during the 1860s, saw the homosexual as the "third sex," as a biological category of equal validity to the male and the female; likewise, some Jews, such as the early Zionists, by the late 1890s began to accept the idea of racial difference as a means of establishing their own autonomy and separation. Such a complex reading of categories of difference is reflected in the response of highly acculturated German and Austrian Jews who were caught between an acceptance of their own difference and a need to conceptualize it in such a way as to make it bearable.

If the "degenerate," the greater category into which the nosologies of the nineteenth century placed the "pervert," was, according to Max Nordau, the "morbid deviation from an original type," the difference between the original type—the middle-class, heterosexual, Protestant male—and the outsider was a morbid one—the outsider was diseased.[54] There is a general parallel drawn between the feminization of the Jew and the homosexual in the writings of assimilated Jews, Jews who did not seek to validate their difference from the majority during the late nineteenth century but who saw themselves as potentially at risk as such a morbid deviation from the norm. Nowhere is this association illustrated with greater force than in an essay written in 1897 by the future foreign minister of the Weimar Republic, Walter Rathenau. Rathenau, who begins his essay by "confessing" to his identity as a Jew, condemns the Jews as a foreign body in the cultural as well as political world of Germany: "Whoever wishes to hear its language can go any Sunday through the Thiergartenstrasse midday at twelve or evenings glance into the foyer of a Berlin theater. Unique Vision! In the midst of a German life, a separate, strange race. . . . On the sands of the Mark Brandenburg, an Asiatic horde."[55] As part of this category of difference, Rathenau sees the physical deformities of the Jewish male—his "soft weakness of form," his femininity—as the biological result of his oppression. It is in the analogous category, that of voice, in which the biological assumptions of pathology and disease are linked. But clearly, as Max Nordau called in 1900 for all male Jews to become "muscle Jews," it is an argument based upon nurture rather than nature.[56]

The male Jews' feminization results from society's oppression even though it has specific biological signs. With the use of the cracked voice of the Jew, the opera points to the nature of the race, a feature read by acculturated Jews (who would have formed Strauss's ideal audience) as the result of a history of persecution. But these acculturated Jews would have projected these stigmata of difference onto a subgroup among the German Jews—the Eastern Jews, understood even by German Jews as quarrelsome, materialistic, and speaking with a clearly different intonation, speaking *Mauschel.*

The charge made against the Jews is that their degeneration is manifested in their perverted sexuality. Thus Herod tries to seduce his stepdaughter because he is an Oriental Jew, a Jew for the new "Orient- und Judenoper," a Jew from the East. And he is understood to be an Eastern Jew, an *Ostjude*, because he is rich and materialistic, and because his voice breaks. The two models of the East are combined in the perspective of the acculturated German-Jewish observer. Herod's stepdaughter is a hysteric, not merely because her stepfather wishes to seduce her, but because Eastern Jews are particularly at risk for such forms of mental illness. Wilde already indicates in the play that Jews are at special risk for that madness which results from incest, for Jews permit a form of marriage, parodied in Wilde's play, which fascinated the Christian by its perversion. Unmarried Jewish men were required to marry their brother's widow, a practice that as early as the seventeenth century was one of the major focuses of Christian accusations of Jewish incest.[57] It is this type of marriage which reappears in *Salome* with Jochanaan's opening solo and its charge of incest against the house of Herod, a charge substantiated more in the relationship between father and stepdaughter than in that between Herod and Herodias. The parodic element comes with the reason for Herod's "incest," his Claudius-like murder of Salome's father and his marriage to her mother.

All of the Jews in the Court are marked by the stain of incest and thus madness, as understood by the Christian viewer. They are as marked by the signs of innate, biological degeneracy as are homosexuals, whatever the cause of their deviance. Both groups reveal their criminal perversion to us not only through their sexual activities, but through their high or breaking voice.

Strauss Creates His Audience

Strauss was indeed reading Wilde against the German grain. For Strauss was subversively working against one of the basic tenets of German anti-Semitism, which saw the Jews of the Bible, especially of the New Testament, as a very different category from contemporary Jewry. As early as the German Enlightenment, there had been complicated attempts to separate the discourse of the New Testament from the language of the Jews heard in the streets of Frankfurt and Berlin. Jesus was really not a Jew, for he spoke a different language, preached in a different discourse. So wrote K. W. F. Grattenauer in 1788.[58] The British, on the other hand, accepted the continuity of contemporary Jewry with the figures of the Bible, including the New Testament.[59] This connection was understood both positively, as in the ability of Christian Hebraists to persuade Cromwell to readmit the Jews as part of a Puritan theology of biblical continuity, and negatively, as in the early twentieth-century anti-Semitic doggerel written by one of the founders of the Fabian movement, G. D. H. Cole:

> Beyond the Baghdad railway
> Thy Chosen people wait. . . .
> They stand, those hills of Judah,
> Completely clothed in Jews
> Selections of the Samuels
> And Leagues of Montagues
> Lord Rothschild ever with them. . . .
> There shines the wig of Reading
> From viceroy-ships released
> And Guggenheim and Mannheim
> And Lewis, Levys, Lowes.[60]

And from yet another perspective, Houston Stewart Chamberlain, Wagner's son-in-law, argued, in one of the most influential presentations of the science of race during the nineteenth century, that the Jews had little or nothing to do with the pure race that had inhabited the Near East during the time of Jesus.[61] The Jews of present-day Europe were a mixed race; they merely inherited the name of a people, whose true cultural ancestors are the Germans.

What sort of an audience would Richard Strauss have had in mind when he selected Oscar Wilde's play with all the rich references to disease and difference which link themselves under the term *perversion*? Why should Strauss signal to his audience that this is indeed an opera about rich, decadent Jews, their crimes and their perversions? And why should he accept a model of the Jews which would have provided a sense of continuity between the Jews of the past and the Jews of the present? How did Strauss construct his understanding of the audience when he undertook to compose *Salome*?[62]

The answer is different from what one might have imagined. In choosing to set Oscar Wilde's play, Strauss is drawing on an ambiguity in German-Jewish self-understanding during the fin de siècle. He is clearly playing on the increased popularity of Wilde's work, fostered to no little degree by Wilde's iconographic role among the German (Jewish) avant-garde as the essential outsider. But he is also echoing the clear association between the Jews, as defenders of homosexual emancipation, and the "perverted" text of *Salome*. The association between the stigmata of degeneration present in Jews and homosexuals, the sign of their criminal sexual perversion, created a category that Strauss's ideal "liberal" (read: Jewish) audience would have understood as the biological result of social prejudice. But they would also have distanced the anti-Semitic charges concerning their own perverted nature by projecting them onto a sub-group of Eastern Jews, much as Kraus read Wilde's representation of the "Jews" as a discussion of the "Pharisees," a distanced subset of that all-encompassing category. The need for the continuity of images from the New Testament to the present day underlies the presumed Jewish under-standing of the stigmata of degeneration as the result of centuries of anti-Jewish attitudes and actions upon Eastern Jews. For the conflation of "Oriental" and "Eastern" was one that acculturated Western Jews of the fin de siècle easily made. It was not the liberal Jews who were portrayed onstage; it was those ancestors of the loud, aggressive, materialistic, incestuous, mad Jews whom the Viennese and Berlin Jews saw every day on streets and in shops; it was the Jews from the East, the embodiment of the anti-Semitic caricatures that haunted the dreams of the assimilated Jews. It was the "Pharisees," those already condemned by Christianity as the "bad" Jews of the New Testament, who now walked the streets of Vienna dressed in their long, black kaftans, gesticulating and arguing.

Strauss believed himself to be appealing to such a German-Jewish au-dience of the avant-garde. It is his fantasy that shapes the text. Strauss was attempting to create an image for himself as the new composer of opera for this idealized "Jewish" avant-garde. He simply accepts the self-hating model of Jewish identity, with its pathological image of the East-ern Jew, and presents a text that fulfills all of the necessary categories for acceptance by this idealized, self-hating audience—a "perverted" text that can also be read as an attack on the nouveau riche, conservative, materialistic, and disputatious (Eastern) Jews of his time. He knew he could not be the new Wagner. This was evident to him in the reception of both his *Parsifal* (*Guntram*) and his *Meistersinger* (*Feuersnot*).[63] But he could become the creator of the new opera for the avant-garde. The Wag-nerians by 1905 had clearly placed themselves in alliance with the politi-cal as well as the cultural anti-Semites, following Wagner's own anti-Semitic views. The uneasy alliance between Jewish advocates of Wagner (such as the conductor Hermann Levi) and the non-Jewish Wagnerians had collapsed by the turn of the century and the house organ of the Wagner Society, the *Bayreuther Blätter,* had become one of the major intellectual mouthpieces of cultural anti-Semitism.[64] This is not to say that Jews as part of the general public, desiring to share in the German cultural patrimony that defined for all Germans their membership in the middle class, did not remain solidly in the Wagner camp. But it was the musical avant-garde, rather than the world of conservative music, that was perceived as Jewish. And it was to this avant-garde that Strauss believed himself to be appealing.

Mahler as Strauss's Ideal Reader

Strauss read his audience extraordinarily well: with the creation of *Salome,* he became the opera composer of the avant-garde. How he appealed to the ambiguity of the acculturated Jews whom he saw as the source of his potential popularity can be seen in his relationship with Gustav Mahler. For German anti-Semites Mahler was one of the essential "Jewish" composers, even though he was baptized in 1897. Even Strauss, recording Mahler's death in his diary on 18 May 1911, refers to him as "der Jude Mahler."[65] And Mahler, the Jewish composer of the avant-garde, as head of the Vienna Imperial Opera, was one of Strauss's (and *Salome*'s) strongest supporters—he attempted unsuccessfully to have the opera produced in his house. The correspondence between Mahler and Strauss shows Mahler's unalloyed enthusiasm for the opera and Strauss's energetic desire to have it produced in Vienna. Mahler clearly thinks of the opera as the major work produced by Strauss up to that time. In his exchange of letters with Strauss he is full of praise for the opera and its libretto.

But if we look at Mahler's personal correspondence other concerns appear. In 1894, prior to his baptism, Mahler writes a long letter to his sister Justine in which he mocks Strauss as the new cultural "pope," the new Wagner, and understands that "his [Mahler's] being Jewish is closing all of the doors" to his advancement.[66] This sense that Mahler was less successful than Strauss because of the prejudice of the society against him as a Jew echoes in Mahler's behavior after his baptism. He would often ask his wife to "stop him when he emphasized his speech with too much gesticulation," a clear sign of his Jewishness.[67] This was clearly a response to his having been labeled the arch-Jewish composer, a composer of "Oriental" music. The arch-conservative music critic Rudolf Louis, in 1909, coupled this charge with a related one:

> If Mahler's music would speak Yiddish, it would be perhaps unintelligible to me. But it is repulsive to me because it *speaks with a Jewish*

accent [jüdelt]. This is to say that it speaks musical German, but with an accent, with an inflection, and above all, with the gestures of an Eastern, all too Eastern, Jew. So, even to those whom it does not offend directly, it cannot possibly communicate anything. One does not have to be repelled by Mahler's artistic personality in order to realize the complete emptiness and vacuity of an art in which the spasm of an impotent mock-Titanism reduces itself to a frank gratification of common seamstress-like sentimentality [*an gemeiner Nähmädel-Sentimentalität*].[68]

Mahler is not only merely a Jew, but his work is Jewish and it is feminine. It appears to be be male and Titanic but is merely the impotent product for (and of) a seamstress's sentimentality. For the fin-de-siècle writer such as Weininger, Jews and women, especially women of the lower class (such as seamstresses), have no aesthetic sensibility. Strauss was quite aware of this ambiguity and played upon it in his setting of *Salome.* Is it merely accident that one of the clearest markers of this "Oriental" music was Mahler's use of the solo oboe, exactly the instrument that for Strauss became the orchestral voice of the Jews? Mahler's nostalgic and sentimental use of that instrumental sonority (understood by his contemporaries as a "typically Jewish" musical tone) is parodied in the harsh and mocking quality of the "Jewish" music in *Salome.*

But there is an even more telling moment in Mahler's internalization of this image of the Jew's hidden, perverse discourse. To his wife Mahler once characterized a journalist in Paris as being so "perverted" that "Strauss might one day set him to music."[69] Mahler had internalized the negative associations between Jews and homosexuals present in *Salome,* a work that overshadowed the first performance of Mahler's Sixth Symphony, produced in the same year. He understood that he remained merely a Jew, with his own "perverted" discourse, while Strauss could capture the essence of this discourse and thus the leadership of the cultural avant-garde through his setting of *Salome.* This was not merely the reading of the difference between the "insider" and the "outsider" by one acculturated (indeed assimilated) Jew. At least one "Jewish" observer saw in the two composers the "eternal conflict between the successful-blond [Strauss] and the fateful-dark [Mahler]."[70] This dichotomy, delineated by one of the coaches at the Viennese Court Opera, Thomas Mann's Jewish brother-in-law, Klaus Pringsheim, points to the internalization (and projection) of Mahler's sense of difference, a sense that heightened his need to see Strauss's *Salome* performed in *his* house to show that he was not merely one of those loud, gesticulating Eastern Jews. Rather, he was part of the world of the avant-garde, distanced from the world of the characters, of their perversion, of their contaminated discourse. In Mahler's case, Strauss's opera magnificently served its function as a litmus test for an assimilated Jewish identity.

Strauss succeeded beyond his greatest expectations. *Salome* became the touchstone of German avant-garde opera. According to his own contemporary testimony, he became the "leader of the Moderns," "the head of the Avant-garde." At the same time, however, he felt the need to retrench, to declare that he really was opposed to modernity, was a "reactionary"; he even denied that the avant-garde existed.[71] True, in this rejection of the avant-garde (read: of his presumed Jewish audience) he still criticized those who would limit opera to Wagner's "Teutonic legends" and who demanded that "biblical topics be taboo." But his retrenchment, and the basic reason for it, is clear. Strauss, the arch-manipulator of audiences, had been overtaken by events: he had become, against his will, a "Jewish" composer, a "pervert." The financial and artistic breakthrough of *Salome* was achieved with a double-edged sword. Strauss had conquered the avant-garde; but in doing so he had engendered a "perverted" creation from which—protest as he might—he could not distance himself.[72]

Constructing the Image of the Appropriate Therapist: The Struggle of Psychiatry with Psychoanalysis

Historical Background

What if Wittgenstein and Popper were right after all? What if psychoanalysis is not "scientific," not by any contemporary definition—including Adolf Grünbaum's—but what if it works all the same?[1] And what if, against all of the views of Habermas, it is not merely a question of hermeneutics? Indeed, what if "science" is defined ideologically rather than philosophically? If we so redefine "science," it is not to dismiss psychoanalysis but to understand its origin and impact, to follow the ideological dialectic between the history of psychiatry, its developing as a medical "science," and the evolving self-definition of psychoanalysis which parallels this history.

We know that Freud divided psychoanalysis into three quite discrete areas: first, a theory, a "scientific structure"; second, a method of inquiry, a means of exploring and ordering information; and last, but certainly not least, a mode of treatment. Let us, for the moment, follow the actual course of history, at least the course of a history that can be described by sorting out the interrelation of psychoanalysis and psychiatry, and assume that we can heuristically view the mode of treatment as relatively independent of the other two aspects of psychoanalysis. What if the very claims for a "scientific" basis for psychoanalytic treatment and by extension the role of the psychoanalyst as promulgated by Freud and his early followers were rooted in an ideologically charged historical interpretation of the positivistic nature of science and the definition of the social role of the scientist? This may seem an odd premise to begin a discussion of the mutual influence of psychoanalysis and psychiatry, but it is no stranger than the actual historical practice.

Psychoanalysis originated not in the psychiatric clinic but in the laboratories of neurology in Vienna and Paris.[2] That origin points to a major difference between the traditional practice of nineteenth-century psychiatry and modern clinical psychiatry in our post-positivistic age. Psychiatry in nineteenth-century Europe, in Vienna as well as in Paris, was an adjunct to the world of the asylum. Indeed, the second great battle (after Pinel's restructuring of the asylum) that nineteenth-century psychiatry waged was the creation of the "alienist" as a new medical speciality. The alienist was the medical doctor in administrative charge of the asylum rather than in service as a medical adjunct to the lay asylum director as had earlier, in the age of "moral treatment," been the practice.

The medicalization of psychiatry, by the closing decades of the nineteenth century, was successful. Its success, however, was due to political factors.[3] In Britain, a series of parliamentary commissions began, in the first decade of the century, to examine the abuses of the asylum, abuses that seemed to provide a rationale for its medicalization. "Reform" was simply not enough. For "madness" came to be seen as "mental illness" in what was understood as a natural extension of the general model of somatic pathology. This view was not based on the actual benefit that medicine had to offer the mentally ill; rather, it was an attempt to place the asylum within the growing sphere of medicine as science. Moral treatment, coming as it did out of a religious (the Tukes and the British Quaker) tradition or a more radical, revolutionary tradition (Pinel and the "freeing" of the insane), was seen as scientifically "old-fashioned" and/or politically "dangerous." This development of the asylum out of the early nineteenth-century "reformed" British asylums with their lay directors relied on a new scientistic definition of the nature of psychiatry. But it also continued the separation of psychiatry as a mode of treatment undertaken in asylums rather than in general hospitals. Thus the new science of psychiatry had been imbued with the status of science, but it was placed in its own ghetto, the asylum, which still isolated it from all of the other medical specialities being practiced in the general hospital.

Psychiatry was rather a unique case in other ways, too. For in accepting the power of the state to control directly the actions of a group labeled as "different" and "diseased," psychiatrists straddled the worlds of politics and science, much like the police doctors, whose area of control, public health, was the inspection of prostitutes. While they laid claim to the status of the world of science through the introduction of the medical model of madness, they were still perceived in their older, nonscientific function as the administrators of institutions of control. This function lowered the prestige of the alienists. It was the search for a higher status within medicine, and thus within the academy, which drove the psychiatrist to lay claim to the status implicit in the world of the anatomically based areas of medicine. But it was also the relatively lower status of psychiatry which enabled individuals viewed as marginal, such as Jews, to enter this new medical speciality.

The German and Austrian situation (if one can generalize over a wide range of experiences and a large number of national variations) was likewise the result of a gradual professionalization of medicine and an extension of this medicalization into those areas of health care delivery, from the running of lying-in hospitals to the direction of the asylums, which were not traditionally seen as part of "medicine."[4] This extension made itself especially evident in the creation in the mid-nineteenth century of the huge centralized state asylum at Bielefeld with its professional staff. But the central focus of all of these movements is the medicalization of the office of asylum director and the concomitant rise in the status of this role. Psychiatry in Germany and Austria was as much the administration of the asylum as the treatment of the insane. Neurology, on the other hand, was often seen as a "pure" medical science, using the positivistic model of late nineteenth-century science, and was seen as quite independent of any "applied" function (at least to the degree that psychiatry had claimed for itself in assuming control over the asylums).

After the mid-nineteenth century, however, neurology and psychiatry shared a set of scientific presumptions that were heavily laced with nineteenth-century racist ideology. Their basis was, indeed, first articulated in the academic forum by Kant in his essay of 1764 on the nature of illness of the head.[5] There he mocks the view that mental illness could have its roots in the emotions, seeing mental illness as inherently somatic. What Kant undertook was to apply to the area of mental illness the rising status of the new French biology and its attempt to explain all aspects of human nature (such as racial difference) through the biological model. It was an attempt to move the understanding of mental illness out of what Kant perceived to be the moralizing tendency of religion, which had labeled madness the result of sinfulness. Madness was a disease and, like all diseases in the age of Jenner, was understood to be somatic. (It was not the wrath of God which caused illness, but the failure of the corporeal machine.) But it is vital to understand that inherent in views such as those espoused by Kant are the racist premises of eighteenth-century French biology and anthropology: the great chain of being, with its implicit hierarchy of the various races, as well as the polygenetic origin of the races.[6] Kant, in his own anthropology, commented that the Jews are a unique group in the West, marked by their own sign—for him the corruption of their discourse—which sets them apart from all other groups.[7]

Kant's view was clearly in the avant-garde of the eighteenth century. But the general view after the mid-nineteenth century was, following Wilhelm Griesinger's standard textbook of 1845, that "mind illness was brain illness," and much attention was given to the description and localization of neurological pathologies.[8] Between Kant and Griesinger, however, lay an epoch that stressed the independent existence of mental illness, rooted in the mechanics of the emotions and their repression. J. G. Langermann in his 1797 dissertation on mental illness cast these views into their most representative form.[9] Langermann presented a theory of the origin of mental illness which not only dismissed the origin of psychopathologies as anomalies of the brain but also stressed the origin of psychopathology in the "spirit." He separated the mind and the body completely. But even more important, Langermann presented a case study of a "psychological" cure. Langermann was not alone. Later "romantic" psychiatrists such as Ideler, Heinroth, Carus, Kieser, and the widely translated Belgian asylum director Guislain stressed the centrality of psychological mechanisms in the manifestation of mental illness.

Such a view was dynamic in that it denied the primacy of human biology in shaping the human psyche and assumed a certain flexibility of human emotions. It was also implicitly racist. Indeed, the most widely read popularization of this view, Christian Heinrich Spiess's *Biographies of the Mentally Ill* (1795–96) had as one of its centerpieces the tale of the "beautiful Jewess" Esther L— and her collapse into madness.[10] Spiess's views are typical of the strain of seeing mental illness as the result of psychological rather than physical disease. Spiess uses Esther L— as his exemplary case of "love madness," erotomania, stressing above all the sexual nature of the Jew and the relation of this psychological weakness to psychopathology. Thus in the formation of both biological and romantic psychopathology, contemporaneous attitudes toward race played a major role.

The domination of the biological model over the psychological was in point of fact the presumptive success of the "scientific" over the "religious," or at least that is how the nineteenth century perceived it. The position taken by late nineteenth-century clinical psychiatry was not merely in line with the sense of the status of medicine as it existed after mid-century but also in opposition to what Emil Kraepelin as late as 1918 felt compelled to dismiss as such "natural-philosophical speculation." Kraepelin's views, however, were aimed not at the "romantic" psychiatrists of the early nineteenth century but at the resurrection of their position in the works of Sigmund Freud.[11]

The Nature of Medical Science in Freud's Vienna and Freud's Early Understanding of the Medical Practice

Sigmund Freud's early work in the laboratories of Theodor Meynert centered about the neurological description of primitive vertebrates, with the hope that such analysis would lead to an understanding of the mechanisms and structures that are also present in human neurological development. His work was aimed at a purely mechanistic description of the nature of human psychology. When he came into contact with Jean Martin Charcot in Paris, Freud maintained his attitude toward the nature and value of such a scientific undertaking, an undertaking that was "pure" science. For Meynert and Charcot shared the patriarchal status of the new scientific medicine, following Claude Bernard's lead. Or so the legend created by Freud is supposed to be read.[12] As I have shown elsewhere, the tradition of French, as well as German, anthropological psychiatry labeled Jews at high risk for specific forms of mental illness.[13] But neurology, the origin of modern psychoanalytic thought, was itself not free from such perversions. And it was in Freud's relationship with one individual—the Berlin ear, nose, and throat specialist Wilhelm Fliess—that the racist overtones of "scientific" medicine were articulated and distanced.

In Freud's correspondence with Wilhelm Fliess, the nature of the scientific undertaking of psychiatry and neurology and the definition of the medical practitioner were drawn into question.[14] Traditionally Fliess is represented as a marginal figure in the history of medicine. He is seen as the mute sounding board for Freud's views. Everyone (up to but not including Peter Swales, who is now writing Fliess's biography) has wondered how Freud, as bright and insightful as he evidently was, could have gotten himself associated with this Berlin quack. It has been accepted that Fliess was a quack—he put forth absolutely mad views such as the intimate relation between the nasal passages and the genitalia and the idea that male as well as female physiology reflected rigid periodic cycles. Quackery, however, implies a misappropriation of the status of scientific medicine, and it is the implication of this misappropriation which can help us understand Freud's gradual redefinition of the science of medicine.

Fliess actually acted on his theories, undertaking surgical procedures on the nose to relieve sexual problems. His surgical ineptitude almost killed Freud's patient Emma Eckstein. He left a wad of surgical dressing in the nasal cavity which caused massive bleeding and infection. Since Fliess operated on Freud's nose (and thus potentially placed his life at risk) during the same stay in Vienna in which he undertook the Eckstein operation, his action, as Max Schur stated when he first revealed this material, must have negatively influenced Freud's understanding of the implications of science, both in the ineptitude it revealed and in the fact that Freud had earlier placed Fliess on an intellectual plane that clearly paralleled the level Freud himself wished to attain.[15] Fliess's assumed role as a "surgeon," the highest of the medical specialities, was only disguised by his label as a "nose" doctor. His actions were those of medical practitioners whose status was clearly higher than that permitted him by the society in which he lived. This denial was based on Fliess's racial identity.

And it is no accident that all of Fliess's patients, Freud included, were Jewish. The isolation felt by the Jewish health care practitioner formed both Freud and Fliess. Both saw in the social status of medicine a chance to establish themselves in a society that rejected Jews but acclaimed academic physicians. Freud and Fliess both sought out specialities that were open to Jews. But they conceptually restructured these areas to reflect the higher sense of status of other medical specialities.[16] Sexual questions were dealt with by the psychiatrist in the role of forensic specialist on deviant behavior as well as by the syphilologist, who, as a dermatologist, occupied the lowest rung in Viennese medicine. Indeed, when Ferdinand Hebra assumed the chair in dermatology (a field nicknamed *Judenhaut*, "Jewskin") in Vienna, he was able to recruit only Jewish assistants! And psychiatry, with its transitional status between administration and practice, had an equivalently heavy and early Jewish representation. Thus Freud and Fliess sought out two areas, psychopathology and sexuality, where Jews were permitted to function on the level of academician. Their meetings, which they dubbed "congresses," were mock academic events. And their desire was to move the study of psycho- and sexual pathologies into a new area—that of neurology.

Freud and Fliess both needed the status of the higher academic specialities. Both sought this status in the area of neurology through which they attempted to ask traditional (in Viennese medicine) "Jewish" questions about sexuality and psychopathology. For Wilhelm Fliess, it was the movement from a concentration of the ear, nose, and throat to the interconnection of all human experience through the nervous system. Now, Fliess was clearly marginal to the Berlin medical community, as was Freud to that of Vienna, but being "marginal" means relating in a direct manner to the center. Both Freud and Fliess oriented themselves to the center of German medicine; both sought after (and Freud obtained) the status of the medical academic. Both functioned in relation to a discourse, that of medicine, that was critical of marginality—and which defined marginality in racial terms.

Fliess's theories, based on the best of late nineteenth-century endocrinological and neurological theory, appear to us as more than slightly mad.[17] But they fulfilled a function for him, as well as for Freud, in creating a sense of the new pathway that medicine, stripped of its overt racist overtones, could take. Let us look at two of Fliess's "mad" ideas—the relation between the nose and the genitalia and his "proof" of male periodicity—in the light of the science of medicine, with all its racist overtones in late nineteenth-century Germany and Austria. It is precisely the implications of even the higher medical specialities, such as neurology, which colored Freud's and Fliess's sense of the status of medicine and the medical practitioner.

The idea that the nasal cavities were anatomically parallel to the genitalia grew out of the study of human embryology during the nineteenth century. As early as G. Valentin's 1835 handbook of human development, the parallels in the development of soft-tissue areas and cavities of the fetus had been noted.[18] By the time of the publication of the standard atlas of human embryological development by Wilhelm His in 1885, the assumption of such parallels was at the center of European embryology.[19] But the history of embryology, and His's very creation of "standard developmental stages," is rooted in the ideology of recapitulation. Nineteenth-century biologists believed that they could see in the development of the human fetus the "highest" form of life, the repetition of all of the evolutionary stages. Central to this biological reworking of the "great chain of being" was the innate superiority of the human as the end of the teleological development of evolution. Biology placed humanity at the epitome of this development and saw in Ernst Haeckel's commonplace that "ontogeny recapitulates phylogeny" the statement of human superiority.[20] But in late nineteenth-century Germany some humans are better than other humans. And it is the implied sense of the hierarchy which is present in German embryology.

Hierarchy in late nineteenth-century German and Austrian science implied the hidden analogy to the science of race—and the key group for this hierarchy was the Jews. Christianity saw in the Jews a stage through which modern humans had progressed. Hegel labeled the Jews as an atavistic structure in Western history. For, once having played a role in history, like other ancient peoples, they should have vanished. Their presence in the society of the West was a sign of how much further modern humans had come. If indeed "ontogeny recapitulates phylogeny," then the Jew was at a lower rung on the "great chain of being." This view was so powerful that it was shared even by Ferdinand Ratzel, the originator of modern geographical anthropology, when he looked at the Jews of Western Europe.[21]

But embryology also proved that the formation of the nasal passages and the incipient genitalia happened very early in the development of the fetus. Fliess, by making this association overt, showed that the "head," as the source of the rational, and the "genitalia," as the source of the irrational, were related on an atavistic level and that the manipulation of one could affect the other. The presumption of a primitive relation between sexuality and the nose is not only bad embryology but bad medicine.

It points, however, to a necessary preoccupation of two Jewish scientists of fin-de-siècle Europe by the significance of this relation between the "nose" and the "genitalia." For Fliess and Freud it served as a sign of universal development rather than as a specific sign of an "inferior" racial identity. The association between the Jewish nose and the circumcised penis was made in the crudest and most revolting manner during the 1880s. In the streets of Berlin and Vienna, in penny-papers or on the newly installed "Litfassäulen," or advertising columns, caricatures of Jews could be seen.[22] These extraordinary caricatures stressed one central aspect of the physiognomy of the Jewish male, his nose, which represented that hidden sign of his sexual difference, his circumcised penis. For the Jews' sign of sexual difference, their sexual selectiveness, as an indicator of their identity was, as Friedrich Nietzsche strikingly observed in *Beyond Good and Evil*, the focus of the Germans' fear of the superficiality of their recently created national identity.[23] This fear was represented in caricatures by the elongated nose. (The traditional folkloric association between the size of the nose and that of the male genitalia was made a pathological sign.[24]) When Fliess attempted to alter the pathology of the genitalia by operating on the nose (in this age before plastic surgery), he was drawing on an accepted sense of the implication of human development joined to the association of the nose and the genitalia in the German biology of race.

This association of the nose and the genitalia did not exist merely in the popular mind. The central sign of male periodicity for Fliess (and for Freud) is male menstruation. And its representation, according to Freud in his 20 July 1897 letter to Fliess, is an "occasional bloody nasal secretion."[25] Later, in his letter of 15 October 1897, Freud traces the implications of male menstruation for himself as well as (one assumes) for Fliess:

My self-analysis is in fact the most essential thing I have at present and promises to become of the greatest value to me if it reaches its end. In the middle of it, it suddenly ceased for three days, during which I had the feeling of being tied up inside (which patients complain of so much), and I was really disconsolate until I found that these same three days (twenty-eight days ago) were the bearers of identical somatic phenomena. Actually only two bad days with a remission in between. From this one should draw the conclusion that the female period is not conducive to work. Punctually on the fourth day, it started again. Naturally, the pause also had another determinant—the resistance to something surprisingly new. Since then I have been once again intensely preoccupied [with it], mentally fresh, though afflicted with all sorts of minor disturbances that come from the content of the analysis.[26]

The editor of the new edition of the letters, Jeffrey Masson, comments on Fliess's observations on male menstruation that it is "highly unlikely that these communications to Freud played any role in Freud's research at the time."[27] Quite to the contrary: had Masson researched a bit into the history of the concept of male menstruation he would have found a lively nineteenth-century medical literature on this topic, by such writers as F. A. Forel and W. D. Halliburton, as well as a fascination with this question in regard to the problem of hermaphroditism as a sign of bisexuality, a fascination that was as prominent in the nineteenth century as it had been in the Middle Ages.[28] With the rise of modern sexology at the close of the nineteenth century, especially in the writings of Magnus Hirschfeld, male menstruation came to hold a very special place in the "proofs" for the continuum between male and female sexuality.[29] The hermaphrodite, the male who menstruated, became one of the central focuses of Hirschfeld's work. But all of this new "science" that used the existence of male menstruation still drew on the image of the marginality of those males who menstruated and thus pointed toward a much more ancient tradition.

The idea of male menstruation is part of a Christian tradition of seeing the Jew as inherently, biologically different. Thomas de Cantimpré, the thirteenth-century anatomist, presented the first "scientific" statement of this phenomenon (calling upon St. Augustine as his authority).[30] Male Jews menstruated as a mark of the "Father's curse," their pathological difference. This image of the Jewish male as female was introduced to link the Jew with the corrupt nature of woman (both marked as different by the same sign) and to stress the intransigence of the Jews. Thomas de Cantimpré recounts the nature of the Jews' attempt to cure themselves. They are told by one of their prophets that they would be rid of this curse by "Christiano sanguine," the blood of a Christian, when in fact it was "Christi sanguine," the blood of Christ in the sacrament, which was required. Thus the libel of the blood guilt, the charge that Jews sacrifice Christian children to obtain their blood, is the result of the intransigence of the Jews in their rejection of the truth of Christianity and is intimately tied to the sign of Jewish male menstruation. The persistence of menstruation among Jewish males is a sign not only of the initial "curse of the Father" but of the inherent inability of the Jews to hear the truth of the Son. For the intrinsic "deafness" of the Jews does not let them hear the truth that will cure them.

The belief in Jewish male menstruation continued through the seventeenth century. Heinrich Kormann repeated it in Germany in 1614 as did Thomas Calvert in England in 1649.[31] And Franco da Piacenza, a Jewish convert to Christianity, reiterated this view in his catalogue of "Jewish maladies," published in 1630 and translated into German by 1634.[32] He claimed that the males of the tribe of Simeon menstruated four days a year! These charges continued throughout the age of Enlightenment in slightly altered form. In F. L. de la Fontaine's survey of the health of the Polish Jews, published in 1792, their sexual pathology is stressed.[33] Jews show their inherent difference through their damaged sexuality, and the sign of that is, in the popular mind, the fact that their males menstruate. Jewish sexuality remained labeled as different even in the fin de siècle. Freud's contemporary, the arch-racist Theodor Fritsch—whose *Antisemite's Catechism*, published in 1887, was the encyclopedia of German anti-Semitism—still saw the sexuality of the Jew as inherently different from that of the German: "The Jew has a different sexuality from that of the Teuton; the Teuton will not and cannot understand it. And if the Teuton attempts to understand it, then the destruction of the German soul can result."[34] The hidden sign, unmentioned by Fritsch, the link between the woman and the Jew is the menstruation of the Jewish male.[35]

Freud and Fliess attempt to change this sign from one of difference to one of universality. Just as Franco da Piacenza tried to remove himself from the "curse of Eve" by claiming that only ancient Jews (and those of one of the "Lost Ten Tribes" at that) menstruated—not of course himself and his contemporaries—so, too, do Freud and Fliess distance this charge from the Jews. The public sign of Jewish identity (from the standpoint of the anti-Semitic society in which they live) is the nose that "menstruates." But its significance for Freud and Fliess, who are desperately trying to escape classification as "Jews" in the racial sense, is as a sign of the universal law of male periodicity which links all human beings, males and females. Thus Freud and Fliess wrought a successful form of resistance to the racist substructure of European medicine. Fliess is not simply a quack; his "quackery" is accepted by Freud since it provides an alternative to the pathological image of the Jew in conventional medicine.

The basic nature of the medical sciences during the late nineteenth century was racist, whether the speciality was a "Jewish one," such as syphilology, or a "non-Jewish" one, such as surgery. Freud's attempt to distance the racism of medicine through his identification with Fliess's neurological theories was an attempt to use the status of science to overcome the stigma of race. Freud could not, neither did he wish to, abandon the status he needed in order to define himself as a full member of his own community. But using the model of medicine and accepting the role of the medical practitioner, whether in psychiatry or neurology, meant that he had to deal with the profession's racist attitudes toward the Jews.[36]

The Changing Concept of the Practitioner

Sigmund Freud was forced to choose from among a series of poisoned alternatives: psychiatry (like dermatology/syphilology) had implicit police functions and a relatively low status; neurology, like psychiatry, was damaged by racist implications. But, of course, psychiatry and sexology (in the guise of syphilology) were medical specialities open to Jews, as was neurology, but only with great difficulty and as long as they remained on the level of laboratory science rather than clinical practice. In the early history of psychoanalysis the desire of the psychoanalyst for the higher status of specific medical specialities competes with the innate understanding that medicine condemns (in labeling as pathological) those groups it perceives as marginal. Thus medicine is initially poisoned for the Jewish physician, whose marginality is linked to racial identity and is thus labeled as part of a group at risk. Jews can be patients, but can they be doctors? In the pre–World War I period, however, medicine is also poisoned for the psychoanalyst who incorporates that sense of marginality stemming from the Jewish identity of the early psychoanalysts as part of his or her self-definition as a mental health professional.

Freud's desire to recruit non-Jewish psychoanalysts, such as Carl G. Jung and Lou Andreas-Salomé, was based in his need to overcome the sense of marginality implicit in the parallel positions of the Jew and the psychoanalyst in the intellectual world of fin-de-siècle Viennese medicine.[37] The psychoanalyst, however, whether Jew or non-Jew, was to the medical profession as the Jew was to society at large—a frightening outsider. Freud's "myths" (to use Frank Sulloway's highly suspect term) about isolation and anti-Semitism had a real basis in the perception of reality shared by nineteenth-century Jewish medical practitioners. This was then transfered to the new "Jews" in Viennese medical circles, the psychoanalysts. In Freud's history of the psychoanalytic movement, there is a tendency to perceive the opposition to the equal access of Jews (and therefore psychoanalysts) in medicine as absolute. It is this sense of the monolithic nature of the medical profession (whether true in detail or not) which shaped Freud's relationship to medicine and medicine's perception of psychoanalysis.

What Freud came to understand by the 1920s was that the status given to him as a medical doctor was not sufficient to counter the hesitancy and animosity directed at him as an outsider—both as a Jew (with the increase of public anti-Semitism in Vienna and Freud's own increased visibility) and as a psychoanalyst. During World War I he began to shuck the various conceptual categories, beginning with those of anthropology, which had given psychiatry its status in the nineteenth century.[38] This was not a difficult thing to do, for by this period the presence of anthropology in psychiatry was viewed as slightly old-fashioned as well as decidedly "French"—two categories that, in fin-de-siècle Vienna, with its stress on the modern and the Teutonic, were quite easily dismissed. He assigned to the anthropologist a negative role as the creator of the idea of degeneration (in which, of course, he was right—Morel had introduced this concept into psychiatry as a means of labeling entire groups perceived as marginal, among which were the Jews).

Freud also began to doubt that the status that medicine had grudgingly granted to psychoanalysis was a positive factor, especially since he saw in psychiatry much of the state control that he feared elsewhere. Psychoanalysis was to be its own master. In 1926, in a court case for quackery brought against Theodor Reik, one of Freud's most orthodox supporters, the question of the relation of psychoanalysis to the status of medicine was raised for the first time within the structures of power which Freud had always associated with medicine. Reik, whose Ph.D. was in German and French literature, had been accused by the American counsel, Hurley, in Vienna of having treated an American by the name of Morti without a medical license. Freud had referred this patient to Reik. When the patient's mental status began to worsen, an American doctor in Vienna by the name of Gross asked the noted Viennese psychiatrist Herschmann to examine Morti. At that point it became clear that Reik had had the patient under treatment, and the American counsel brought charges of quackery and fraud against Reik. The Viennese medical establishment, represented by such figures as Julius Werner-Jauregg, came out strongly against the idea of lay analysis. Freud, and a number of his supporters in the Viennese Psychoanalytic Society, undertook Reik's defense with the argument that it was not necessary to be a medical practitioner in order to be a psychoanalyst.

Although the charges against Reik were eventually dropped for lack of evidence, Freud used that occasion, in a memoir written for Julius Tandler, the city's health minister, in support of the defendant, to examine the relation between the expanding status of psychoanalysis and the more evident racism of medicine. He states his position quite directly: "Doctors have no historical claim to the sole position of analysis."[39] He continues by defining (or actually redefining) what a quack is by dismissing the need for state control ("possessing a state diploma to prove he is a doctor") and stressing the "knowledge and capacities necessary" to undertake treatment. The shadow of Fliess stretches over this view of the primacy of "knowledge" over certification. "Knowledge" is, however, not to be understood as the knowledge of the "science" of medicine. For it is precisely this type of "knowledge" which Freud dismisses, rejecting the "doctor" as the ideal practitioner, just as he had rejected the anthropologist:

His [the doctor's] interest is not aroused in the mental side of vital phenomena; medicine is not concerned with the study of the higher intellectual functions, which lies in the sphere of another faculty. Only psychiatry is supposed to deal with the disturbances of mental functions; but we know in what manner and with what aims it does so. It looks for the somatic determinants of mental disorders and treats them like other causes of illness.[40]

Psychiatry is but medicine; medicine is but biological science; and (we can add) biological science is racist. But Freud could not cavalierly abandon the status of science which he had so painstakingly acquired. He continued his argument with the (in recent years) oft-quoted passage: "In view of the intimate connection between the things that we distinguish as physical and mental, we may look forward to a day when paths of knowledge and, let us hope, of influence will be opened up, leading from organic biology and chemistry to the field of neurotic phenomena."[41] This future time also will mark the period when purified science no longer needs to label the marginal as diseased. In his micro-autobiography *cum* mini-history of the psychoanalytic movement which he appends as the 1927 postscript to the publication of his essay on lay analysis, Freud outlines this sense of marginality within science without giving actual voice to its racist implications:

In my youth I felt an overpowering need to understand something of the riddles of the world in which we live and perhaps even to contribute something to their solution. The most hopeful means of achieving this end seemed to be to enroll myself in the medical faculty; but even after that I experimented—unsuccessfully—with zoology and chemistry, till at last, under the influence of Brücke, who carried more weight with me than anyone else in my whole life, I settled down to physiology, though in those days it was too narrowly restricted to histology. By that time I had already passed all my medical examinations; but I took no interest in anything to do with medicine till the teacher whom I so deeply respected warned me that in view of my impoverished material circumstances I could not possibly take up a theoretical career. Thus I passed from the histology of the nervous system to neuropathology and then, prompted by fresh influences, I began to be concerned with the neuroses. I scarcely think, however, that my lack of a genuine medical temperament has done much damage to my patients.[42]

Freud's postscript concludes with an eye cast toward the American scene. He condemns the American psychoanalytic community's 1922 rejection of lay analysts (spearheaded by I. H. Coriat) while acknowledging that "local conditions" may alter the reputation of the lay analyst, as was the case with Fliess in Berlin. Nevertheless, Freud maintains his newly articulated position, rejecting the medicalization of psychoanalysis.

The status of psychoanalysis in Vienna by 1926 had been grounded in public acceptance as well as academic opinion.[43] Freud had been granted his academic position at the University of Vienna, and he had acquired a series of major academic disciples, among them Eugen Bleuler. Training institutes had sprung up throughout Europe—all of them created after the pattern of academic institutions. Freud saw that psychoanalysis no longer depended on the status of medicine. Indeed, the inability of the "brain mythologists" of the 1890s to localize the anatomical lesions purported to lead to most forms of mental illnesses had brought their work into some disrepute by the 1920s. (The work by Kurt Goldstein during World War I on aphasia avoids any discussion of mental processes other than strictly observable ones, such as the disruption of speech and movement.) Freud no longer needed the status of medicine, even though he still did not feel himself free to abandon its protection completely.

There is a hidden, private dimension to the question of lay analysis, one that was rarely mentioned publicly during the late 1920s. This was the involvement of the redefinition of the analyst as part of Freud's search for his eventual successor as the head of the psychoanalytic movement, as his intellectual heir. Freud initially sought out his protégé from among the medical establishment, preferably the Christian medical establishment (e.g., Jung). But none of these potential medical psychoanalysts proved to be a reliable successor. From 1918 to 1921 Freud twice analyzed his youngest child, his daughter Anna, a young woman with minimal professional credentials, except for an interest in pedagogy.[44] Her analysis by her father was not, on its surface, that unusual. Many of the early analysts undertook prophylactic analysis of their own children. Without a doubt the best known of these were those of Anna Freud's later chief rival, Melanie Klein.[45] But Klein's children were very young at the time of their analysis; Anna Freud was a young woman.

Sigmund Freud, unlike the other analysts who practiced on their own children, had a secondary interest in his daughter's analysis. He began to see her, at least in the late 1920s, as his heir apparent—but an heir without any pretensions to medical training, without the imprimatur of state and profession. To no little degree, the very thought of Anna Freud as the potential successor to the leadership of the psychoanalytic movement made it imperative that lay analysis be the wave of the future.

One further note to the case of Anna Freud's central position in the question of lay analysis must be the implications of her own analysis. It is clear that Melanie Klein's analysis of her children was conducted in the light of her clinical interest in early childhood development. This process was much more in line with earlier attempts to record (and analyze) childhood changes, the earliest being Charles Darwin's detailed account of his oldest child's development. But the analysis of an adult female by the father who must—given Freud's own theoretical position—figure so very largely in her own fantasy life was clearly much more problematic, particularly in the context of such basic issues as transference with a beloved parent. The implication is of a type of psychological incest, a doubling of roles in a socially unacceptable manner. This potential charge is one that cannot be taken lightly, certainly not by a Viennese Jew who knows that one of the labels he wears is as an individual at risk from mental collapse as a result of his incestuous inbreeding.[46] For Freud, this charge must have at least been lurking in the background of his analysis of his daughter. And the suspicion of Jewish incest would have charged the idea of lay analysis with a great deal of covert political tension.

It is evident that Anna Freud, given her own complex relationship with her father, her gender, and her lesbian sexual identity, needed to find a female analyst, and that, at least by proxy, she did with Lou Andreas-Salomé. But by then the role of the heir had become part of her identity. Her own ambiguity concerning the question of lay analysis can be judged by her careful political position once she moved to Great Britain in 1938. She never challenged the second-class status of lay analysis which permitted her to practice (like all lay analysts in Great Britain after 1927) only under medical supervision. She quickly became the ally of Ernest Jones, an M.D., who wished to maintain this dual definition of competency within the profession of psychoanalysis in Britain. Better the ability to practice legally with fetters than not to practice at all, as in the United States. Such a position, given her own role in defining the nature of lay analysis, is not unexpected. But it did point to her awareness of her role in conflict with a masculine world that defined its power in terms of its professional, medical standards. The irony is that Anna Freud's medical supervisor in London, Willi Hofer, became her surrogate in many ways, including his role as president of the International Psychoanalytic Society. Hofer became an extension of the power that she had assumed as Freud's designated successor, just as she was assumed to be an extension of his medical status.

In 1933 Theodor Reik fled the Nazis from his position in the psychoanalytic institute in Berlin, first to The Hague and then, in 1938, to New York. New York remained the bastion of opposition to lay analysis. The secretary of the New York Psychoanalytic Society, C. P. Oberndorf, informed the International Psychoanalytic Society (i.e., Freud) in 1924 that the membership of the New York organization would remain open, as it had since 1922, only to physicians because of the importance of the status of psychoanalysts as doctors. He noted that many of their members held important positions in hospitals and medical schools. In 1926 the New York Psychoanalytic Society again, and this time unanimously, refused to consider the idea of non–medically trained psychoanalysts. In response to the case against Reik, the American psychoanalytic establishment, at the meeting of the international training committee of the International Psychoanalytic Society, which took place at Innsbruck on 2 September 1927, firmly and officially rejected Freud's proposal to have the analytic institutes train lay candidates. In 1938, the year Reik arrived in New York, the question of lay analysis was again raised before the American Psychoanalytic Society's "council on professional training."[47] A "majority resolution" was proposed "against the future training of laymen for the therapeutic use of psychoanalysis" which definitively banned the training of lay analysts except for "non-therapeutic purposes" such as "research and investigation in such nonmedical fields as anthropology, sociology, criminology, psychology, and education, etc." (This resolution excluded, among others, Theodor Reik from ever becoming a full-fledged member of the American Psychoanalytic Association.)

From that moment, what had been a general policy became a specific rule, one that exists today. But it was not sufficient. In February 1939 Sandor Rado proposed to the same committee a "numerus clausus" on the admission of analytic candidates to the American Psychoanalytic Association. The extraordinary move of limiting the number of qualified medical practitioners admitted to candidacy, following the exclusion of the nonmedical practitioners, bears examination. It documents the high status of the "new" science of psychoanalysis among the medical profession. For the three fellowships at the Boston institute in 1938, there were seventy-five inquiries and twenty-five actual applications from qualified applicants. But who were the individuals whom Rado wished to exclude—and why?

The minutes of the 26 February 1939 meeting, chaired by Franz Alexander, the director of the Chicago training institute, summarized Rado's proposal: "Advisability of a date as a limitation of registration for students in each institute each year. For frank attention to the problem of social and financial deterioration of any professional medical group. Necessitates a limitation of students on social, intellectual and economic grounds." Bertram Lewin saw this as a problem specifically in the New York Psychoanalytic Institute: "They [the students in New York] work under exceptional economic pressure. They are primarily interested in earning a living and not in academic or scientific work. They hold meetings like county medical politicians." This is an extraordinary statement given the influx of Jewish, Viennese-trained psychotherapists in the

United States. Lewin stresses the image of the psychoanalyst as a scientist, but as scientist in a mode both attractive to as well as clearly rejected by Freud. For inherent in this image, as stated by Freud in his postscript, is the image of the scientist as a well-to-do individual undertaking science as an extension of an haut-bourgeois identity. The image of the analyst as money-grubbing practitioner is thus contrasted with that of the pure scientist, pure in a number of senses of the word—pure as unsullied by filthy lucre, pure in devotion to an abstract science.

But Lewin picked up the thread of racism present in Freud's rejection of science. It was Theodor Billroth, one of Freud's teachers, who put the case against the admission of Jews to the Viennese medical faculty most directly (and most publicly), in his survey of medical education in the German-speaking countries:

> Young men, mostly Jews, come to Vienna from Galicia and Hungary, who have absolutely nothing, and who have conceived the insane idea that they can earn money in Vienna by teaching, through small jobs at the stock exchange, by peddling matches, or by taking employment as post office or telegraph clerks in Vienna or elsewhere, and at the same time study medicine. These people, who present to anyone not acquainted with Viennese conditions a most puzzling problem, who are not seldom inherently queer, but whose numbers are fortunately diminishing year by year, could hardly exist anywhere else. So this outcast [the Jewish student] in the Viennese world must first of all look for pupils, but he finds that the lesson hours conflict with the lectures. Still, he must live before he can study; the private lessons that he is to give cannot be postponed; he must accept them, and therefore cannot attend his classes.[48]

The image of the student as Jew and its extension, the urban psychoanalytic candidate as Jew, is thus part of the idea of the Jew as incapable of *Bildung*, the type of culture represented by the abstraction of science in nineteenth- and early twentieth-century Vienna. For Lewin, it was the Eastern Jew who filled the conceptual category of the "money-grubbing Jew" in European anti-Semitic rhetoric. In a rejection of this image, status is associated with the idea of pure science, an idea that in many ways, as we have shown, for the Jews involved is corrupted by racism.

During the succeeding decades psychoanalysis was transferred from the anti-Semitism of European science to the United States, where the racism of science had another, more accessible object, the black. The status of the Jewish psychoanalyst was tied to the status of European science, and Freud's attempt to loosen these bonds ran counter to the need of the exiled or emigrant psychoanalysts to call upon the status of

European science to establish themselves within the closed world of American medicine. In Europe, the specter of racism, which had haunted psychoanalysis because of its questionable reliance on the status of Viennese medicine, undermined the status of the psychoanalyst. In terms of the perspective of the European, especially the German and Austrian of the 1930s and 1940s, the psychoanalyst no longer had the status of medical practitioner; rather, the very term *psychoanalyst* became a sign of quackery. In the United States the case was quite different. Jewish medical practitioners, once they were certified to practice in the United States, entered into a world where medicine not only had high status, but where continental medicine had even higher status. And one of the medical specialities most representative of continental medicine was psychoanalysis. In 1930 Franz Alexander became the first professor of psychoanalysis at the newly founded University of Chicago Medical School, and in 1932 Hanns Sachs, a lay analyst, received a similar position at the Harvard Medical School. The psychoanalyst was free, at least momentarily, from the blemish of race; but of course, as we have seen, that blemish remained within the psychoanalysts' sense of themselves and their profession.

The high status of medicine in the United States was still tied to the biological definition of medicine and an acceptance of the medical model in defining medical practice. Psychoanalysis encouraged this attitude in part during the 1940s and 1950s with its enthusiasm for "general medicine" in the form of psychosomatics. As Robert Michels cogently observed: "In fact, for a time, one of the appeals of psychoanalysis to psychiatry was that it seemed to offer a chance for psychiatry to join the mainstream of medicine. Surprising though this may seem today [1981], psychoanalytic ideas concerning psychosomatic illness marked the first legitimatization of the return of the alienist-psychiatrist to the general hospital and the medical community—in many ways playing the same sociological role in the 1940s that neurobiology and psychopharmacology played in the seventies."[49] With the introduction of psychotropic drugs in the 1960s, the centuries-old division between the definition of psychiatry as the treatment of the brain versus its definition as the treatment of the mind reappeared, and at that point the question of the status of psychoanalysis became ever more tenuous.

Even with the perceived decline in the status of psychoanalysis in the 1970s and 1980s, the debate about who was to be given the title of psychoanalyst continued. The American Psychoanalytic Society put a series of committees in place—on professional standards, on the feasibility and desirability of the training of lay analysts. And this debate marked another turning point in the relation between the now firmly entrenched biological psychiatrist and the ever more isolated psychoanalyst. One marker of this sense of dissolution and separation was Robert Michels's address, referred to above, to the fiftieth anniversary celebration of the Washington Psychoanalytic Institute in December 1980. Michels, chair of the Department of Psychiatry at the Cornell Medical College, spoke on "Psychoanalysis and Psychiatry—the End of the Affair" and saw the pressure for lay analysts as the potential watershed that marked the dissolution of the relationship between psychiatry and psychoanalysis. Contemporary psychoanalysis (represented by Klein, Schafer, Ricoeur, and Lacan) has consciously moved away from the older, "biologically rooted" psychoanalytic model toward "the study of language, symbols, and meaning." Michels thus sees the movement away from psychiatry as a parallel movement toward the humanities and the social sciences, replacing the older model of the *Naturwissenschaften*, positivistic science, with the antithetical model of the *Geisteswissenschaften*, hermeneutic interpretation. It is understood as a movement from science to its antithesis. And this movement takes place even though "psychoanalysis continues to be the dominant paradigm organizing the way that psychiatrists think about patients and treatment." Michels sees this "end of the affair" as moving both fields "to a more open, less monogamous, but more honest, relationship, and I believe a far more promising future as a result."[50]

The separation of practice from theory has become absolute. Freud saw the need to distance himself from the corruption inherent in the medical model, with its image of domination (and the racist implications of the model of control). But the risk he took was to distance himself, at least tenuously, from the status of medicine. The debates that this position caused centered around the marginal position of psychoanalysis in the 1980s. This is especially true in the United States. To address the question of who is or is not to be considered a psychoanalyst would be to write a history of modern American psychoanalysis. Innumerable committees set up by the American Psychoanalytic Association as well as study groups set up by the various institutes of psychoanalysis chronicled the growing sense of defensiveness brought about by the redefinition of the status of psychoanalysis in the age of the re-Kraepelinization of American psychiatry, the age of DSM-III-R.

The objections to the training of lay analysts which grew out of the altered sense of the psychoanalyst's status before World War II are slowly being overcome within the profession. As late as 1985 the debate about who could be a psychotherapist raged within the psychiatric and psychoanalytic communities. But the imperatives of status are now quite different. For within the psychoanalytic institutes, the lack of M.D.s to train reveals the diminished attraction of psychoanalysis for the medical practitioner. The institutes are now turning to other areas, such as social work, for their potential students. But the opposition is loud and shrill. A letter written to *The New York Times* on 19 May 1985 by Seymour C. Post, associate clinical professor of psychiatry at Columbia's College of Physicians and Surgeons, bemoans the coming age of the "barefoot psychoanalyst."[51] He objects to the introduction of "lay psychotherapy" into psychiatry, which "threatens to denude the country of its only wholly qualified line of defense against mental and emotional illness: the physician trained both in biological and psychodynamic psychiatry." For Post, the villains are clear—the professionals, but especially the psychoanalysts: "And Freud was the first psychiatrist, but not the last, to train a member of his family (his daughter Anna) to do psychotherapy or psychoanalysis. Conflict of interest makes it difficult to speak frankly. Absence of criticism has emboldened lay therapists."

We have now come full circle—medicine, represented by clinical psychiatry, first accepted psychoanalysis to purge itself of the last vestiges of the stigma of political control and thus moved psychiatry back into the general hospital. Rejected by Freud because of its inherent racism, of its need to marginalize the mentally ill, medicine continued to draw on the status of the new science of psychoanalysis, to the degree that psychoanalytically oriented psychotherapy became the norm even for those practitioners who rejected psychoanalysis. With the introduction of psychotropic drugs in the 1960s, medicine began to loosen itself from the theory of psychoanalysis, while maintaining the model of treatment. Psychoanalysis wished to rid itself of medicine and its pretensions. But psychoanalysis (like osteopathy), now firmly established within the status of Western medicine, worked to preserve its sense of centrality by retaining a pre-Freudian definition of the appropriate (or competent) psychotherapist. Thus the question of whether Freud's theories are scientific may well rest on a definition of science quite different from that debated on by the philosophers of science—it may well rest on the sociology of status (and its relation to definitions of centrality and marginality) within the greater culture.

Constructing Schizophrenia
as a Category of Mental Illness

Defining Schizophrenia

How can we define the illness we label "schizophrenia"? As there seems to be no clear and definite answer to this question, I have assumed here the existence of a nosological category called "schizophrenia" and have also assumed that this category was constructed historically.[1] Thus our present diagnostic criteria for schizophrenia evolve out of a constant analysis and restructuring of other concepts, which are formed to create the category of schizophrenia. Unlike most other disease entities in psychiatry, "schizophrenia" is still a label in search of a structure; it is a category applied to a rather large group of symptoms with an almost equal number of etiologies proposed for it.

Some histories of the concept of schizophrenia have tried to push this disease entity into the distant past in order to prove its historical uniformity. Nowhere is this inherently futile attempt more radical than in the brief history of schizophrenia prefacing the clinical discussion of the concept in Freedman, Kaplan, and Sadock's *Comprehensive Textbook of Psychiatry* (1976). They begin "as early as 1400 B.C." with "a Hindu fragment from the Ayur-Veda" which describes "a condition, brought on by devils, in which the afflicted is 'gluttonous, filthy, walks about naked, has lost his memory, and moves about in an uneasy manner.'"[2] The authors make no attempt to understand that this description is the projection into the historical past of mid-twentieth-century diagnostic criteria. To admit this is not to reject such documentation as evidence for a set of symptoms. Such a set is clearly linked by this text. What Freedman, Kaplan, and Sadock undertake is to define the disease schizophrenia in such a manner that this association of symptoms becomes the disease entity schizophrenia. Such a process assumes some type of inherent continuity, not in the language used to describe the illness but in the illness itself. This assumption pushes the concept of schizophrenia into the company of somatic pathologies, which is where, as I shall show, midtwentieth-century psychiatry would very much like to place it. It assumes that the perception of the illness is constant across space and time, does not reflect the presuppositions of culture, is in no way colored by the associations with the stigma of mental illness (or its glorification), and is basically invariable. The wide variation in the symptoms ascribed to this disease and their seeming alteration over time tends to argue against such views. Like the presentation of hysteria in nineteenth-century Vienna, certain "classic" presentations of schizophrenia have become clinical rarities. "Waxy flexibility," for nineteenth-century psychiatry one of the most salient proofs of the existence of that disease entity called "catatonia" and which became (as I shall show) part of the definition of schizophrenia, has all but vanished from the late twentieth-century presentation of the disease. Neither shall I assume that "schizophrenia" is merely a label for the social control of those perceived as at variance with the norms or goals of a society. Schizophrenia is an illness, in its social manifestations; it is most probably a disease (rather than a syndrome), but the structure of that disease must yet be shown.[3]

I shall thus begin my history of the concept of schizophrenia with the caveat elegantly expressed by Henry Monro in an essay published in 1856 entitled "The Nomenclature of the Various Forms of Insanity," that the terminology applied to psychopathologies alters the perception of the illness itself. He observed that "a philosophical and sufficient nomenclature for the various forms of Insanity is still a desideratum, and must, I fear, remain so, until the physiology and pathology of the brain are better understood, and the relationship of mental with cerebral phenomena more accurately determined."[4] To this one can add, in the closing decades of the twentieth century, that such a sufficient nomenclature for schizophrenia may also depend on a greater understanding of the psychological phenomena that certainly also play a substantial role in shaping, if not causing, that illness or family of illnesses labeled "schizophrenia." Eugen Bleuler, in his classic monograph on schizophrenia, argued much the same point in his desire to abandon the designation of "dementia praecox" for the new label of "schizophrenia."[5]

I shall examine the history of the concept of schizophrenia, that is, the nosological category that was coined at the beginning of the twentieth century and which builds on nineteenth-century psychopathologic categories. This view will run counter to such positions as that taken by Jane M. Murphy on the parallel existence of similar modes of behavior, perceived as abnormal, across many cultures. Indeed, such studies of medical anthropology use a normative definition of psychopathology generated by combining specific sets of signs and viewing them as symptoms of a unified disease entity. The creation of such a "disease entity" called "schizophrenia" is, however, an artifact of the ideologies implicit in nineteenth-century European and American medical nosologies.[6] It is not the semiotics of an "objective" set of symptoms which is of interest to the historian of schizophrenia, but rather the ideology associated with the entire structure of disease which is extrapolated (correctly or incorrectly) from this set of phenomena. Thus the cultures that Jane M. Murphy (and other scholars of comparative medical anthropology) has examined reflect different conceptual structures in organizing their understanding of signs into comprehensible patterns.[7] It is the ideology ascribed to these perceived patterns (and the implication of this ideology for patterns of treatment) which is central to any history of the concept of schizophrenia. Thus H. Tristram Engelhardt is quite correct to see schizophrenia as a pattern of explanation rather than as a disease in itself or as an eidetic type of phenomenon.[8]

The very choice of the term *schizophrenia* as the designation of what has come to be the central focus for the study of mental illness in the course of the twentieth century was an attempt to create an innovative category out of the ideological presuppositions inherent in the various component categories subsumed by Bleuler into his new disease entity schizophrenia. It is the background to the creation of this term and the influence of this term which shall be the subject of my history.[9]

The Background of the Concept of Schizophrenia

While some may wish to trace the origins of the illness labeled "schizophrenia" back into the mists of time, it is clear that the central conceptual paradigm that schizophrenia replaced was dementia praecox. Indeed, Eugen Bleuler's first major book on the topic of schizophrenia, published in 1911, is entitled *Dementia praecox; or the Group of the Schizophrenias*.[10] He presented the shift in labels as central to the paradigmatic shift he perceived in the title of his book, from the older "dementia praecox" to the new label "schizophrenia." Schizophrenia was no longer to be understood as the dementia of adolescence, even by the remotest association with the term *dementia praecox*. It is therefore in the tension between the concept of the dementia of adolescence and its antitheses, dementias of age and mid-life, that the first stage of the history of schizophrenia must be sought.

While specific psychopathologies of youth had been assumed as early as Thomas Willis's *Two Discourses Concerning the Soul of Brutes* (1672), it was only in the mid-nineteenth century that the category of early dementia, dementia praecox, became the focus of attention. Willis sketched the course of the disease: young, lively, indeed even brilliant, individuals at the onset of puberty become stupid and morose. Late eighteenth-century "mad doctors" such as William Perfect, in his *Select Cases in the Different Species of Insanity and Madness* (1791), continued the image of a "puberty-neurosis." (Indeed, even Jean-Jacques Rousseau believed in a "folie d'adolescence.")[11]

It was only in the nineteenth century that the category of a psychopathology of adolescence became embedded in a more highly evolved medical nosology. To the early nineteenth-century observer it was clear that there was a dementia of old age (*dementia senilis*) and a dementia of mid-life (*dementia paralytica*). Or at least some nineteenth-century medical nosologies saw these two categories as parallel, based on the seemingly shared symptoms of dementia. Thus the missing link for a comprehensive psychopathology of aging was the dementia of youth; or more specifically, since senile dementia and general paralysis of the insane were illnesses that appeared on the border of perceived shifts of states (from youth to mid-life, from mid-life to old age), it was necessary to create a category of adolescent dementia, dementia praecox. It is important to understand that the category of adolescent dementia incorporated *all* categories of psychopathology which appeared during this period of development. Thus as late as 1888 Thomas Clouston, in his presidential address to the Medico-Psychological Association (London), could speak of "adolescent insanities" and mean all psychopathologies that affect youth. In the early and mid-nineteenth century the syndrome of primary dementia, that is, dementia following endogenous mania or melancholia, was set off from secondary dementia, that is, the dementia associated with general paralysis of the insane. The focus of these commentators, such as J. E. D. Esquirol, was on the manifestations of the symptoms rather than the course of the illness. Dementia in general was, however, defined by writers such as Etienne Georget (Esquirol's student) as the terminal state of all incurable psychoses.[12] Built into the concept of a dementia of youth, then, was the implication of a negative outcome linked to early onset. This link is quite different from the implications for the other two segments of this trinity of developmental psychoses, since negative outcome and early onset had also been connected in another category, that of masturbatory insanity.[13]

Masturbatory insanity, with all of its influence on the psychiatric nosology of the nineteenth century, helped color the early discussions of dementia praecox. One of the central links between the two categories lies in the fact that the masturbator, like the patient suffering from dementia praecox, was considered to be overly intelligent. Indeed the charge that the act of reading caused masturbation is paralleled by the implication, in the early discussion of dementia praecox, that a child of extraordinary intelligence became "demented" through some unexplained means. Adolescence, as Patricia Meyer Spacks has detailed in her study *The Adolescent Idea*, focuses on the sexuality of youth. This focus is implicit in the category of dementia praecox but explicit in the category of masturbatory insanity.[14] We can turn to the first "case study" of dementia praecox, or at least the first case study that employed the label "dementia praecox," to examine the connections between this form of dementia and other psychopathological categories in nineteenth-century medicine.

Bénédict-Auguste Morel, best known for his popularization of the concept of degeneration during the mid-nineteenth century, seems to have been the first to have used the label "dementia praecox," in 1860:

An unfortunate father consulted me one day about the mental state of his 12- or 14-year-old son, in whom a violent hatred for the originator of his life had suddenly replaced the most tender feelings. He was despondent at being the smallest in his class, despite the fact that he was always the first in his compositions, and that without effort and almost without work. It was, so to speak, by intuition that he comprehended things, which he organized in his memory and his intelligence. He gradually lost his cheerfulness, became gloomy, taciturn, and showed a tendency toward solitude. His mother was psychotic and his grandmother eccentric to an extreme degree. I ordered the interruption of the child's studies and his confinement in an institution for hydrotherapy. A most happy change occurred in the bodily state of the child. He grew considerably but another phenomenon as disquieting as those I have mentioned came to dominate the situation. The young patient progressively forgot everything he had learned; his so brilliant intellectual faculties underwent in time a very distressing arrest. A kind of torpor akin to hebetude replaced the earlier activity, and then I concluded that the fatal transition to the state of *démence précoce* was about to take place. This dreadful diagnosis is ordinarily far from the minds of parents and also physicians who care for these children. Such is, nevertheless, in many cases the sad termination of hereditary insanity. A sudden paralysis of the faculties, a *démence précoce*, indicates that the patient has reached the end of his intellectual life that he can control.[15]

Morel's case study of démence précoce is revealing because it stresses the relationship between extraordinary intelligence and the endogenous nature of the disease. The higher the native intelligence, it seems, the more predisposed one is to the manifestation of the illness. Morel sees early onset dementia as a constitutional problem.

Seeing the patient as a member of a marginal group, here the highly intelligent, defined to a degree by its heightened potential for disease pertained also to the category of masturbatory insanity. Morel suggests the removal of the patient from intellectual stimulation as part of his course of treatment, a process that parallels the removal of sources of stimulation, such as novels, from the masturbator. But Morel also introduces the concept of heredity into the initial discourse about dementia praecox—not unexpectedly, given Morel's general views concerning the relation between inherent characteristics and environmental stimuli. But its introduction at the very inception of the category démence précoce provides the matrix for the later nineteenth-century discussions of the concept. The disease of adolescence becomes one of the keys to an understanding of the cyclical patterns of psychopathology within human development. To isolate the scientific observer (who, of course, would be undergoing a parallel development) from potential inclusion in this category of marginality, a further qualification is introduced. The links among "genius," "heredity," and "psychopathology" are thus present in the earliest discussions of the concept of dementia praecox.

Morel's initial case can provide a model for examining other mid-century discussions of the psychopathology of adolescence, even though it is rarely cited until much later in the century, when the formulators of the concept of dementia praecox were searching for the historical context of their new nosological category. The term *infantile dementia* was coined by J. T. Dickson in 1874 (following earlier English models) and Morel's "démence précoce" actually reappeared in the title of G. C. Gauthier's 1883 Paris thesis.[16] The concept is a commonplace in late nineteenth-century nosologies, retaining many of Morel's implications. Richard von Krafft-Ebing, in his standard textbook of psychiatry, raised the insanity of adolescence to the rank of touchstone for late nineteenth-century psychopathologies (replacing "general paralysis of the insane" as this became increasingly understood as a neurological rather than a psychiatric category):

> I answer the question 'what is the typical form of insanity' by saying that the insanity of adolescence is the typical form, because it most frequently ends in typical secondary dementia, without any other function being affected but mentalization, and because in its course we have all the forms of psychosis represented. . . . Almost all pure cases of secondary dementia will be found to have begun in the developmental (pubescent and adolescent) insanities. . . . Undue and unphysiological means through a forcing-house mode of education during adolescence without

regard to the hereditary capacity and weakness of the organism tend toward dementia. The constant changes in each generation of modern civilized environment and the special efforts thus rendered necessary by the struggle for existence tend towards dementia through the strain they put on the most delicate of all organized tissues.[17]

Here it is not masturbatory insanity but the identical categories of that "disease," transferred to the "modern" disease of "neurasthenia," which color the category of "dementia." Again note that it is education and intelligence (or in this case the relative lack of intelligence in relation to the pressure of the educational system) that provide the etiology for the psychopathology of adolescence. By 1891 when Alois Pick, professor of psychiatry in Prague, published his standard paper on dementia praecox (the paper that established this term as the accepted nosological label for the psychopathology of adolescence), the concept as well as the term was fully accepted.[18] Pick points to Morel and Gauthier as his forerunners. With Pick's paper the dementia of adolescence became the standard label for "secondary dementia," and it remained part of the vocabulary of psychiatric nosology until the turn of the century.

Toward a Synthetic Concept of Schizophrenia

The stage was thus set for the synthesis of a set of related concepts into the greater category of dementia praecox. The signifying signs of the dementia of adolescence remain constant, however. Following Morel's application of the classical dramatic unities to medical nosology (unity of cause, course, and outcome tied, if possible, to special lesion), the late nineteenth century provided a vocabulary of images for dementia praecox. One set of images was generated by Karl Ludwig Kahlbaum, whose 1863 psychiatric nosology set the stage for the development of a general clinical psychopathology in the German-speaking lands.[19] Kahlbaum (and his friend and collaborator of many years Ewald Hecker) described two clinical entities, *hebephrenia* (from the Greek for "frenzy" of youth) and *catatonia* (from the Greek "tension against"), which were later to be integrated into the overall category of dementia praecox. "Hebephrenia" was Kahlbaum's label for pubertal psychoses; "catatonia" was employed to characterize a cyclic pattern of dementia, which passed through a manic, melancholic, and paranoid state and had a negative outcome. (Kahlbaum was quite open in paralleling catatonia to *vesania progressiva*, his designation for general paralysis of the insane. He saw in catatonia a set of particular motor tensions as specific for that disease as those of tertiary syphilis are for general paralysis of the insane.

Here he drew on the work of Antoine Laurent Jessé Bayle, who in 1822 stressed the association between syphilis and derangement, and Jean Pierre Fabret's concept of *folie circulaire*.) Like Morel's case study of démence précoce, Kahlbaum's nosology was little read by his immediate contemporaries. It was only the writings of Emil Kraepelin and L. Daraszkiewicz which fixed Kahlbaum's categories as components of an age-bound designation of dementia.[20] (Indeed, Kahlbaum's categories became so firmly associated with this disease entity that one term for dementia praecox in France became the "maladie de Kahlbaum."][21] By this point it was clear that the complex of categories, although loosely associated, spelled out a disease called dementia praecox; and, using Kahlbaum's designation, it was perceived to be a *paraphrenia*, a disease that is age specific.

Kraepelin's resuscitation of Morel's label in 1893, following Alois Pick's lead, marked a most fascinating shift in the meaning and implication of this disease. For in employing an older, latinate term *(dementia)* to form a cognitive superstructure for the various *phrens* evolved by Kahlbaum, Kraepelin signified a movement away from the idealization of Greek categories of mind which had dominated much of the latter half of the nineteenth century. I mentioned Morel's adaptation of the concept of the classical unities, which are aesthetic categories, for his definition of disease. Kahlbaum created or revived a number of Greek (or at least Greek-sounding) terms for related, though independent, psychopathologies. Among them was the term *paranoia*, in use from the eighteenth century and of importance in the nosological systems of the German Romantic psychiatrists, such as Johann Christian August Heinroth. "Paranoia" was revitalized by Kahlbaum as the designation for the primary form of systematized delusions.[22] Kraepelin, in using "dementia," pointed toward a new set of images for the concept of dementia rather than Kahlbaum's set (while employing the structure of Kahlbaum's nosology). Even Freud saw the vocabulary of Greek aesthetics as an appropriate one for the discussion of psychopathology. He borrowed the term *catharsis* from the writing of Jakob Bernays, one of the leading classicists of the period.[23]

The vocabulary of the intelligentsia in the German-speaking countries during the latter half of the nineteenth century was peppered with Greek words or neologisms based on Greek. Greek had, following Johann Joachim Winckelmann and the rise of German neoclassicism in the late eighteenth century, the aura of being the tongue closest to the roots of human experience.[24] Especially in the area of psychopathology, where the parallels to the literary world of the Greeks seemed self-evident, Greek stood for the hidden truth revealed by the observer, a truth rooted in history. Kahlbaum's terminology (like Freud's later use of Greek myth) revealed his reliance on the status of the language.

When Kraepelin subsumed the *phrens* to the Latin *mentalis,* he consciously announced a change in the conceptualization of dementia praecox. Indeed he debated the question of the appropriate designation of the disease in his early writing, rejecting the Italian "demenza primitiva" or subsuming one of the existing labels such as "dementia simplex" to his more general category before deciding on "dementia praecox." What is important is that, even though Kraepelin adopted Morel's designation, he did so while abandoning much of its traditional associations of late nineteenth-century French psychopathology. For Valentin Magnan had stressed Morel's association of this (and other) disease entities with the etiology of degeneration. What Magnan called "délire de persécution à évolution systématique," a chronic delusional state, is Morel's démence précoce; it is related by Magnan to a degenerative process. Kraepelin avoids all such oversimplification. The political undercurrents that set German and French psychopathology in consciously different directions following 1872 also shaped Kraepelin's "reading" of Morel, his restructuring of Morel's views to fit his own concept of the disease.

To trace Emil Kraepelin's concept of dementia praecox is a complex undertaking. It is perhaps best linked to an understanding of the category of "deterioration," which, at least in retrospect, seems central to his restructuring of the concept of dementia praecox. Kraepelin introduced the category of dementia praecox in a paper entitled "The Diagnosis and Prognosis of *Dementia Praecox"* at the twenty-ninth congress of Southwestern German psychiatrists in 1898. But he had begun reformulating this concept in his compendium of psychiatry published in 1883. In that edition "dementia praecox" was used in a narrow sense to refer to those patients who fitted Kahlbaum's and Hecker's definition of hebephrenia. Paranoia and catatonia were perceived as independent entities. By the fifth edition (1896) of his comprehensive handbook of psychiatry (which was the dominant textbook on psychopathology for the period through World War I) dementia praecox, catatonia, and dementia paranoides were subcategories of "processes of dementing" (*Verblödungsprozesse*). This trinity of interlocking diagnostic criteria replaced the independent categories of hebephrenia, catatonia, and paranoia. Also, Kraepelin's earliest formulation of the etiology of dementia praecox pointed to its prior association with the psychopathologies of puberty and adolescence, especially masturbatory insanity. Dementia praecox was, for Kraepelin, a "degenerative" pathology. This classification tied into Morel's more general category for démence précoce and keyed it to a continuation of the understanding of this disease as having a somatic etiology. Kraepelin saw dementia praecox as the result of some type of "self-poisoning." (Kraepelin himself sets this term off in quotation marks.) But it is a "self-poisoning" related to sexuality, or at least, to the sexual organs:

Here it must be first pointed out what in the clinical descriptions must ever again be emphasized, that in our patients very frequently a lively sexual excitement exists, which makes itself known in onanism, debauches, and tormenting sexual ideas of influence. Especially of male patients one learns with striking frequency that for many years they have constantly masturbated. Formerly therefore certain morbid pictures belonging to hebephrenia were simply described as the "insanity of masturbation"; perhaps also part of the widespread ideas about the terrible consequences of onanism is connected with such experiences.[25]

As Kraepelin developed his category of dementia praecox he shifted his attention from "deterioration" (another category closely associated with the sexual etiology of diseases such as masturbatory insanity and general paralysis of the insane) to the phenomenology of the disease. Kraepelin's understanding of the phenomenology of this disease category was relatively sophisticated if static. It was he who incorporated (even if in response to other views) the linguistic phenomena that are classically associated with later discussion of schizophrenia. For Kraepelin did not merely dismiss the altered language (and thought processes) of the patient as "word salad." He described "derailing" of thought processes, using the written and artistic products of his patients to document it. And he described the structural changes of the patients' language, including their use of stereotypy and neologisms.

The concept of negative outcome was also altered in the course of Kraepelin's development of the concept of dementia praecox. Deterioration came to mean a marked loss following the onset of the active psychosis, rather than, as it had earlier implied, resultant idiocy and eventual death. But Kraepelin tied even this more marginal loss to some type of disruption of brain function, implicitly seeing it in some ways as parallel to the general paralysis of the insane. Kraepelin saw the disease as endogenous, as did Morel and others who employed the term *dementia praecox*. But the ideological implications of this seemingly basic manner of perceiving dementia praecox at the close of the nineteenth century had shifted from the time of Morel. For Kraepelin was at pains to contrast this disease entity with neurasthenia, that disease of "civilization" which so dominated the nosologies of late nineteenth-century psychiatry.

By the eighth edition (1909–13) of Kraepelin's handbook, which had grown to four volumes, dementia praecox was covered in a segment of over three hundred pages. The disease had become a "special disease unit." It is important to note that by the date of this edition, general paralysis of the insane had moved from the stormy waters of psychiatry into the safe harbor of neurology. Kraepelin's restructuring of dementia praecox placed it, however, center-stage in the concerns of the psychiatrist. But Kraepelin, in this definitive presentation of his views, also attempted to change dementia praecox from a somatic, degenerative illness (bearing the stigmata of masturbatory insanity, even by analogy) and place it in the realm of the new psychology. He made the distinction, which he borrowed from Paul Julius Möbius, between endogenous and exogenous causes of dementia praecox. For Kraepelin, shortly before World War I, dementia praecox became a "peculiar destruction of the internal connection of the psychic personality." The etiology of this "destruction" could lie either within or without the patient. This movement toward a new psychology of dementia praecox was due to the rise of the psychoanalytic view of psychopathology, and specifically to the competing view of dementia praecox as having a psychogenic rather than a somatic etiology.

The Appearance of *Schizophrenia*

The eighth edition of Emil Kraepelin's handbook of psychiatry reflected the publication, in 1911, of Eugen Bleuler's now classic study *Dementia Praecox; or the Group of Schizophrenias*. Bleuler, director of the famed Swiss teaching hospital of the Burghölzli in Zurich, was one of the first followers of Sigmund Freud to apply the "new" teachings of psychoanalysis to the major psychoses.[26] Both Bleuler and Freud viewed dementia praecox as an organic or constitutional disease, as did Kraepelin, but both placed renewed emphasis on the meaning and organization of symptoms. In one of Freud's first psychoanalytic papers (1894), he had suggested that "unbearable ideas" gave rise to hallucinatory psychoses by means of repetition of the idea as a hallucinatory wish-fulfillment.[27] In 1896 this concept allowed Freud to develop a dynamic interpretation of a case of chronic paranoia,[28] a case in which he formulated the concept of projection latent in his earlier interpretation of psychosis. In general, these early theories reflect Freud's belief that psychopathology is the consequence of the conflicts arising from the faulty repression of drives. Freud uses the term *dementia praecox*, or its various constituent parts (e.g., paranoia), as the nosological label for some of the psychopathologies he was examining. It was only in 1911 that Freud turned to a detailed analysis of a case of dementia praecox, and that case study, together with Bleuler's monograph, determined the direction of much of the psychological literature on schizophrenia for the next three decades.

Bleuler broke, at least overtly, with the descriptive accounts of dementia praecox as provided by Kraepelin. Indeed, his monograph was perceived by himself and by his contemporaries as a total break with the clinical psychiatry of the later nineteenth century. Bleuler focused in on the question of "deterioration" and its supposed centrality to Kraepelin's understanding of dementia praecox:

> There is hardly a single psychiatrist who has not heard the argument that the whole concept of *dementia praecox* must be false because there are many catatonics and other types who, symptomatologically, should be included in Kraepelin's *dementia praecox*, and who do not go on to complete deterioration. Similarly, the entire question seems to be disposed of with the demonstration that in a particular case deterioration has not set in previously but only in later life.[29]

Thus Bleuler rejected not only the term *dementia praecox*, but also *dementia dessecans, dementia sejunctive, dementia primitive, dementia simplex, dementia apperceptive,* and *paradementia.* He coined the new term *schizophrenia*, which he considered analogous to Kraepelin's *dementia praecox.* He defined it as "a group of psychoses whose course is at times chronic, at times marked by intermittent attacks, and which can stop or retrograde at any stage, but does not permit a full *restitutio ad integrum.* The disease is characterized by a specific type of alteration of thinking, feeling, and relation to the external world which appears nowhere else in this particular fashion." Bleuler's discussion of "deterioration" is not, however, that much different from Kraepelin's. What is different is that he wished it to be perceived as a much more "liberal" definition than Kraepelin's and that he shifted the burden of the disease that he calls "schizophrenia" from its full symptomatology to the much more limited focus of "thought, feeling, and the relation to the external world." The focus of this interrelationship for the turn of the century is to be found in the patient's language. Freud had drawn attention to the various modes of language present in the conscious and subconscious, and through his very introduction of the "new" language of psychoanalysis provided a mode of treatment which was itself language-based. Language disruption thus becomes for Bleuler, following Freud, the central marker of the schizophrenic thought process.

But why does Bleuler choose "schizophrenia" as the label for this "new" entity? Partly as an attempt to relate his nosological category to those generated by Kahlbaum and to isolate Kraepelin as a "blind alley" in the history of the disease; partly as a homage to Freud, whose use of Greek terms reflected the Viennese fascination with the tradition of Greek neoclassicism and the readings, not of Latin myth, but of the "more original" world of Greek mythology. Latin had a relatively low status, associated as it was with the language of imperial expansion and royal corruption, states all too familiar to late nineteenth-century inhabitants of Austria and Germany (which saw itself as the new Imperium).

Rome, represented by its language, was too much in mind among liberals in pre–World War I Europe; Greece, with the German myth of its role as the originators of Western civilization, could be called upon to free the mentally ill from the Roman chains of dementia praecox and its "inevitable deterioration." German (and indeed, Swiss) popular mythology, which in the late nineteenth and early twentieth centuries called on Greece for the origins of liberalism, could be incorporated into the new disease entity, the "splitting" of the "psychic functions," *schizo-phrenia*. The power of this avant-garde designation, lodged to no little degree in the very fact of its newness, was such that it immediately captured the popular fantasy.[30]

The return to Greek paralleled Kraepelin's early flight from Greek into Latin. With Bleuler's return to the more ancient language, there was a natural sense of continuity between the older pre-Kraepelinian categories and the new label. Despite the attractiveness of the "modern" label, with all of its "classical" associations, the Greek "schizophrenia" did not immediately drive the Latin "dementia praecox" out of the marketplace. These two labels competed in various spheres until mid-century, when "schizophrenia" finally prevailed. The standard American survey of the work done on this disease entity was first titled *Dementia Praecox. The Past Decade's Work and Present Status. A Review and Examination* even though it was first published in 1948. Subsequent editions employed the term *schizophrenia*.[31] Even though the universal replacement of "dementia praecox" by "schizophrenia" took almost half a century, the ideological importance of Bleuler's break with Kraepelin can be measured by observing who used the label "schizophrenia" and how early that term was employed by any given researcher. Indeed, as early as 1913, when Karl Jasper's phenomenological overview of psychopathology appeared in Germany (and created a new school of psychiatry) and used the term *schizophrenia*, this label came to be the accepted designation for the syndrome among those psychiatrists who saw themselves as true innovators, whether "Freudians" or "phenomenologists."[32]

Bleuler, however, maintained much of Kraepelin's understanding of the disease. He divided it, as did Kraepelin, into a limited set of component segments—Kraepelin's paranoia, catatonia, and hebephrenia—and gives independent status to Kraepelin's simple schizophrenia. But Bleuler also created a hierarchy out of Kraepelin's more static description of the status of the various symptoms of schizophrenia. He designated one set of symptoms as primary or "fundamental." All of these are related to the alteration of language. These symptoms are, for Bleuler, necessary but not sufficient for the diagnosis of the disease. By 1973, in the World Health Organization's *International Pilot Study of Schizophrenia*, only 10 percent of the patients examined showed the classic Bleulerian thought disorders. The shift may well parallel the disappearance of "waxy flexibility" from the clinical picture of catatonia or may reflect Bleuler's embeddedness in the Freudian model, which stressed the centrality of language.

Bleuler makes a distinction between these primary symptoms and "basic" symptoms, which are necessary for the diagnosis of schizophrenia. For Bleuler, "basic" alterations in association, affectivity, and ambivalence (as well as autism), all illustrated by linguistic examples in his text, were the *Grundsymptome,* or basic symptoms; the more "classic" symptoms such as hallucinations, illusions, and catatonic stupor were relegated to incidental (or "accessory") roles.

It was the question of the reliability of Bleuler's "basic symptoms" which led Kurt Schneider to propose a series of so-called "first-rank" symptoms as early as 1925.[33] Each of these symptoms (e.g., auditory hallucinations, somatic passivity, disturbed thinking) had pathognomonic value and reflected the more traditional conceptualization of the symptomatology of schizophrenia. Schneider therefore stands as much in the tradition of Kraepelin as does Bleuler. For even though he accepts the importance of the psychological component, he stresses the importance of the patient's symptoms as an indicator of the disease rather than of its outcome. He moves away from the category of "deterioration" and into the "pure" phenomenology of the disease. His more conventional set of symptoms formed the basis for the post–World War II phenomenological category of schizophrenia in Great Britain and the United States.

Eugen Bleuler stressed a continuum between the "normal" and the "psychopathological," seeing the appearance of "schizophrenic" symptoms even among non-schizophrenics (e.g., in the form of displacement). He emphasized the totality of the psychological setting. Bleuler, following Freud's lead, saw schizophrenia as a psychopathology represented by a loss of harmony among the various groups of mental functions and expressed in linguistic malfunction. Like Kraepelin, he believed that the ultimate etiology for the disease (or group of diseases) would most probably be metabolic, but that personality structure and psychogenic factors determined the form of the symptoms. Unlike Kraepelin he dismissed any distinction between endogenous (for Bleuler, "process") and exogenous (for Bleuler, "reactive") forms of schizophrenia. In abandoning this distinction, Bleuler also abandoned any attempt to distinguish the origin of the disease.

Bleuler took the discussion of schizophrenia into the sphere of dynamic psychiatry. Kraepelin's image of the illness was inherently static; Bleuler wished to understand the symptomatology of the illness in terms of its psychological content, as well as its appearance. Thus he perceived the "loosening of associations" as the central symptom. This loosening was a sign of the "splitting" of the basic functions of the personality. While focusing on the symptoms (which he saw as psychogenic) he avoided (indeed, as did Freud) any discussion of the etiology of the disease. Bleuler's central role in the discussion of schizophrenia was to move the disease entity ever more in the direction of a psychological category.

Sigmund Freud, in his classic study of dementia paranoides, written in 1911, suggested that dementia praecox was the result of a complex set of projections.[34] The psychopathology of Daniel Paul Schreber, the German jurist, was interpreted by Freud as the rejection of Schreber's deep-seated homosexual wish and its projection onto the world in a negative form. Later, in his paper on narcissism (1914), Freud refined this concept, applying his libido theory and seeing paranoia as the result of an early libidinal fixation at the autoerotic stage.[35] The disease is thus the "return of the repressed," or at least of the attachment of libido (and associated drives) to the ego.

For Freud the question of dementia praecox had become a question of psychological mechanisms at work. When, in the adult, sexual frustration forces the patient to regress to the earlier point of development at which the fixation had taken place, an abnormal narcissistic state is created which generates paranoia. Paranoia, that subcategory of schizophrenia, becomes for Freud an overarching category. Bleuler, writing at more or less the same time as Freud, comes to quite different conclusions, even though both men are departing from quite similar objects. For, just as Bleuler's study is laced with images and words taken from the schizophrenic, Freud's study departs from a reading of Schreber's autobiography. The literature on the "Schreber case" is extensive.[36] Suffice it to say that Freud used the literary product of the schizophrenic as the key to an understanding of the disease. Rather than having the patient before him, he had the patient's published account of his illness—published, one might add, as part of Schreber's attempt to be released from the institution in which he was being held. (Freud was evidently introduced to the text by Carl G. Jung.) For Freud the language of the schizophrenic becomes the necessary substitute for the patient. Since schizophrenic patients cannot be approached through an external erotic attachment (they are thus incapable of using the language of transference), it is through their writing that an understanding of the disease process can be had: "Since paranoics cannot be compelled to overcome their internal resistances [hence free association proves most difficult], and since in any case they only say what they choose to say, it follows that this is precisely a disorder in which a written report or a printed case history can take the place of a personal acquaintance with the patient." It is not merely, as with Bleuler, that language is the primary (or one of the major) signs of this illness; rather it is only through the fixed representations of the language of the patient that any insight into the illness can be had. Freud shaped much of the discussion concerning the concept of schizophrenia during the early decades of the twentieth century. His understanding of the mechanisms of regression and projection provided much of the formal framework for the reinterpretation of the central structures of this disease.

Freud's view shaped and colored much of the concern with the products of the schizophrenic which dominated the literature (and its reception into the wider public domain) during the coming decade. In Heidelberg Karl Jaspers devoted a large segment of his discussion of schizophrenia to the products of the schizophrenic—to their speech, art, and writing. While there had been a literature on the writing and art of the schizophrenic during the late nineteenth century, much of it had been devoted to an antiquarian interest in the products of the insane as representatives of another (inherently inferior) culture, analogous to the objects collected for ethnological museums from among colonized peoples.[37] With the Heidelberg school, specifically in the work of Karl Willmanns and two of his assistants, Hans Prinzhorn (in 1922) and Wilhelm Mayer-Gross (in 1924), there was a shift to an understanding of these objects as keys to the existential world view of the schizophrenic.[38] Thus the object, whether painting, poem, or autobiography, became the representation of the altered perception of the world, as discussed in Chapter 6. It became the key to an understanding of the disease schizophrenia and, indeed, became *pars par toto* the disease itself. The representation of altered communicative states became the key for an insight into the disease.

It is in the work of Carl G. Jung, perhaps even more than in Bleuler's, that the movement from a primarily descriptive to a dynamic understanding of dementia praecox takes place.[39] In his 1903 *Psychology of Dementia Praecox* Jung, still closely allied to Freud, postulated the importance of the conception of dissociation for the formulation of his understanding of this illness.[40] Using word association tests, Jung saw the ideas dissociated by the patients as dynamically determined. He saw the deep structure of the illness as a series of "complexes" that determined the physiognomy of the disease. But he viewed the complexes of dementia praecox as inherently different from those of other psychogenic illnesses such as hysteria. Language revealed to Jung the psychogenic origin of the complexes associated with dementia praecox; to explain the etiology of the disease (and why it did not respond to the "talking cure"), Jung relied on a quite different model. He saw the complexes present as producing a toxin that influenced brain action. In this way he accounted for the inherently negative prognosis in the disease. (This notion was, of course, contrary to Bleuler's view, who postulated some brain toxin as the cause of the disease.)

Jung refined his theories, incorporating into them the sense of the inherent predisposition. In 1913, his work on dementia praecox led to his differentiation of various psychological types, since in trying to distinguish between the categories of "hysteria" and dementia praecox Jung needed to find further differences between these two illnesses, rooted, as he perceived them, in complexes.[41] It was only well after his break with Freud, in the early 1920s, that the fragments of Jung's understanding of dementia praecox coalesced in his work on the collective unconscious. This was the most important development in the direction of the aesthetic interpretation of schizophrenia. As we have seen, the focus on the aesthetic production of the schizophrenic is an important feature of nineteenth- and early twentieth-century psychiatry.

Jung uses the objects as well as the concepts of the schizophrenic to point to the archetypal structure of the disease. For the schizophrenic's view of the world revealed an unencumbered image of the primal structures of perception shared by all human beings. These mythopoetic structures, similar to Freud's own use of myth, represent a collective sense of self. The schizophrenic may well be able to present these collective perceptions in a less mitigated manner than the non-schizophrenic. The schizophrenic thinks archaically. Schizophrenics are thus atavistic, at least in the formulation of their world view. And this primitivism is reflected in their production of words and art. Jung returns to a nineteenth-century model of madness, one subscribed to by, among others, Charles Darwin in his study of expression (in which the insane reveal the psychological ontogeny of the genus *Homo sapiens*).[42] But Jung relies on the linguistic and artistic manifestations of illness, not the expression of the emotions of the insane, for the basis of his theories. The schizophrenic may be ill, but he or she may also be "closer" to the wellsprings of human experience: it is this notion that helps shape the post–World War II view that the schizophrenic is perhaps more a seer than a patient.

From *Parergasia* to the "Divided Self"

If there is a "mainstream" in the development of the concept of schizophrenia, then it is rooted in the debate between Kraepelin (and those who see Kraepelin as having had a purely somatic understanding of the disease) and Bleuler (and those who see Bleuler as having had a purely psychogenic understanding of the disease). It is evident that the dichotomy traditionally perceived between Kraepelin and Bleuler is an artifact of the reception of their views (and the need for later theories to rewrite the

history of this concept to give them a sense of historical embeddedness].
In truth, these two major views were tempered by a series of theories,
many departing from the two "rootstock" theories, which, however,
shaped the later evolution of the concept and which must therefore be
examined in any history of the concept of schizophrenia. Surely the most
influential, at least during the lifetime of its promulgator, was the further
redefinition and relabeling of schizophrenia as "parergasia" by the Swiss-
American psychiatrist Adolf Meyer.

With Adolf Meyer we move our concern with European theories of
schizophrenia across the Atlantic Ocean.[43] Meyer, who like Bleuler studied with the chairman of the department of psychiatry in Zurich, August
Forel, made his reputation in the United States. He paralleled Bleuler in
rejecting Kraepelin's conceptualization of dementia praecox; and, like
Bleuler, attempted to abandon that designation through the introduction
of a new term—*parergasia*, literally "incongruity of behavior."

Meyer's understanding of parergasia had a great influence on the formulation of later definitions of schizophrenia, at least in the United
States. He believed that the illness had to be understood holistically and
traced its presence throughout the development of the individual up to
the moment of its actual onset. He also saw exogenous causes as playing
a central role in the etiology of the disease. It was Meyer who later coined
the term *schizophrenic reactions* to place emphasis on the origin of the
illness outside of the patient. While Meyer labeled his categories "dynamic," as they traced the development of the disease over time, he also
saw them as "psychobiological," since he considered biological as well as
psychological aspects of the disease. He traced the progress of the disease,
however, in the accumulation of "bad habits" and the inability to make
any constructive adjustment of these habits. The view that parergasia is
but an accumulation of bad habits stressed the continuity with the earlier life of the patient.

Meyer wished to abandon the "European" rigidity that he found in
Kraepelin's theory of dementia praecox. Relying on neither specific
pathognomonic signs nor "deterioration" as the certain indicator of the
disease, Meyer's subtypes proliferated, especially in the 1952 *Diagnostic
and Statistical Manual* of the American Psychiatric Association. Numerous categories such as "pseudoneurotic schizophrenia" (coined by Hoch
and Polatin in 1949) and "pseudopsychopathic schizophrenia" (coined by
Hoch and Dunaif in 1955) were generated under Meyer's influence.[44] The
image of schizophrenia as a disease of development still haunts Meyer's
formulation, but, even more importantly, the image of the schizophrenic
as unable to deal with the daily realities of the world and thus taking
refuge in the world of madness lays the groundwork for one of the more
interesting critiques of the concept of mental illness, that of Thomas

Szasz, which appeared decades after Meyer's death in 1950.[45] But Szasz's critique of the concept of schizophrenia, like his more general critiques of the conceptualization of mental illness, rests on the question of the volition of the patient. Szasz, trained in a world in which Meyer's views dominated the "official" discourse of American psychiatry on schizophrenia, simply carried Meyer's views to their extreme. For Szasz mental illness is the mask that some individuals use to disguise their bad habits.

Concurrently with Meyer, Harry Stack Sullivan, who died a year before Meyer and had a status among many American psychoanalysts equivalent to the position that Meyer had among American psychiatrists, evolved his own understanding of the dynamics of schizophrenia.[46] Sullivan abandoned the drive-repression theories of Freud, and saw the development of schizophrenia in the interpersonal sphere. Disease results from faulty interpersonal relationships rather than the repression of drives. Sullivan, like Meyer, studied schizophrenia in an asylum setting; it led him, however, unlike Meyer, to evolve a truly psychodynamic definition of the disease. Basing his view on the work of Bleuler and Freud, Sullivan saw the disease as organized around a framework of interpersonal dynamics. In many ways Sullivan began the twentieth-century interest in the role of the family in the genesis of schizophrenia. The creation of the schizophrenic personality happens (as Meyer observed) over the course of the individual's development, but, rather than resulting from the inability of the individual to deal with the faulty habits (or repressed drives) that arise with intrapersonal development, the schizophrenic personality results from the patient's response to the "reflected appraisals" coming from the parents. If a child is exposed to "uncanny" experiences, resulting from poor care, a tension state occurs which is internalized as the sense of the "bad" self. This tension, which may be repressed, surfaces in the first stage of the disease and results in the collapse of the personality. He writes in 1924 that the regression:

> to genetically older thought processes—to infantile or even prenatal mental functions—[attempts] successfully to reintegrate masses of life experiences which had failed of structuralization into a functional unity, and [which] finally led by that very lack of structuralization to multiple dissociations in the field of relationship of the individual not only to external reality, including the social milieu, but to his personal identity.[47]

Sullivan, like Bleuler, sees schizophrenia as primarily a disorder of thought processes. But Sullivan stresses the origin of the disease in the life history of the patient rather than attributing it to a specific etiology. Thus he set the stage for the later theories of R. D. Laing.

Like Freud, Sullivan relied on the subjective perception of the patient as the determinant of the structure of the disease. Indeed, one of the richest sources for our understanding of Sullivan's work is his cases, not retrospectively compiled by him but recorded as a dynamic process and then published. According to Sullivan's concept of schizophrenia the dissolution of the initial experiences of the patient had to be undertaken by a participant analyst rather than by a merely passive one. But for this the language of the patient had to be understood, as well as respected. Sullivan distinguished between thought processes and the social or communicative device of language. He sees in the language of the schizophrenic the magical, autistic language of childhood. Sullivan's views on the language of the schizophrenic paralleled the increasing interest in the language of psychopathology.

The work of Kurt Goldstein was initially on brain-damaged patients; then, in a seminal volume (to which Sullivan also contributed) on the language and thought of the schizophrenic edited by J. S. Kasanin (1944), he applied his earlier model to discussions of the schizophrenic's loss of the "abstract attitude" of thought and language.[48] In that same volume a classic paper by E. von Domarus postulated schizophrenic language as a regression to a "paralogical" stage of thought (parallel to Jung's search for a paralogical set of universals in the thought and language of the schizophrenic).[49]

These two views, that the language of the schizophrenic reflected either earlier stages of social development or a pre-logical state of language, manifest the influence of L. S. Vygotsky, whose ideas on concretization of schizophrenic language were introduced into the English-speaking world by E. Hanfmann and J. S. Kasinin in 1936.[50] Vygotsky, using an object-sorting test, saw a parallel between the concept formation of normal adolescents and adult schizophrenics in the manner by which they grouped objects. They shared a set of "pseudo-concepts" that are used inconsistently, relying on an incomplete or incorrect sense of the meaning of the concept. Schizophrenics are, according to those interested in their language, merely incomplete adults—flawed, as are adolescents.

Thus Sullivan continued to associate schizophrenia with its nineteenth-century origin in the debate about age-specific definitions of disease. In his *Conceptions of Modern Psychiatry* (1953) Sullivan qualifies his postulate that schizophrenia is a result of early childhood experiences.[51] He returns to the view that this disruption can take place during adolescence as well. The individual who is constantly rebuffed during this period, whose character is formed through a series of negative experiences, can become just as disordered as the infant rejected by its mother. Adolescence like childhood a fragile state of development, is perceived by Sullivan as a point at which the individual is potentially endangered. The result of the disease is a return to the infantile (or adolescent) state, at which point the roots of the disease had established themselves. This view, expressed as early as his first paper (1924) on the topic of schizophrenia, stressed the relation between symptoms and early developmental errors. But linked to this understanding of the relation between adolescence and illness is yet another echo of past views. For in this paper Sullivan states "that there is a hereditary predisposition to the schizophrenic dissociation." Thus, while Sullivan stresses the interpersonal error that results in the disease, the fact that any number of individuals could have experienced similar maltreatment and not have become schizophrenic is accounted for by some type of genetic predisposition.

It is in the work of Frieda Fromm-Reichmann that the concept of schizophrenia suspended between the world of Freud and Sullivan is most elegantly revised.[52] She traces the etiology of the disease in the "schizophrenogenic" parent (specifically the mother) and the course of the disease as a regression to an earlier period to find an autistic sense of security. Her work reflects Sullivan's view that the schizophrenic is indeed capable of forming a transference. The patient, while desiring contact, seems to withdraw from it, signifying a basic hostility. This hostility is mirrored in the transference. The image of a positive outcome in the disease, indeed the myth of a necessarily positive development through the model of schizophrenia offered by Sullivan and Fromm-Reichmann, had its apotheosis in Hannah Green's novel and the resultant film *I Never Promised You a Rose Garden* (1964), which chronicles a therapy for the treatment of schizophrenia at Chestnut Lodge Sanatorium in Washington, D.C.[53] It was here that the family of the schizophrenic became the subject of study (as later, at R. D. Laing's Kingsley Hall). The novel and the film had a remarkable role in altering the popular concept of schizophrenia with its image of a negative outcome and, indeed, linking it to an image of a positive outcome.

In the work of the British object-relations school of psychoanalysis around Melanie Klein, the evolution of Freudian (or at least neo-Freudian) concepts continued in a quite different direction.[54] Indeed, the entire evolution of object-relations theory concerning schizophrenia provides a case study for the extraordinary diversity of views within a single "school" of thought, itself rooted in one aspect of Freud's theories. For Klein's views expanded the dialogue concerning the etiology of schizophrenia in early life experience and its dynamic recapitulation of these experiences in the disease process. Although some of the members of this "school" stress the primacy of repression (as does Klein) while others (such as W. R. D. Fairbairn, D. W. Winnicott, and Harry Guntrip in Britain, and in the United States Otto Kernberg) stress the interpersonal nature of the etiology of the disease, all center their views on the earliest stages of infancy. Klein sees the schizophrenic as rooted in the "paranoid-schizoid" stage of infantile development, situated during the first three months after birth as the infant "splits" its focus, creating an idealized "good" object in the world through the projection of its own libido and a "bad" object, projected onto the denying mother. In normal development, the "good" fantasies dominate; in the abnormal (schizophrenic), the "bad" dominate, owing to the presence of a nongratifying mother. This view is picked up by Gregory Bateson in a series of articles on the mode of transmission of the sense of distance from the nongratifying mother to the infant, a mode that Bateson labels the "double bind."[55] Klein sees in the anxieties produced in the infant the source (and the parallel) to the later symptomatology of the schizophrenic. She extrapolates the existence of "pathological envy" as part of this modality.

Within the Kleinian school, the model of schizophrenia quickly assumed the central focus for the study of all psychopathology. Specifically, W. R. D. Fairbairn saw schizophrenia, or at least the "schizoid personality structure," as the basis of all psychopathology.[56] For Fairbairn the infantile "ego" (actually a version of Freud's libido) searches for objects in reality. The dynamics of human development are thus always set in relation to external realities, as these realities reinforce or deprive the infantile ego. The external objects must remain "good" and are internalized. Fairbairn sees the development of the individual in three stages: infantile dependence, with its identification through the internalization of the object; a transitional stage (adolescence), in which the struggle for autonomy is undertaken; and the final stage of maturity, with its differentiation between the self and the other. The fixation at either the earliest stage or the transitional stage is due to the actual (rather than fantasized) relationship with the mother.

D. W. Winnicott's views parallel these issues.[57] He stresses the ability to draw the line between the sense of self and the image of the other. For Winnicott, however, the source of the infant's anxiety is the sense of the potential destruction of the self. This view, which is rooted in Klein's understanding of the source of infantile anxiety, is in direct contrast to the interactional model postulated by Sullivan (and later Bateson and Laing). For Winnicott the "good enough" mother is sufficient to shield the infant from this overwhelming sense of its own fragility.

R. D. Laing, whose work spawned a cult of the "schizophrenic as victim," is rooted very much in the tradition of seeing the schizophrenic as the result of a long process of pathology, in which the patient played a basically marginal role.[58] Laing's theories, while contemporary with the work of the object-relations theorists, are much more concerned with the family structure as the source of pathology. His work, beginning with *The Divided Self* (1959), stressed the "mystification" within families that rely on the denial of the experience of one of its members in order to preserve the sense of control.[59] In calling his work "the divided self," Laing reinterprets the implications of *"schizo–phrenia,"* which by the 1960s had ceased to be a technical term. While Bleuler had introduced the term to stress the fragmentation of mental functions, Laing anglicized it to remove it from the jargon of medical science (as employed in popular usage) and stressed the "splitting" of the object. Thus the term *schizophrenia*, which initially had reference to the damaged language of the patient, came to imply a sense of "truthfulness" in the communication of the schizophrenic, at least in regard to the illness being a statement on the damaged world in which the patient developed. A cult of the "schizophrenic as seer" evolved from Laing's work—both indirectly, as in a series of novels and plays about the inner world of the schizophrenic (such as Heinar Kipphardt's *März*), and in the work of Laing's collaborators, such as Joseph Berke and his "pet" patient Mary Barnes.[60] The image of the schizophrenic as artist which dominates the discourse of both Berke's account of Mary Barnes's therapy and her own self-image (clearly patterned after her analyst's expectations) relates both to the older, romantic image of the mad as creative individuals and to the newer image of the "schizophrenic as seer." The schizophrenic sees differently, but more incisively, into the confusions of the world and can reproduce this sense of confusion in works of expressive quality. That Mary Barnes was most probably not schizophrenic, even by Laing's broad definition, but rather mimicking her brother's schizophrenic symptoms has been suggested.[61] Nevertheless, Laing's view dominated the popular understanding of the illness during the 1960s.

Laing's work must be understood within the greater context of the "adolescent" model for the disease. Even though Sullivan had stressed the "interpersonal" nature of the origin of the disease, it was only in the 1950s that concentrated effort was focused on the families of the schizophrenic. Carried out at Yale (under the leadership of Theodore Lidz), the National Institute of Mental Health in Washington (under the leadership of Lyman C. Wynne), and Stanford (under the leadership of Gregory Bateson), these studies attempted to place the disease within the family as an illness of development.[62] Lidz centered on the question of the emotional instability of the family of the schizophrenic and the parents' orientation toward their own family of origin.[63] It is the family that fails to provide the necessary support structure during development, providing instead faulty models of identification.

The child is placed by the family in a "double bind" situation (as Bateson labeled it). The parent expresses two orders of messages simultaneously which, however, contradict one another (e.g., the baby is brought lovingly to the breast, at which point the mother recoils from the baby's touch). The disease is thus viewed as part of a pathological family structure of which the individual labeled "schizophrenic" is but the victim.

Wynne's work began with an eye toward the organization of such family roles.[64] He outlined the pattern of relationships among the members of the patient's family. Based on an understanding of the nature of development as contradictory—moving both toward the establishment of individual identity and toward relating with other individuals, Wynne sees three possible models for human interaction: mutual, nonmutual, and pseudo-mutual. It is the "pseudo-mutual" category that for Wynne serves as the basis for the schizophrenic personality, revealing a faulty sense of interpersonal relationship. Thus the schizophrenic's family is highly rigid and completely determined by assigned roles. Wynne then turned to a series of studies (together with Margaret Singer) to show the link between patterns of family structure and schizophrenic thought disorder.[65] They found that the patterns of interaction within the schizophrenic's family were determined by erratic and inappropriate types of distance and closeness, a sense of meaninglessness and emptiness, as well as a consistent denial of reality. During the 1970s Wynne turned to the question of the genetic and biochemical basis of schizophrenia, a shift that seems to parallel the general fascination with the biological model during the late twentieth century.[66] The implications of this model and the research undertaken to support it will form the final section in our history of the concept of schizophrenia.

The Genetics and Biology of Schizophrenia

The 1970s saw the virtual abandonment of innovative interest in psychoanalytic and family theorizing on the etiology of schizophrenia.[67] Freud's theories became more the subject of literary and historical interest and less the impetus for further work on the nature and origin of the psychoses. This change in direction was due in no little part to the dominance of the biological model for the definition of disease in general and the need felt on the part of the psychiatric community to situate itself within the "mainstream" of the Western medical model.[68] A general sense of the "decline" of psychoanalysis set in, echoed by the popular press, and there was a renewed interest in the biology of schizophrenia, reinforced by the patterns of research funding in the United States and Great Britain. This general social trend, coupled with a fairly idealized understanding of the nature of genetics as the antithesis of "nurture" theories of illness, placed biological schizophrenia research, which had been conducted in parallel with development of psychoanalytic models, in the center of late twentieth-century concerns.

Two major questions were raised within this research: the first related to the role genetics had in the transmission of the disease, the second to the actual biochemistry of schizophrenia.[69] While neither necessitated an understanding of the other, the two aspects of the "biology" of schizophrenia became linked in many attempts to reconceptualize (or "rescue") schizophrenia from the dominant psychoanalytic model. But as we have seen, the "psychoanalytic" model in all its diversity was itself never totally free from a biological component. For in the early theories of dementia praecox (in Kraepelin, Freud, and Sullivan, for example) there was always an assumption that there was a constitutional factor in the disease. It was with the epidemiological work of the father of psychiatric genetics, Ernst Rüdin, who assembled statistical evidence for advocating the eugenic sterilization of schizophrenics, that this approach began to achieve some type of scientific predominance.[70] Rüdin, however, as early as 1916 noted that any simple pattern of "dominant" or "recessive" genetic transmission (founded on the somewhat primitive Mendelian model available to him) could not explain the patterns of occurrence.

The basic work on this question, work that dominated the German- as well as the English-language scholarship, was the studies of schizophrenic twins undertaken by one of Rüdin's students, Franz Kallmann.[71] As late as 1983, Kallmann's "twin study" was cited in Harry Munsinger's *Principles of Abnormal Behavior* as *the* historic study of the incidence of schizophrenia.[72] In Kallmann's work many of the fundamental problems associated with the ideology of genetic studies of pathology (or indeed, of the "normal" as in Cyril Burt's I.Q. studies) can be examined.

Based on a detailed statistical analysis of the family histories of schizophrenics from 1893–1902 (comprising a huge sample of 1,087 schizophrenics and 12,777 of their relatives), Kallmann concluded in 1938, shortly after he was forced to leave Nazi Germany because of his "racial" identity, that there was a substantially greater risk of the disease reappearing within these families than appearing in other groups.[73] To sharpen his focus he began to limit his sample only to twins in order to measure the genetic predisposition for the syndrome. In 1946 Kallmann reported his first twin study, a survey of 691 pairs of twins, of which 174 were monozygotic. Kallmann's total pool of information extended to the relatives of these twins, so that he had information on 5,804 subjects.[74] Kallmann's study revealed that if one member of a pair of identical twins was schizophrenic, there was approximately an 86-percent chance that the sibling would also be impaired, while there seemed to be only a 15-percent chance of fraternal twins both manifesting the illness. The figures also revealed that if both of the parents were schizophrenic, there was a 68-percent chance of the child being impaired. Since there was not a higher concordance between inheritance and illness, Kallmann suggested that the transmission of schizophrenia was caused by a single recessive gene together with specific (but multifaceted) constitutional factors. Thus all schizophrenics had this recessive gene, but not all of those who possessed the gene became schizophrenic. This factor would account for the discordant 40 percent of identical twins of whom at least one sibling did not become schizophrenic.

Kallmann's study "proved" to a large number of researchers that there was indeed a recessive gene that was directly responsible for the disease. Two major questions have recently been asked of Kallmann's research.[75] The first has to do with the relationship between the twins. Since there was no independent verification of their relationship, it could well be that the figures reflected a set of biases of the informants. Parents or siblings would repress the actual nature of the relationship between the siblings, if there was a greater chance of the non-schizophrenic child's being stigmatized as at risk. More important, there is the question of the definition of *schizoid* in Kallmann's work. He never provided a clear definition of his diagnostic criteria, observing only that schizophrenics are "an unceasing source of maladjusted cranks, asocial eccentrics and the lowest type of criminal offenders." His answer to the definition question is found in the ideological association of the study of genetics and the eugenics movement: "In this way psychiatry would accomplish its part in making the biological quality of future generations an important matter for medical concern and activity, by decreasing not only the number of schizophrenic patients, but also the number of heterozygotic taint-carriers, such as schizoid eccentrics, criminal adventurers or other members of the lunatic fringe."[76] For Kallmann social behavior and therefore social control were the determinants for the definition of the schizophrenic.

The problems raised by Kallmann's study, and by the later attempts to see the perceived patterns of schizophrenia occurring within families, are evident. While later researchers, such as Böök, followed through Kallmann's views with some variations, it was in the so-called "Danish twin" study, which began in 1962 and was headed by Seymour S. Kety, that the most conclusive proof of a genetic predisposition was thought to be found.[77] These studies have been pointed to over and over again as "proof" of the genetic basis of the disease. The researchers traced the relatives of a group of hospitalized schizophrenics who had been adopted as children. They then compiled a parallel control group of individuals matching the psychiatric patients who had never been hospitalized. A detailed search of the Danish records was undertaken to compile a family psychiatric history of each group. Records were found on 150 relatives of the 34 index cases and on 156 relatives of the control group. It was discovered that there was a substantially greater relation between the occurrence of the disease in the index group and its relatives. Indeed, 8.7

percent of the relatives of the index group showed impairment, while only 1.9 percent of the relatives of the control group did. Again the figures seemed to indicate the absolute genetic determinism of the illness. In point of fact, Kety's study so expanded the definition of schizophrenia (to include such diagnoses as "inadequate personality," for example) that no true correlation could be shown. Recently it has been argued that the social placement of these children may well have played a role in the appearance of the disease, as the Danish placement structure tended to match socioeconomic backgrounds when referring children to potential adoptive parents.[78] It should also be noted that although Kallmann found a much higher incidence of the occurrence of the disease (a fact that Kety criticized), the problem of definition haunts his work as well. "Absolute" relations between illness and inheritance depend on the definition of the illness.

The inability to pinpoint the "schizophrenic gene" led some researchers to seek a model that proposes the liability for schizophrenia, rather than the disease itself, as inherited. The work of P. E. Meehl is typical of this search.[79] He sees schizophrenia as the social result of the existence of an inherited neural deficit. Thus the illness has a somatic cause but manifests itself over time. Such attempts to span the "nature-nurture" division cannot be shown to be accurate until the reality of the "neural deficit" can be proven.

In the history of the concept of schizophrenia, the belief that there must be some constitutional cause for the disease becomes closely linked to the mechanisms by which the disease is produced. As early as Kraepelin's belief that dementia praecox was a metabolic disorder, there has been a desire to pinpoint the mechanism by which the symptoms are generated, even if no firm etiology could be found. The discovery of a specific enzyme deficiency, caused by a specific gene, as the etiology of phenylketonuria in 1934 provided another historical model (analogous to the influence of the model of the general paralysis of the insane on late nineteenth-century theories of dementia praecox). Indeed, the power of this model was such that even Kraepelin's metabolic theory was countered completely only with the work of S. S. Kety, who in 1969 argued that the metabolic errors found in schizophrenics were artifacts of the poor diet and lack of exercise of the asylum setting.[80] Similarly, the identification of a schizophrenic body type (the domination of the "pyknic" type) by researchers such as Kretschmer and Sheldon may well have its roots in the sequelae of asylum life rather than in the nature of the disease process.[81]

The irony is that while there was an attempt to follow through with the assumption, rooted in the very core of the concept of schizophrenia, that the illness has some type of genetic mode of transmission as well as

228

a specific somatic presentation, it was in the practical question of treatment that one of the most startling indicators of the somatic basis of the disease was found. (The importance of this discovery lies in the fact that the somatic roots of the disease may reveal the mechanism by which the genetic error causes the symptoms.) It was found that antipsychotic neuroleptics had an effect on the presentation of the symptoms associated with schizophrenia. The reason was the subject of much speculation. Earlier theories of a fault in brain chemistry, such as Osmond and Smythies's proposal that schizophrenia was the result of an error in the metabolism of the neurotransmitter norepinephrine, had had a specific cultural dimension.[82]

With the rise of the "drug" cult after World War II and the introduction of LSD (lysergic acid diethylamide) and other hallucinogenic drugs such as amphetamine, atebrin, and mescaline as cult drugs, the possibility of establishing a biochemical error as the root of schizophrenia was raised. The similarity between the chemical configuration of LSD and the methylated derivatives of neurotransmitters even led the form to be labeled "psychotomimetic," as if the hallucinogens were producing psychological states identical to schizophrenia. Later work, influenced by R. D. Laing's views of the "prophetic" aspects of the disease and linked with the cultic aspects of LSD use, led to the view that the body produced its own endogenous hallucinogens as a means of escaping the conflicts of family and the confines of society. The search for this endogenous hallucinogen moved from norepinephrine to the metabolism of serotonin, again because of the supposed similarity between known hallucinogens (such as bufotenine) and serotonin.[83]

Studies of brain chemistry during the 1960s, which ignored brain structure and concentrated on the biochemistry of the brain, proposed other errors as the root of schizophrenia. There was interest in the catecholamines, specifically in the presence of DMPEA (3,4-dimethoxphenylethylamine) found in the urine of an index group of schizophrenics (but not in the urine of a control group).[84] Again, what seemed to be a specific quality of the biochemistry of schizophrenia revealed itself to be an artifact of hospitalization. For the index group was not on a controlled diet, and the biochemistry of their urine reflected this fact rather than any specific metabolic error in the group. Indeed, studies that attempted to correct for this biochemical error in the patient population showed that even with additives being given to supplement the "missing" biochemical factors, there was no change in behavior.[85] Later studies that attempted to correct for the discrepancy in diet brought the entire theory further into question.[86] In fact, Lewontin, Rose, and Kamin characterize the search for the schizophrenic gene and the apparent discovery of schizophrenic urine as a reductionist search for the holy grail of the disease, for the simple and direct answer that will provide a unified field theory for the disease. Many other such reductionist theories have been offered: Stein and Wise's 6-Hydroxydopamine hypothesis, which links the disease to specific neural systems; Murphy and Wyatt's theory of lowered monoamine oxidase activity; Heath's theory of the existence of an abnormal blood protein, taraxein, in schizophrenics.[87]

None of these has proven to be the single answer. And the difficulty inherent in this reductionist position, given the protean nature of the various concepts of schizophrenia, is evident. Manfred Bleuler, the son of Eugen Bleuler and a major researcher of the nature of schizophrenia in his own right, observed that the very definition of schizophrenia, as a "natural process" of disintegration, causes the contemporary scientist to avoid confronting the essence of the syndrome and flee into the search for other, less frightening, explanations.[88] Indeed, it is this fear of the amorphous nature of the disease, of the schizophrenic process, which drives the biological scientist to evolve a specific, limited (and limiting) understanding of the disease.

The complexity of the psychological presentation of the disease, its shifting from age to age in terms of its manifestations, does not lend itself quite as simply to such a reductionist approach. But, as we have seen, the most "scientific" conceptualizations of the disease have always reflected the intellectual and cultural presuppositions of their age. In our times, so dominated by the biological model with its one-to-one relation between cause and effect, it is no little wonder that such views have come to hold center stage.

I began my history of the concept of schizophrenia with the caveat that I was going to sketch how a group of blind fakirs saw that elephant they all agreed was called "schizophrenia." Each described the part that he grasped and could not understand how the others could be so foolish as to fail to perceive their own segments in the same manner. Sadly, when we look at the various descriptions and theories of schizophrenia, it is clear that no elephant can be constructed from the often contradictory views proposed and held. Rather there is a dialectic at work in the construction of the disease concept. Theories react to other theories and to the position of various models in the culture of a specific place and time. No composite theory of schizophrenia can be proposed and perhaps none will even be generated, certainly not one that will unify all of the views discussed here. Thus the best we can do is to understand how the various concepts have evolved historically—and how, on one level or another, they relate to each other.

CHAPTER THIRTEEN

Seeing the Schizophrenic:
On the "Bizarre" in Psychiatry and Art

We have now seen how the general category of "schizophrenia" was constructed over a period of almost a hundred and fifty years. The close relation between external forces and our fantasies about disease is evident. What may not be so evident is how closely the discourse about schizophrenia is linked to the aesthetic discourses existing in our culture. For Western culture understands disease, even mental illness, in aesthetic terms. Our discourse about the ugly is also our discourse about disease.

When we address the question "How do psychiatrists write about their patients' illnesses?" we can gather some sense of the complex link between the image of disease and the language of aesthetics. It is clear that little attention has been paid to the vocabulary applied to psychopathologies by contemporary psychiatry. Although some interest has been shown in the signifiers of psychiatric nosology, only Michel Foucault has examined the roots of the vocabulary in which the various nosological categories are expressed.[1] As he indicated, the inherent structures of the nosological systems in medicine are determined to no small degree by the clinical vocabulary. In studying how psychiatrists perceive and represent their patients, especially within the published literature on mental illness, we can document their underlying presuppositions concerning mental illness and the nature of the patient. These presuppositions are found often to contradict the practitioner's own expressed intent.

Bizarre, the term taken from the language of aesthetics which serves as the focus of this chapter, seems at first glance to be outside the "scientific" vocabulary of modern psychiatry. And yet, when the history of this term is examined within the context of twentieth-century discussions of schizophrenia, it becomes clear that the term has acquired a specific significance in the debates concerning the nature of the disease. This is not to say that *bizarre* was not a term applied to mental illness before the fin-de-siècle debate about schizophrenia between Emil Kraepelin and Eugen Bleuler. Indeed, B. A. Morel, best known for his formulation of the concept of "degeneracy," wrote an essay on "general considerations of the eccentricities, bizarreness of the character and taste, and violent passions, in regard to madness" in 1853.[2] But it has been only in the twentieth-century context of clinical psychiatry that the term *bizarre* has acquired a complex function as a signifier. Morel's general usage gave way in the course of this century to a specific set of meanings that qualified the language production of those patients diagnosed as "schizophrenic." The application of the term *bizarre* to the classification of one aspect of schizophrenia did not, however, imply that this quality was pathognomonic. The very use of this term, in fact, reflected the debate over the nature of the disruption of communicative functions in schizophrenia.

Bizarre as a Technical Term in Psychiatry: An Objective Quality of Schizophrenia

In the second draft of the *Diagnostic and Statistical Manual of the American Psychiatric Association (DSM-III-R)*, which appeared in August 1986, schizophrenia was described as characterized by "bizarre delusions (i.e., involving a phenomenon that the individual's subculture would regard as totally implausible, e.g., through broadcasting, being controlled by a dead person)."[3] These delusions were one of the necessary symptoms for the diagnosis of the disorder. In the earlier (1980) edition of *DSM-III*, which the 1986 draft intended to improve, the "content of thought" in schizophrenic patients was described as evidencing "delusions that are often multiple, fragmented, or bizarre (i.e., patently absurd, with no possible basis in fact)."[4] Whereas the qualities of "multiplicity" and "fragmentation" are left undefined, the authors of this entry found it necessary to limit the meaning of the "bizarre" in the nature of the delusional systems of the schizophrenic. The major difference between these two statements is the authors' attempt in the revised draft to contextualize the quality of the "bizarre," labeling it as an artifact of the culture in which the patient resides. This is a major shift to an understanding that bizarreness is a culturally determined quality of perception (and stigmatization) and not a universal of human understanding.

The first published draft version of *DSM-III* had left all three terms undefined.[5] However, the official *Case Book* as well as the *Quick Reference to the Diagnostic Criteria from DSM–III* both listed "bizarre delusions" as the *first* diagnostic criteria for schizophrenia.[6] Although it should in no way be understood as an exclusive or pathognomonic sign for this illness, its presence in all of the standard definitions of schizophrenia does give the term *bizarre* the strength of a major signifier. The term *bizarre* has had a long history within the official terminology of American psychiatry. *DSM-I,* published in 1952, applied it to the quality of the communicative structure of "schizo-affective" disorders which "may show predominantly affective changes with schizophrenic-like thinking or bizarre behavior."[7] *DSM-II* (1968) employed *bizarre* to categorize the behavior of schizophrenics in general.[8] Although the movement from "bizarre behavior" to "bizarre delusions" may seem substantial, the adjective was still used within the phenomenology of schizophrenic communicative structures, whether kinetic (behavior in the observable sense) or semantic (the presentation of systematic delusions through written or spoken language).

Parallels to the application of the term *bizarre* to the communicative aspects of schizophrenia can be found in an extensive range of methodological traditions in twentieth-century psychiatry. In his 1932 essay on the artistic production of schizophrenics, Hans Bürger-Prinz described the character of the schizophrenic thought process as containing a "richness of bizarre notions."[9] Walter Benjamin, the Marxist critic who collected, among other things, psychopathological literary products, employed the same phraseology when in 1928 he described the content of such works as "bizarre."[10]

The German tradition of the clinical use of the concept "bizarre" was transplanted to the United States when Bleuler's classic monograph on schizophrenia appeared in English. Bleuler had, of course, emphasized the primacy of the thought disorder in clinically defining schizophrenia. He had, however, defined the nature of the thought disruption as *ungewöhnlich*, "unusual."[11] In the extraordinarily influential English translation this became "bizarre."[12] Thus, for example, when Carney Landis wished to characterize schizophrenic thought processes, he simply cited Bleuler's categories and labeled the thinking of the schizophrenic as "illogical, confused, bizarre."[13] Bleuler's influence on American clinical definitions of schizophrenia is wide-ranging. David Forrest, in an insightful essay on the phenomenology of schizophrenic language published in the 1960s, characterized the "flight of ideas, self-references, neologisms and idiosyncratic associations" as "bizarre."[14] Harold J. Vetter described the delusional structure of paranoid schizophrenia as "highly fantastic, . . . inconsistent, illogical, bizarre, with a good deal of mysticism, persecutory and grandiose notions, and various hallucinations."[15] Silvano

Arieti also labeled the loosened associations of the schizophrenic thought process as "bizarre."[16] In Freedman, Kaplan, and Sadock's basic textbook of psychiatry, the definition of schizophrenia includes the observation that "one of the most characteristic features . . . is the pronounced symbolism expressed in the patient's often bizarre behavior, ideation, and speech."[17]

This Bleulerian view runs through much of modern clinical psychiatry, including the work of some of the formulators of the *DSM-III* definition of schizophrenic delusional structures, such as Nancy Andreasen.[18] Their view is that the key to the nature of schizophrenia is inherent in the nature of the alteration of communicative structures, what Bleuler called the "altered simple function" of "association." But even non-Bleulerian psychiatrists have adopted the label "bizarre" for a quality of that illness called "schizophrenia." Richard Hunter and Ida Macalpine, in their major revisionist essay on the Schreber case, published in 1953, described Schreber's delusions as "bizarre or grotesque."[19] At the other extreme, in his programmatic volume *The Divided Self*, R. D. Laing characterized the socialization of the schizophrenic as "merely a trick, a technique. His own view of things, the meaning they have for him, his feeling, his expression, are now likely to be at least odd and eccentric, if not bizarre and crazy."[20]

The use of *bizarre* to describe a quality of schizophrenic thought and communicative disorders places this term within a wide range of related terms: *fragmented, absurd, illogical, confused, fantastic, grandiose, grotesque, eccentric, and crazy.* But *bizarre* more than all others maintained itself within the vocabulary applied to the nature of schizophrenia. Indeed, by the late 1970s *bizarre* became a code word in discussing schizophrenia. Stephen Gerson, Frank Benson, and Shervert Frazier, in a widely cited essay following up earlier work by Kurt Schneider, characterized the major difference between schizophrenia and posterior aphasia as "bizarre themes . . . present in schizophrenia but absent in posterior aphasia."[21] A central quality of the language products of the schizophrenic is their "bizarre" content, and it alone is sufficient to distinguish schizophrenia from other communicative disorders.

The Bizarre Perception of Schizophrenia

Since as early as 1940, when L. Kerschbaumer's essay "Poetry in Schizophrenia and Other Psychoses" was published, there has been a parallel tradition of labeling the perception of schizophrenic language production as "bizarre." It is not the language itself, but the incongruity between it and the listener's (or reader's) expectations which causes the sense of the "bizarre." Kerschbaumer, a Viennese psychiatrist in exile in the United States, wrote that poetry in most psychoses, neuroses, and psychopathies does not necessarily appear "mental," whereas in schizophrenia, with perhaps the exclusion of the very early stage, creative output, be it poetry or drawing, is experienced as "abnormal"—queer, odd, fantastic, bizarre, freakish—even by the inexperienced.[22] In Wilhelm Mayer-Gross's textbook of psychiatry, which holds the same position in Great Britain as Freedman, Kaplan, and Sadock's does in the United States, this tradition is continued. Mayer-Gross also sees this alienation of the "normal" from the "abnormal" in the reaction of the non-schizophrenic toward the patient and his or her utterances, ideas, and actions. The words *queer, bizarre,* and *absurd (verschroben, zerfahren,* and *verrückt* are some equivalents in German) are used to convey it.[23] The term *bizarre,* then, becomes the label used to describe the neutral observer's own reaction to the language of the schizophrenic. This may seem to be a continuation of the initial category of the use of *bizarre* as a means of labeling the innate quality of schizophrenic language. But, in fact, it shifts the ground of this category, placing the emphasis on the reception of this language.

The "bizarre" sense in the observer of the schizophrenic has been seen as resulting from what has come to be labeled the "praecox feeling," a term coined by H. C. Rümke. Rümke observed that as a diagnostician he is "guided by the 'praecox feeling' which arises in the examiner, or perhaps the 'praecox experience,' for it is no true feeling. Only highly experienced psychiatrists can employ this compass." For him the observation of the psychopathology is central to the diagnostic experience: "In Athens and in Helsinki, in Paris and in London, in Mexico City and in Toronto we meet with the same 'genuine schizophrenes,' often recognizable at a glance."[24] W. Th. Winkler has attributed this awareness to a specific type of countertransference inherent in the syndrome of schizophrenia, a countertransference that relies on earlier subjective contact between the diagnostician and other schizophrenics.[25] And, in his study of transference and countertransference, U. H. Peters has emphasized that the praecox feeling is not an emotional reaction to the patient but rather is rooted in the "nonrational" memory of the psychiatrist.[26] These views of the praecox feeling stress that it is the application of a diagnostic label based on cumulative experience in observing schizophrenics. That this feeling is the result of the interpretation of phenomenological clues may be the source of Peters's observation that the more one knows the patient, the less reliable is the praecox feeling as an indicator of schizophrenia, for the accumulation of other data will tend to mask the initial impression of a psychopathology.

The nature of the impression made on the observer is qualified as "bizarre" and is placed in a similar semantic field to that of the objective qualification of schizophrenic communicative disorders. Here, the reaction of the observer to the schizophrenic's communicative structure is "abnormal," "queer," "odd," "fantastic," "freakish," "absurd," or "bizarre." These are not the objective qualities of the schizophrenic but rather of the "praecox feeling."

A Faulty Label for Schizophrenic Communicative Disorders

Although the rejection of Kraepelin's labeling of the products of schizophrenic language as "word-salad" appears to be post-Laingian, Laing's views are but the most recent articulation of an earlier tradition. The view that the language of the schizophrenic possesses the potential for interpretation reaches back to the early twentieth-century reevaluation of the role of language in schizophrenia by Freud and Bleuler. Typical of the psychiatrists who rejected the concept of "word-salad" was William A. White, who as early as 1928 dismissed such labeling of schizophrenic language:

> In the past, the language of the schizophrenic patient, because of its frequently bizarre and incoherent aspects, was supposed to correspond to thought processes that were similarly bizarre, meaningless and incoherent. It has been only in recent years, since the comparative method has come to be applied in psychopathology and since the surface of thought has not been accepted as final for its structure, any more than the surface of the body has been considered as offering a full explanation of its anatomy, that there has arisen an appreciation that what may appear to be without meaning may, as a matter of fact, be full of meaning. The language of the psychoses and its interpretation is not without analogy to the inscriptions of unknown languages and their final translations.[27]

The sense that the language of the schizophrenic is merely discourse on another plane rather than confused or disrupted discourse is to be found throughout the 1940s and 1950s. Widely cited papers, such as that by E. von Domarus on schizophrenic logic (1939), assumed that rules for understanding schizophrenic language could be generated.[28] Much as Michael Ventris had deciphered the hidden language of Linear B, so too could the psychiatrist or linguist find the key to the nature of schizophrenic language production, and communication would be reestablished. Such interpretation of the term *bizarre* as meaning "incomprehensible" and its subsequent rejection continued throughout the antipsychiatric movement of the 1960s and 1970s.

Sherry Rochester and J. R. Martin begin their *Crazy Talk* with a two-page refutation of the Bleulerian view that loosened associations are mirrored in the "confused and bizarre" flow of thought.[29] Rochester and Martin, like John Neale and Thomas Oltmanns in their parallel study,[30] survey (and subsequently condemn) the theories that hold the nature of the disruption in schizophrenia to be "bizarre." For they take the very term *bizarre* to apply solely to an inherent fault of the thought processes of the schizophrenic (and seem oblivious of the theories that describe the communicative relationship between listener and speaker as "bizarre" or alienated). These two studies, from the late 1970s, continue the attempts to see a parallel but unique structure of communication in schizophrenic speech, only they reject the label of "bizarre" for this parallel linguistic or conceptual world. For Rochester and Martin, as for Neale and Oltmanns, the labeling of schizophrenia, or the group of the schizophrenias, as "bizarre" is closely linked to the perception of the communicative malfunction as the central, indeed, necessary quality of the illness. In their view, the very use of the term *bizarre* places the schizophrenic speaker into a special category, one that is inherently separate from the observer, in terms of the use of language. This ambiguous use of the term *bizarre* is but a reflection of an even more complex web of semantic structures inherent in the word itself.

The Etymology of *Bizarre*

The roots of the word *bizarre* are shrouded in the Etruscan past of ancient Italy.[31] The first modern appearance of the word, however, is most revealing. In the eighth canto of the *Inferno* Dante and Virgil enter the fifth circle. A spirit, covered in the mud of sinful rage, addresses them. It is the spirit of Filippo Argenti degli Adimari of Florence, who had been known for his violent temper:

Whilst we were running through the dead channel there rose before me one full of mud, and said: "Who are thou, that comest before thy time?"

And I to him: "If I come, I remain not; but thou, who art thou, that hast become so foul?" He answered: "Thou seest that I am one who weeps."

And I to him: "With weeping, and with sorrow, accursed spirit, remain thou! for I know thee, all filthy as thou art."

Then he stretched both hands to the boat, whereat the wary Master thrust him off, saying: "Away there with the other dogs!"

And he put his arms about my neck, kissed my face, and said: "Indignant soul! blessed be she that bore thee.

In your world, that was an arrogant personage; good there is none to ornament the memory of him: so is his shadow here in fury.

How many up there now think themselves great kings, that shall lie here like swine in mire, leaving behind them horrible reproaches!"

And I: "Master, I should be glad to see him dipped in this swill, ere we quit the lake."

And he to me: "Before the shore comes to thy view, thou shalt be satisfied; it is fitting that thou shouldst be gratified in such a wish."

A little after this, I saw the muddy people make such rending of him, that even now I praise and thank God for it.

All cried: "At Filippo Argenti!" The *bizarre* Florentine spirit turned with his teeth upon himself.

Here we left him, so that of him I tell no more; but in my ears a wailing smote me, whereat I bent my eyes intently forward.[32]

"Bizarro" is the label Dante gave to that quality which had already been described by Aristotle as psychopathological brutishness of spirit. Filippo Argenti is the choleric madman. This image is codified within Dante's labeling as "bizarre" the icon of the madman devouring himself, the mute image with which Filippo Argenti slips out of sight. This is a traditional image of the madman. It is a gesture that typifies the irrational and inexpressible anger that Seneca ascribed to the madman when he portrayed him as having "a bold and threatening mien, a gloomy brow, a fierce expression, a hurried step, restless hands, an altered color, a quick and more violent breathing."[33] Filippo Argenti's anger ends in inarticulate madness.

The image of inarticulate madness which dominates Dante's understanding of the "bizarre" becomes part of the visual vocabulary of insanity in Europe. Indeed, in the only work of art that can be paralleled to Cibber's statues at Bedlam, the 1686 cornerstone of the asylum at 's-Hertogenbosch, the image of the inarticulate insane is placed opposite that of the madman eating the "bread of iniquity," the medieval icon of sloth (Plate 38). The contrast here is between the active, aggressive, self-destructive madman, the visual icon of Dante's image, and the passive melancholic. The "bizarre" madman is thus on one level the image of the

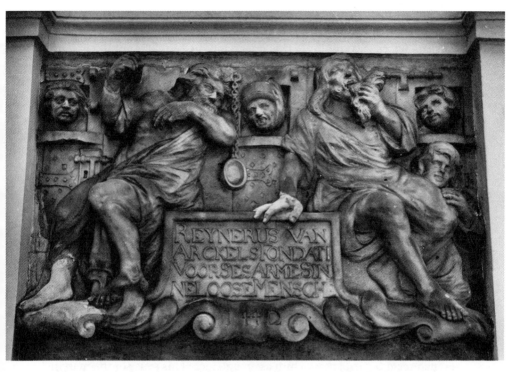

38. The cornerstone of the asylum at 's-Hertogenbosch (1686) (Rijksdienst voor de Monumentenzorg, Zeist, Netherlands).

bestial madman, robbed of speech, able only to consume himself in his rage. When later images of the "bizarre" insane recur, inherent in their subtext is the association with such visual images of bestiality and self-destruction.

In the very use of these images is the representation of the confinement of madness. For such images, at least beginning in the seventeenth century, are associated with images of the asylum. This association continues throughout the eighteenth century, as is testified by the figure of raging madness in Hogarth's *Rake's Progress*. Madness is thus contained within an image that itself represents containment. Dante not only places the inarticulate madman in the inferno but contains him within the slime that represents his mortal sin. When this image of raging madness is transferred to the portal of the Dutch asylum, it is to signify the containment of such madness within the walls of the institution. In this way, from its very inception the association of the idea of madness with the quality of the "bizarre" points to the labeling of madness as contained, as captured within an aesthetic representation of control.

The "bizarre" becomes a code for the representation of the loss of control within strict artistic bounds. Both the frightening quality of the madman and his inarticulateness are captured by Dante's use of the word *bizzaro*. Boccaccio employed this image and the term in a similar manner in the *Decameron*.[34] In the eighth novella of the ninth day, Ciacco uses Filippo Argenti's unreasoning anger and brute strength to avenge himself on his friend Biondello. Here, too, the frightening strength and inarticulate anger of the "bizarre" madman are compassed by Boccaccio's use of this term.

The "bizarre" underwent a transformation in the Renaissance. Giordano Bruno used the term to characterize not only the choleric but also the unique and repulsive.[35] And Lope de Vega added to it the quality of the capricious.[36] The combination of qualities remained throughout the seventeenth century. In the first appearance of the word in German during the seventeenth century, in the comic poetry of Johann Lauremberg, the term is used to characterize the unusual but is made into a sign of the repulsive by being embedded in the mangled German-French of one of the figures.[37] Here the confused, garbled, "bizarre" language traditionally ascribed to the insane became the context for the first use of the word *bizarre* in German. But the figure who uses this word is not mad; he is rather comic by being eccentric, a borderline figure between the linguistic worlds of the "real" languages of German and French. He does not belong to either world, and thus his language (including his use of the French term *bizarre*) marks him as an outsider. This sense of the marginal, eccentric quality of the "bizarre" is found contemporaneously in England in the work of John Dryden.[38]

By the Enlightenment the original meaning of the word with its semantic core of the aggressive and the inarticulate had been overlaid with the sense of the marginal. Traditionally, the marginal within the literary sphere has been represented by the figure of the insane; *bizarre*, from Dante to Dryden, is an aesthetic rather than a scientific term, but included within its semantic field are associations with the insane. With the Enlightenment, in Condillac's *Dictionnaire des synonymes*, the bizarre also becomes part of the discourse of science. Condillac made a logical distinction among the mad (*lunatique*), the fantastic (*fantasque*), the capricious (*capricieux*), and the bizarre (*bizarre*). The bizarre is "that which acts and thinks in an extraordinary manner."[39] This coupling of the bizarre with eccentric thought and action is a continuation of Dante's original paradigm but appears here within the realm of scientific discourse. Thus Condillac's sense of the "bizarre" as the extraordinary continued the older, aesthetic tradition of the eccentric.

By the end of the nineteenth century *bizarre* had become a "scientific" term. As such it bore the stamp of the new and powerful medical discourse that, stemming from the new biology, dominated the century. It was a new discourse of power, represented to no little degree by the ability of the alienist (the physician-psychiatrist) to control the "bizarre." And, coupled with the scientific implication (and power) of psychiatry, the "bizarre" underwent a cultural transvaluation. For the Romantics, the "bizarre," the "extraordinary," came to have a positive connotation. Since Romantic writers saw themselves as consciously marginal, they also proclaimed that their art was "bizarre." As a result, they saw their aesthetic production as sharing the status of the linguistic and artistic productions of that traditional marginal group, the mentally ill, while at the same time they demanded power over their lives and artistic production. The Romantics expropriated *bizarre*, a term associated with mental illness, from the medical sciences of the nineteenth century and returned it, altered and hardly recognizable, to the vocabulary of aesthetics. By the middle of the century the "bizarre" had become the hallmark of creativity, but genius, as the Italian forensic psychiatrist Cesare Lombroso had argued, was but a form of madness. Charles Baudelaire cast this view in positive terms in 1855:

The beautiful is always bizarre. I do not mean that it is deliberately, coldly bizarre, for in that case it would be a monster that has jumped the rails of life. I mean that it always contains a little bizarreness, an artless, unpremeditated, unconscious strangeness, and that it is this strangeness that gives Beauty its specific character. It is its official stamp, its characteristic. Reverse the proposition and try to imagine a commonplace *beauty*! Now, how could this bizarreness—necessary, incompressible, infinitely varied, and determined by milieu, climate, custom, race, religion, and the artist's temperament—ever be controlled, improved, rectified by the Utopian rules that are conceived in some ordinary little scientific temple on this planet, without mortal danger to art itself? This admixture of bizarreness which constitutes and defines individuality, without which there can be no beauty, plays in art the role of taste or of seasoning in foods (may the accuracy of this comparison excuse its triteness), since apart from their usefulness or their nutritional content foods differ from one another through the idea which they reveal to the palate.[40]

Baudelaire's positive use of the term *bizarre* as a means of distinguishing between true and banal art gave the "bizarre" a quality of truth. The real truth of beauty was not the "bizarre" in its eighteenth-century sense, that is, as the unique, the distanced. Rather, the nineteenth-century mind saw the "bizarre" as the wellspring of that greatest truth of art, the expression of the individual rather than the mass psyche. The "bizarre" was seen as transcending all societal laws or rules, containing within itself the laws for its own expression.

When we move from the implications of the word *bizarre* in the general culture to its seemingly contradictory use within twentieth-century psychiatry, certain patterns can be discerned. Central to the idea of the "bizarre" is its original meaning, which referred to the psychopathological alteration of communicative structures. The earliest usages of the word, in Dante and Boccaccio, stress this, and this meaning remains embedded in the history of the word. Present also in its roots is the sense of the "bizarre" as the unique, as the unusual that stands beyond societal norms of expression. In the nineteenth century this quality was given a positive implication. Echoes of all these models are found in modern psychiatry. Disruptions of communication are perceived as inherently "bizarre" if they are seen as placing the patient beyond normal modes of communication.

Even those who attribute the "bizarre" quality of the schizophrenic to his or her perception by the non-schizophrenic incorporate this sense of distance. In refusing to acknowledge the "bizarre," what is rejected is not the sense of the pathological in the alteration of communicative functions, but rather the implication that such alterations produce gibberish. But the "bizarre" is never nonsensical. Rather, it contains within itself the qualities that are ascribed to the schizophrenic, whether or not the term *bizarre* is the appropriate one to describe those illnesses labeled "schizophrenia."[41]

It is not merely within the Bleulerian criteria for the definition of schizophrenia that the language of the schizophrenic can be perceived as "bizarre." One of the most striking qualities ascribed to the stereotype of the "Other" is his or her altered language and behavior. Whether they are perceived as the sympathetic Other or as the fearsome Other, the mad have always been perceived as possessing a special quality of language. Indeed, the very essence of the stereotype of madness can be summarized as a disruption of cognition and language. Whether this disruption is seen as threatening, as prophetic, or merely as inchoate, it is a quality that is inherent to our perception of insanity.

The term *bizarre* is rich enough to be applied in all of these areas. Its protean nature, mirrored in its rich historical past, provides any number of potential qualities for the labeling of schizophrenic language. There is one further ramification inherent in the application of the term *bizarre* to the language of the schizophrenic.

Bizarre is a term from the realm of the aesthetic. It limits the flux of madness to a definable world, that of the mad. The frame for this world is the frame of art. The image that Dante chooses for the representation of the inherent nature of inarticulate madness, of the damaged discourse of the "brutish of spirit," is that of the self-consuming and bizarre madman. This image is located within the world of art, of the *Inferno*. Likewise, when later images of madness label the language of madness as bizarre, they draw a line between their own creation of texts that define madness and mad texts. The line is clear. We, who stand apart from the world and language of the insane, who define ourselves as "mentally healthy," are in no danger of having our language, the language that marks the bounds between ourselves and the insane, labeled as "bizarre." The "bizarre" is precisely the line between our "objective" and "normative" language and the decay into the "monstrous and uncanny," to use Manfred Bleuler's terms.[42] This is an arbitrary line that defines the difference perceived (and represented) between the pathological and the normal.

For Western culture this line is drawn within the text as well as in society when the culture defines the bounds between the observer's stability and the instability of the observed. The vocabulary of psychiatry is but an extension of the common culture. Our Western fascination with the aesthetics of the "bizarre" has provided modern psychiatry with a range of semantic nuances, positive or negative, pejorative or evocative, within which this term is able to categorize the difference of the schizophrenic. All of these meanings center around our perception in the late twentieth century of the centrality of language in defining the essence of madness.

But this is an attempt to comprehend the complexity of a disease (in the sense of the social manifestation of an illness) through the implied centrality of one of its manifestations. The language of madness has long held center stage as that quality of the insane which defines madness in and of itself. From the inarticulate anger of Dante's madman, through the incorporation of this icon as the literal sign of madness on the cornerstone of the asylum, through to twentieth-century definitions of that most central and ambiguous label for madness, "schizophrenia," the "bizarre" language of the insane has characterized the abyss between the normal and the pathological. It was only with the World Health Organization's 1973 *International Pilot Study of Schizophrenia* that an attempt was made to document the "reality" behind this stereotype.[43] It was found that only 10 percent of those patients examined actually showed the classic thought (and therefore, language) disorders associated with "schizophrenia." Thus the age-old association between the representation of madness and its reality can be shown to rest more on the fears of those who have created the representations than on the phenomenology of madness itself.

Seeing the schizophrenic as "bizarre" is our means of drawing a line about our own sense of wholeness. For whether we distance ourselves from it, or whether we adopt it as our mask, we use the *bizarre* as our sign of our own completeness. In the first case we demarcate our sense of self from the Other; in the second, we consciously adopt the external label of difference as a means of showing our control over the world. *In both cases we know we are not different.* We play a role, and that role defines difference as that which lies outside of ourselves. Thus we use the stereotype of the bizarre language of the schizophrenic as a means of defining our own sanity.

CHAPTER FOURTEEN

Seeing the AIDS Patient

Images without End

During the summer of 1986 many Americans read the *Newsweek* cover story on Gerald Friedland of Montefiore Medical Center entitled "The AIDS Doctor."[1] I begin my discussion of the construction of the image of the individual living with AIDS during 1986 and 1987 with this essay—which is in the style of the "new journalism," very personal and very informal—and examine its authors' desire to alter the dominant manifestation of this image and their inability to accomplish their intended goal. The opening sentence of the essay sets not only its tone but its agenda: "One day in April 1985, Dr. Gerald H. Friedland found himself at the bedside of a young woman named Maria, letting her know as gently as he could that she was going to die." Disregarding the self-conscious echo of the opening of Dante's *Inferno*, we can read in this sentence what is clearly a desired shift in the image of the AIDS patient—from that of the male patient to that of the female, with all of its implications for the spread of AIDS through all elements of society. The authors, Peter Goldman and Lucille Beachy, have introduced us to an exemplary AIDS patient—one who is, however, a woman. Maria was not only female but she was a medical anomaly: "Nothing in her medical history marked her as a candidate for AIDS, not at first glance." She should have been a noncombatant in the AIDS invasion of North America. She was not one of the "4-H's": homosexuals, heroin addicts, hemophiliacs, and Haitians, the four categories labeled as being "at risk" for AIDS through the early 1980s.[2] She was an incidental victim, infected by her former husband, an IV drug user, who had subsequently died of AIDS.

The short but frightening history of the reception of the image of the AIDS patient links many of the concerns expressed in this study, including the close relation perceived, in the construction of the image of the patient, among somatic, emotional, and mental illnesses as well as the seemingly independent life of the images in the work of art, images that reappear throughout history, attaching themselves to various and sundry diseases (real or imagined). The *Newsweek* cover story is part of a recent shift in the public image of the nature of the patient infected with AIDS. With over twenty-two thousand cases, about one per million of the population in the United States, and a present case fatality rate of over 50 percent, it is not trivial to ask how these patients are (and have been) perceived.[3] To explore the semiotics of the disease means to understand not only the overt level of meaning but also the complex confusions that permeate the image of the AIDS patient.

AIDS as a Sexually Transmitted Disease

The construction of the image of the AIDS patient has taken the past nine years to reach its present stage. In 1979 Alvin Friedman-Kien of New York University Medical Center identified a group of patients suffering from a rare dermatological disease, Kaposi's sarcoma, which has a striking visual presentation, bluish or purple-brown nodules that appear on the skin. The normal course of this disease is seldom fatal, but this group of young patients were dying within eight to twenty-four months after their diagnosis. Other physicians reported similar patterns during 1979.[4] By June 1981, twenty-six such cases were reported in the Center for Disease Control's (CDC) *Morbidity and Mortality Weekly Report (MMWR).*[5] Parallel to this, five cases of *Pneumocystis* pneumonia, an illness caused by a ubiquitous protozoan parasite which usually manifests itself only in those individuals with depressed immune systems, appeared in Los Angeles. By the time of the report, two of these patients had died. Shortly thereafter, ten new cases of *Pneumocystis* pneumonia were diagnosed, and two of these patients also had Kaposi's sarcoma.[6]

The initial appearance of this pattern in the United States led the investigators at the CDC to try to comprehend its nature, to construct an image of the patient.[7] The epidemiologists perceived a cluster of common attributes: these patients were living in large urban areas (New York, Miami, Los Angeles, and San Francisco), and they were all young men.

By 1981, however, another element had become central to the CDC's image of the AIDS patient—the patient's sexual orientation. As early as the 5 June 1981 report in the *MMWR*, it had been noted that "two of the five [patients] reported having frequent homosexual contacts with various partners" (p. 251). The centrality of sexual orientation as a factor can be further seen in the operational categorization of the AIDS patient during the first quarter of 1982 as suffering from "G[ay] R[elated] I[mmune] D[eficiency] S[yndrome]." This label structured the idea of the patient suffering from AIDS in such a marked manner that the patient was not only stigmatized as a carrier of an infectious disease but also placed within a very specific historical category. For *AIDS*, a term officially coined in the fall of 1982, was understood as a specific subset of the greater category of sexually transmitted diseases, a disease that homosexuals suffered as a direct result of their sexual practices or related group-specific activities—the use of drugs such as "poppers" (amyl or butyl nitrite), for example.[8] The idea of the person afflicted with sexually transmitted disease, one of the most potent in the repertory of images of the stigmatized patient, became the paradigm through which the AIDS patient was categorized and understood. This notion persisted. Even though the *MMWR* began, in late 1982, to record the appearance of the disease among such groups as hemophiliacs and IV drug users, groups that could be defined by qualities other than sexual orientation, sexual orientation remained the salient characteristic used to exemplify the person living with AIDS.[9]

Indeed, the gratuituous appearance of the disease during the late 1970s linked two (at that time) unrelated social concerns: first, the perception of the increase of sexually transmitted diseases in society (following a long period of perceived decline), signaled in 1975 by the National Institute of Allergy and Infectious Diseases declaring research in sexually transmitted disease to be the number one priority of the Institute; second, the growth of the public awareness of the homosexual emancipation movement, at least in large urban areas, following the so-called Stonewall riot in Greenwich Village in 1969, in which there was a violent protest against police harassment of homosexuals.[10] From the beginning the person living with AIDS was seen as a male homosexual suffering a sexually transmitted disease and thus as different from the perceived normal spectrum of patients—but different within very specific structures. We must stress that the AIDS is caused by retroviruses, now labeled "H[uman] I[mmuno-deficiency] V[iruses]," spread by direct contact with infected body fluids, including blood and semen. Sexual contact is not necessary to contract the illness.[11] It is a viral disease that can be transmitted sexually but also can be transmitted by other means. The ambiguity of this fact meant that the disease could have been categorized in many different ways—it was characterized not as a viral disease, such as Hepatitis B, however, but as a sexually transmitted disease, such as syphilis.

The Iconography of Syphilis

The initial categorization of AIDS as a sexually transmitted disease (albeit in a very specific context) strongly marked the initial construction of the disease. One can best document the parallels between the visual history of syphilis, especially the history of the disease during its first decade, and the iconography of AIDS by juxtaposing a series of visual images of AIDS patients published in the popular press during the past few years with representations of the syphilitic patient. The images of the AIDS patient are taken from a press sympathetic in general to the patient suffering from AIDS, not from the papers and journals of the religious right, which have, since the nineteenth century, condemned such patients, as Allan Brandt observed, "as [suffering] an affliction of those who willfully violated the moral code . . . a punishment for sexual irresponsibility."[12] And yet the stigma of sexually transmitted disease maintains itself even in these self-consciously supportive journals of public opinion.

The context for these portraits of the AIDS patient is to be found in the almost five-hundred-year-old iconography of the syphilitic. There one can document how the boundaries of syphilis were constructed during the initial outbreak of the disease and during its subsequent history. This is not to outline the social history of the disease, as Allan Brandt has so admirably done, but rather to sketch the image of the patient as a key to the shift in the boundaries of the image of the disease. We can thereby in turn define the qualities visually associated with persons living with AIDS, qualities resulting from the labeling of AIDS as a sexually transmitted disease limited to a strictly defined group.

The visual image of the syphilitic has its roots in the very first years after the spread of an especially virulent form of syphilis began when Charles VIII of France entered the besieged city of Naples in 1495. Spread by the French armies, the "Mal de Naples," "Morbus Gallicus," "Malafranzcos," or "Franzosenkrankheit" soon appeared in the German states.[13] On 1 August 1496, the first visual representation of the syphilitic appeared, a broadside by Theodoricus Ulsenius, with an illustration by Albrecht Dürer (Plate 39). The broadside assigns the origin of the disease (for even then we were obsessed with finding the origin rather than discussing control) to the ill-fated appearance of five planets in the sign of the Scorpion (the zodiacal sign that rules the genitalia) in 1484. What strikes the viewer initially is the representation of the isolated sufferer, revealing to the viewer the signs and symptoms of syphilis like the stigmata of a parodied Christ. It is a male figure echoing the position of the exemplum of masculinity, the suffering Christ. But note the enormous, plumed hat, the abundant cloak, the broad-toed, slashed shoes,

39. Albrecht Dürer's image of the syphilitic (1496) (private collection, Ithaca, N.Y.).

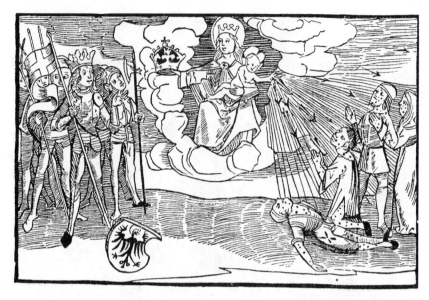

40. The title page vignette to Sebastian Brant's 1496 pamphlet on syphilis, from Karl Sudhoff, *Zehn Syphilis-Drucke aus den Jahren 1495–98* (Milan: Lier, 1924).

and the long, flowing hair. This is the German's caricature of the sufferer as a fop, as a Frenchman, as the outsider already associated in German myth with sexual excesses and deviancy. Even so, the victim of syphilis is portrayed here as the victim of the signs of the zodiac which determine his affliction.[14] From the first, then, the syphilitic is seen as isolated, visually recognizable by his signs and symptoms, and sexually deviant.

The fact that women as well as men suffered from the new epidemic of syphilis is reflected in many of these early images of the sufferer. But always there is a shift that separates the active suffering of the male from the passive suffering of the female. The sense of isolation of the male sufferer can be seen in a reworking of one of the earliest images of the syphilitic. On the title page of a broadside on the new epidemic (1496) by the famed jurist and author of the *Ship of Fools*, Sebastian Brant (Plate 40), there is an image of a closed community of syphilitics, three male and one female.[15] They are being punished by the *flagellum Dei*, the whip of God, for their sexual transgressions. The arrows also signify the martyrdom of the sufferer, suffering for Eve and Adam's fall. The figure of the Christ child indicates, however, the potential for cure. In the parallel vignette, in Joseph Grünpeck's 1496 commentary on Brant, a visual interpretation of the image that introduces Brant's pamphlet, the figure of the male sufferer is brought forward and isolated (Plate 41).[16] This visual shift in emphasis creates the illusion that the male represents the exemplary sufferer, central in his suffering to any understanding of the nature

℄ Ein hübscher Tractat von dem vrsprung
des Bösen Franzos. das man nennet die
Wylden wärtzen. Auch ein Regiment wie
man sich regiren soll in diser zeyt.

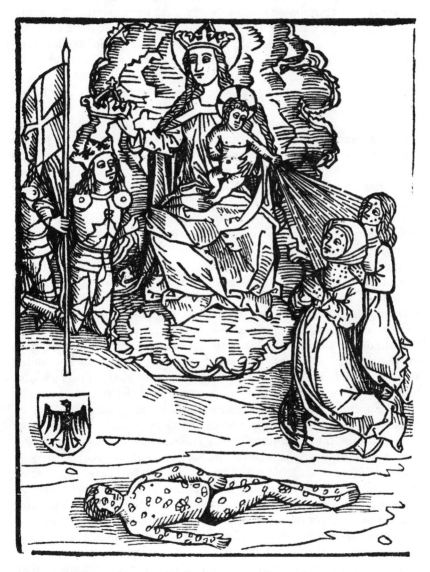

41. The vignette from Joseph Grünpeck's commentary on Brant's syphilis pamphlet
(1496), from Sudhoff, *Zehn Syphilis-Drucke.*

of the disease. In this image the male sufferer is portrayed as the primary victim of the disease rather than its harbinger.

In Amico Aspertini's image in the Oratoria of St. Cecilia in Bologna, dated to 1506, of the decapitation of St. Valerian and his brother, the exemplary image of the syphilitic is that of the isolated male portrayed in the older, established iconographic tradition of the leper. He bears his signs of disease to the world, a disease given a specific sexual reference by the sign of the scorpion on his banner (Plate 42). By the sixteenth century, leprosy no longer was endemic in Western Europe. While the disease had all but vanished, its iconography remained as part of the popular store-house of images of disease and pollution and was immediately attached to the new disease of syphilis. His image, too, is of the isolated sufferer as the victim of forces, such as the signs of the heavens, over which he has no control.

But it is not merely "vacant" constructions of disease which influence the representation of the new illness. In a broadside prayer of ca. 1500 the image of the syphilitic is presented in the classic pose of melancholia (Plate 43).[17] The figure is that of the syphilitic as embodied by the pre-figuration of Job "smote . . . with sore boils from the sole of his foot unto his crown" (Job 2:7) by Satan. The syphilitic is portrayed in the ico-nographic position of the melancholic, elbow on knee, head on hand, a gesture of passive submission and reflection as well as despair.[18] But central to this image is also, as in the earlier images found in Brandt and Grünpeck, the image of cure. It is, of course, a cure for melancholia (as we saw in the discussion of the Greek concept of the cure of madness in Chapter 5). His friends come and play their instruments, attempting, as David did for Saul, to cure his melancholy madness through music. The conflation of such images of existing "diseases," where there was a per-ceived cure, with the new disease of syphilis, provided a vocabulary of images through which to understand and, thus, limit a disease under-stood as boundariless. But the anonymous author of this broadside also located the other contemporary understanding of the source of the dis-ease in another biblical prefiguration—he prays "that you [God] re-member Abraham's prayer for Sodom and Gomorrah and save me from such a painful, horrible plague." Abraham's prayer was that if ten right-eous men be found in these sinful cities, God would spare them. They, of course, were not to be found (Genesis 18 and 19). Given our earlier discussion (in Chapter 3) on the implications of the phrase "Sodom and Gomorrah" for the Renaissance, it is evident that the author is indicating the sexual source of the new pollution of syphilis. But it is the male, the Job figure, who represents the sufferer, and even with the sexual source of the disease, it is the male who is understood as the victim.

Only in the Enlightenment does the image of the syphilitic patient shift from male to female, but then only with the female as the image of

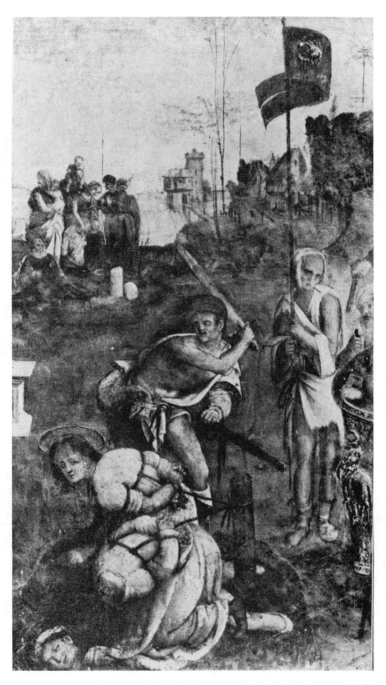

42. Amico Aspertin's portrait of St. Valerian and his brother, from Sudhoff, *Zehn Syphilis-Drucke.*

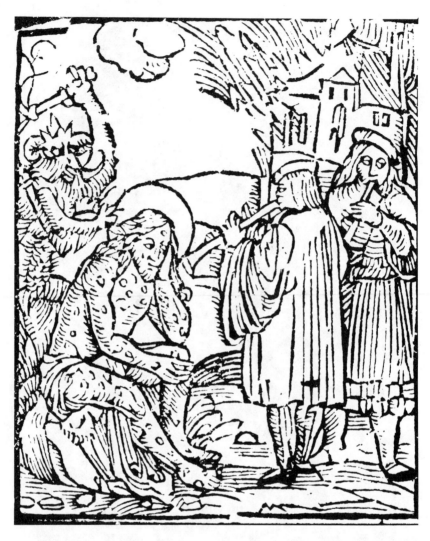

43. A broadside "On the Pox Called Malafrantzosa," 1500, from *Archiv für die Geschichte der Medizin* 1 (1907).

the source of infection. In the high Middle Ages, woman was already understood to be both seductive and physically corrupt, as in the image of "Madam World" from the St. Sebaldus Church in Nuremberg (seen from the front and the back) (Plate 44). By the eighteenth century, the image of the patient, the individual bearing the signs and stigmata of syphilis becomes that of the corrupt female, as, for example, in a late eighteenth-century popular representation of the decayed head of a syphilitic pros-

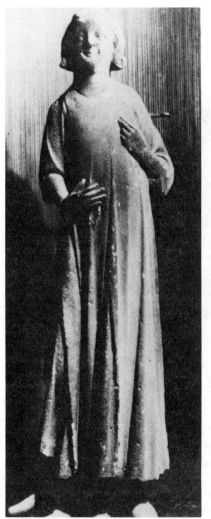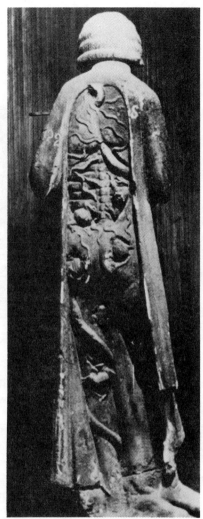

44. "Frau Welt," from the portal of the St. Sebaldus Church in Nuremberg (fourteenth century) (private collection, Ithaca, N.Y.).

titute (Plate 45). (The change here is also from the innate corruption of the female to the potential for the corruption of the male.) It takes over two hundred years for the image of the syphilitic to shift from the male "victim" of the disease to its female "source." In the Baroque, for example, as in Luca Giordana's *Allegory of Syphilis* (1664), the victim is male. But by the time we come to William Hogarth's *Marriage à la Mode* (1745), both the money-hungry aristocrat and the title-hungry alderman's

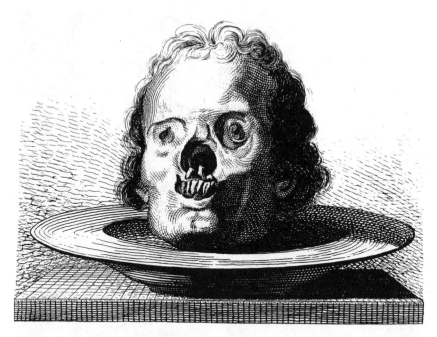

45. The head of a syphilitic prostitute (eighteenth century) (Wellcome Institute for the History of Medicine, London).

daughter are represented as syphilitics. The gradual development of this shift from the male to the female as the exemplary syphilitic can be seen in Hogarth's well-known series. This popular image of the woman as the exemplary patient even permeates the medical literature of the early nineteenth century. For example, Jean-Louis Alibert, one of the founders of modern dermatology, represents all of his syphilitics as women in his great atlas of skin diseases of 1806.[19]

The image of the seductress as the source of pollution can be seen even more strikingly on the title page of a mid-nineteenth-century French edition of the poem *Syphilis* by Fracastoro, which gave the disease its name in the sixteenth century (Plate 46). This image is a nineteenth-century variation of the Baroque emblem representing the choice of Hercules, tempted by Voluptas, the vice of luxury, behind whose mask the temptress hides her ugliness. The difference here, of course, is that by the nineteenth century "vice" becomes "disease," seduction becomes infection. The movement here is to continue the tradition (as in Dürer's very first such image) of depicting the sufferer of a sexually transmitted disease as the outsider (initially the foppish or French male), the sexual deviant. The female is seen as the source of pollution, but also as the outsider, the prostitute, the socially deviant individual.

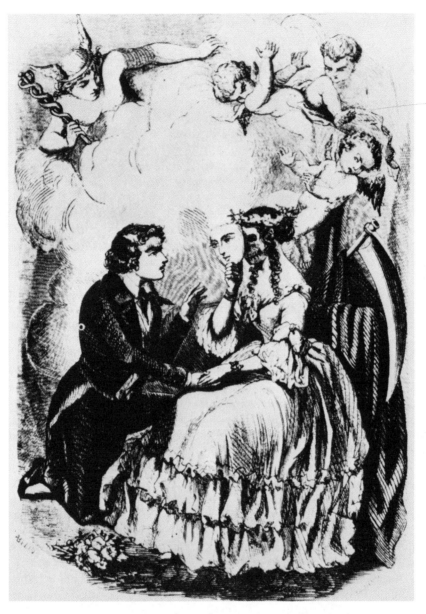

46. The title page vignette of the nineteenth-century French translation of Fracastoro's poem *Syphilis* (Wellcome Institute for the History of Medicine, London).

The Image of the AIDS Patient

It is important to understand that the association of the image of the AIDS patient with the iconography of syphilis is not random. It is clear that the initial association rests on that population of AIDS patients, homosexuals, and society's perception of them as having suffered a sexually transmitted disease. But it is also clear that the "taming" of syphilis and other related sexually transmitted diseases with the introduction of antibiotics in the 1940s left our culture with a series of images of the mortally infected and infecting patient suffering a morally repugnant disease but without a sufficiently powerful disease with which to associate these images. During the 1970s there was an attempt to connect these images with genital herpes, but even though it is a sexually transmitted disease, its symptomatology was too trivial to warrant this association over the long run. AIDS was the perfect disease for such associations, even if it was not a typical sexually transmitted disease.

If we turn to an image of the AIDS patient which appeared in *The New York Times* of 23 December 1985, we find a construction parallel to that of the Brandt and Grünpeck broadsides: the image of the isolated patient in relation to the act of healing (Plate 47). The physical sense of distance is palpable; the observers are as far away from the patient as they can be without being in another room. Although this is a "typical" image of medical treatment, like many late nineteenth- and twentieth-century photographs of physicians at work, the ground provided for the observer of the image is the tension communicated—not by the treatment of the patient—but by the implications associated with the patient's disease. *The New York Times* in 1985 (and subsequently) was full of articles on the anxiety of health workers who treated AIDS patients. And this image corresponded, for the reader of the *Times*, to the anxiety in the general public concerning the transmission of the disease. By 1985, the significance of the single male patient for the readers of *The New York Times* was self-evident: this is the patient as homosexual male. The male is not only the sufferer but also the source of his own pollution. Here we have the conflation of the male and the female images traditionally associated with sexually transmitted diseases such as syphilis.

Another set of images of AIDS patients, such as a group of photographs taken from the Long Island newspaper *Newsday* on 4 August 1985, begins to show the attempt on the part of the "liberal" media to soften the image of the AIDS patient (Plate 48). The uppermost image is of the hemophiliac sufferer, a male, like the central figure in Brant's broadside, but like him within a mixed-sex group, the family, a potential source of more sufferers. The heterosexual male is seen here as both the victim (of a polluted blood supply) as well as the source of pollution (for his family).

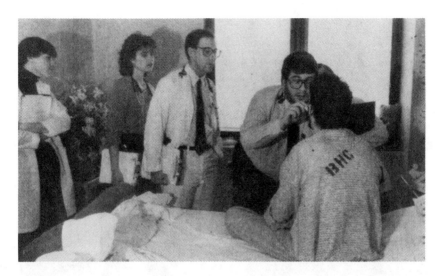

47. The AIDS patient being examined by his physicians (*The New York Times*, 23 December 1985).

The second image, of the sociopathic "drifter and drug user," stresses the visual stigmata of disease. But the final two images return to the association of the AIDS patient with the traditional iconography of sexually transmitted diseases and the resultant despair of contagion and death. They are marginal men, marginal sexually and "racially" presented as visually isolated, especially in the context of the first image of the family, and are depicted within distinctive iconographic traditions of representing the patient of sexually transmitted disease. The two of them, as in Dürer's broadside and Grünpeck's revision of the Brant image, show us their stigmata, Kaposi's sarcoma.

The final image represents the individual living with AIDS as isolated, his very position echoing the classical iconographic position of melancholia, an association, as we have seen, already made with syphilis during the first decade after its first documented appearance. The association of the image of the AIDS sufferer with the traditional iconography of melancholy or depression is an extraordinarily powerful one, reappearing as the first illustration in a major update on AIDS in the popular scientific journal *Discover* in September 1986.[20] In an essay subtitled "still no reason for hysteria," which attempted to counter the evident fear that AIDS was becoming a danger to heterosexuals, John Langone's editorial intent was to combat the growing sense that AIDS was a potential danger for everyone (Plate 49). The iconography of depression, with its emphasis on the body, stresses the age-old association between the nature of the mind (here, the "mental illness" that is depicted as resulting from homo-

The Burk Family

Patrick Burk, 28, of Cresson, Pa., has AIDS, as does his 1-year-old son, Dwight. His wife, Lauren, 24, has AIDS-Related Complex, an early stage of the illness. The virus was in a blood by-product that Patrick was injecting into himself weekly for hemophilia. He passed the virus on to his wife, who passed it on to her son when she was pregnant. They are seen here in the spring with their daughter, Nicole, who is healthy. Lauren works three days a week as a registered nurse, supporting the family. The three were diagnosed as having AIDS when their son became very ill. "At first I couldn't believe it," Lauren says. "And maybe I still cannot."

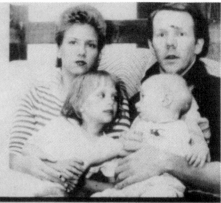

Photo by Frank Fournier/Contact

Alfredo Vega

A drifter and drug user born in New York to a poor Puerto Rican family, Vega, 25, says he got AIDS from his girlfriend, who has since died and who, he says, was a prostitute. Shown here amid medicine in a photo taken in April, he is dying and his body has turned brown in many places. "My family wanted me to stay with them, but my sister was afraid for her three children. So I went to sleep in the hallway for a week [in December]. Then my brother's wife called me. But my brother didn't want me. So I was staying at their place in the daytime and sleeping on the roof at night." He is living now in a Manhattan hotel.

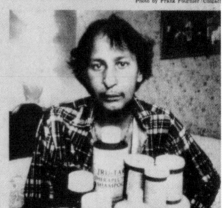

Photo by Alon Reininger/Contact

Victor Bender, Horacio Benegas

A fashion designer from Buenos Aires, Benegas, 36, in photo at right taken in April, is seriously ill with Kaposi's sarcoma, an AIDS-related disease. He lives in a three-story house with a terrace and a neatly tended garden owned by Victor Bender, 39, left, who also has Kaposi's sarcoma. Bender, shown at the Gay Men's Health Crisis Center in Manhattan, where he works on a hotline, is now staying at his mother's house because of the constant activity of crisis-center volunteers taking care of Benegas. "They are doing as much as they can," he says, "but it does not look good."

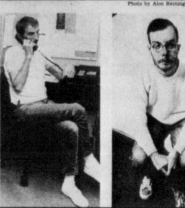

48. Four images of people living with AIDS (*Newsday*, 4 August 1985).

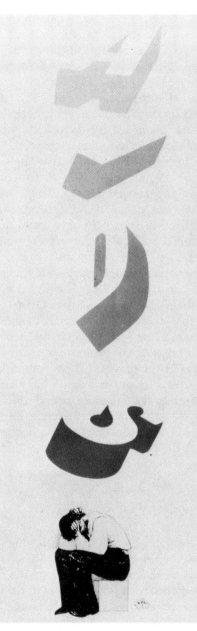

d with the infection caused by n elusive retrovirus known s HTLV-III, HTLV-III/LAV, IIV, or ARV are a vicious omplex of maladies. They to-lly cripple the immune sys-em. They can invade the rain, and have so far resisted ll treatment. Out of a total of 3,000 patients diagnosed in he U.S. so far, 18,000, nearly ll of them in the well defined isk groups, will have died by he end of the year of a disease hat was identified only five ears ago. In 1991 the death oll is expected to reach be-ween 149,000 and 201,000. Jut these figures pale beside hose of cancer, which can trike anyone, in or out of so-alled risk groups, and will kill n estimated 472,000 Ameri-ans this year alone. Moreover, inlike influenza and some oth-'r viral diseases, AIDS isn't asy to contract. It isn't spread hrough casual exposure. Nor loes infection by the virus nec-essarily lead to the disease alled AIDS, which is the end tage of the whole spectrum f HTLV-III-caused diseases. The Centers for Disease Con-trol, or CDC, has estimated that in the U.S. between one million and one and a half mil-lion people are infected with the virus, as indicated by the presence of antibodies in their systems, but only 20 to 30 per cent are likely to get AIDS.)

For the disease to be trans-mitted, it's believed that the vi-rus must be present in the do-nor's blood or semen. It must be alive and stable. And the victim's immune system must be unable to resist the on-slaught of the virus, so that it can successfully invade certain white blood cells that serve as master controls of the immune system. In the U.S. the most likely candidates for infection are: 1) male homosexuals and bisexuals who are the recipi-ents during anal intercourse with an infected partner, a

practice that can damage the fragile, blood vessel-lined tis-sue of the rectum; 2) drug ad-dicts who share contaminated needles; 3) homosexuals and bisexuals of either sex who are also IV drug users; and 4) recip-ients of frequent blood transfu-sions, like hemophiliacs.

The CDC's projections for 1991 don't significantly alter the risk picture. By that time 270,000 people will have been diagnosed as having AIDS. More than 70 per cent of them will be homosexual and bisex-ual males, and 25 per cent IV drug users (about eight per cent of them homosexuals). Of the new cases in 1991, about ten per cent—some 7,000—will be classified as hetero-sexuals, some of them also IV drug users. (The correspond-ing number this year is 1,100.) The projected total seems high, but it represents an increase of only three per cent of hetero-sexual cases. This category includes people who've ac-knowledged contact with ei-ther an infected person or with a member of a risk group. Moreover, the CDC doesn't define what it means by het-erosexual transmission, or het-erosexual contact, nor can it say whether the cases will be spread through vaginal sex, anal sex, or sharing contami-nated needles. In spite of the authoritative ring of these fig-ures, the U.S. Public Health Service (PHS) said in June "Current information is insuf-ficient to predict the future in-cidence of HTLV-III/LAV in the heterosexual population."

The spread of AIDS almost equally among men and women in Africa, reportedly through conventional male female sexual relations, is of-ten cited as a reason to ex-pect widespread heterosexual transmission of the disease in the U.S. But the African expe-rience with AIDS may not be applicable to Americans. As

49. The person living with AIDS as melancholic (*Discover*, September 1986).

sexuality) and the body (here, the icon of sexual deviance). The image of the body becomes the message. The AIDS patient remains the suffering, hopeless male, both the victim and the source of his own pollution. The AIDS patients are represented iconographically as depressed males, with their sense of their marginality stressed even in those media that are not overtly condemnatory of their sexual identity.

There is an additional dimension to the use of the image of the melancholic in this illustration from *Discover*. For in tone the essay is condemnatory of the "hysteria" about AIDS present within the American media because of what is labeled the "unfounded" fear of AIDS crossing into the non–IV drug using, heterosexual community. The image of the person living with AIDS is, on the most overt level, associated with the stigma of mental illness because the fear of impending death, the *momento mori*, is represented by the figure of the melancholic, a figure who has capitulated to despair. But the *Discover* image not only draws the analogy with the despair over impending death; it also, through a broader analogy extended to the general population, which now suffers from an "unwarranted" AIDS phobia, sees the person living with AIDS as the representation of the mental illness (read: fearful fantasy) of an entire nation. This association of AIDS with mental illness is a critique of the claim (which the *Discover* essay is aimed to refute) that AIDS is a danger to the entire community. The image of the person living with AIDS as a melancholic is only marginally related to the fact that one of the more frequent syndromes recently associated with AIDS in the press is "AIDS dementia." In such images what is being represented is not the "reality" of mental illness, such as AIDS dementia, but rather the stigma of mental illness, a stigma implied through the visual association of the representation of the person living with AIDS with one of the most powerful of all stigmatizing diseases, mental illness. Thus the boundary between the "normal" and the hysterically feared "abnormal" is drawn.

Toward a Geography of the AIDS Patient

One aspect of the iconography of AIDS which points to the complexity of the construction of the image of the AIDS patients is the "geography" of the disease. It is clear that we need to locate the origin of a disease, since its source, always distant from ourselves in the fantasy land of our fears, gives us assurance that we are not at fault, that we have been invaded from without, that we have been polluted by some external agent. In the late fifteenth century, syphilis was initially understood as resulting from the malevolent influence of the zodiac. But it quickly became associated with another major occurrence of the 1490s, Columbus's voyage of discovery to the Americas. Whether or not syphilis was actually imported by Columbus's sailors from the New World is not important. Syphilis was understood as society's punishment for transgressing against God-given boundaries of human endeavor, the divine scourge for the collapse of the rigid feudal class system, the rise of capitalism, and the desire to find new worlds to feed this new economic system. So Sebastian Brant labels it in *The Ship of Fools*.[21] In the nineteenth century, in an age of colonialism and black slavery, a counter-explanation arose, placing the origin of syphilis in Africa and predating Columbus. As the need to locate the origin of the disease shifted with time and circumstance, so did the presumed locus.

AIDS presents a similar story in the 1980s. In the United States we have labeled AIDS an "African" or "Haitian" disease.[22] Whatever the reality of the origin of the disease, this assumption is, of course, very much in line with the white American sense that blacks have a basically different relation to disease because of their inherent difference. Blacks were assumed for over a century to have a much higher rate of mental disease because of their inability to cope with civilization.[23] Indeed, it was also assumed that American blacks had a greater immunity against syphilis because of the "African" origin of the disease. This notion led to the horrors of the Tuskegee syphilis experiment, in which black patients infected with syphilis were observed, without any medical intervention, until their death.[24] The irony, of course, is that American blacks were indeed at special risk for AIDS because of the nature of treatment for sickle cell disease, through transfusions. It was the polluted blood supply that placed American blacks, at least those suffering from such genetically transmitted diseases, in the forefront of those who were at risk.[25] But they were not understood as being in the same category as hemophiliacs. For blacks were deemed to be at risk because of their perceived sexual difference, their sexual practices, their hypersexuality. Black sexuality, associated with images of sexually transmitted disease, became a category of marginalization, as it had been in the past.[26] It is interesting that in the 1980s, after white America was made aware of the intolerable state of blacks in this country through the civil rights movement in the 1960s and 1970s, one could no longer as easily localize the source of disease among American blacks, as had been done in the Tuskegee experiment. Rather, the perceived source of pollution was shifted to foreign blacks, black Africans and Haitians, thus assuaging American "liberal" sensibilities while still locating the origin of the disease within the paradigm of American racist ideology.

For the French, at least in 1981, it was clear that AIDS was an American disease. With the rise of American cultural models and practices among the homosexual community (the French homosexual community even adopted the Anglicism "gai"), it was initially believed that the disease was the result of the excessive use of contaminated "poppers" imported from North America.[27] Even today, the popular image of the disease in Europe is as one born, along with jeans and rock, in the USA. This fact is nowhere clearer than in the German reception of the disease. In a recent title story on AIDS in the German weekly news magazine *Der Spiegel* (9 February 1987), the central images are taken from American political cartoonists, even though the essay purports to be about AIDS in the Federal Republic.

For the Soviets it is clear where the geographic origin of the disease lies—the HIV virus was manmade by the biological warfare specialists at Fort Detrick, Maryland, in conjunction with the scientists at the CDC (Plate 50). In the Soviet view, AIDS is an American biological weapon gone amok and destroying its creator.[28] Their image of AIDS, drawn for *Pravda* by D. Agaeva, reflects the complexity of national images of the AIDS patient. His cartoon shows an American general paying for a test-tube of AIDS virus supplied to him by a venal-looking scientist. Swimming about in the test-tube, representing the power of the AIDS virus, are a multitude of tiny swastikas; the dead, the victims of AIDS, appear in the cartoon as concentration camp victims, their bare feet echoing the death camp photographs of bodies stacked like cordwood with only their feet showing. This attempt to place the blame for AIDS on the United States worked only until the spring of 1987, when the Soviets, in the climate of *glasnost*, admitted that they too had indigenous cases of the disease. But during 1985 and 1986, the Soviets were picking up a thread in the Marxist-Leninist image of the United States as fascist, degenerate, and therefore sick. Indeed, the "orthodox" view was that homosexuality was a pathological reflex of the late forms of capitalism which would (and did) vanish once the Soviet state was created. Thus AIDS was defined as a Western disease, a reflection of bourgeois government and society.

Part of the construction of the image of the AIDS patient in the United States does incorporate the idea of geography—which included the search for the "African" or "Haitian" connection. Indeed, the recent withdrawal of the label of "risk group" from Haitians followed a period of severe persecution, both direct and indirect, of Haitians in the United States. Being Haitian in New York City meant that you were understood to have AIDS. The irony is that it seems evident, given the most recent epidemiology of the disease in Haiti, that the disease, limited to the large urban areas on the island, was a result of contact between HIV seropositive American tourists and Haitian men, who passed the disease to their female sexual partners and children.[29] In the United States, Haiti was viewed as one of the original sources of the disease, specifically because it

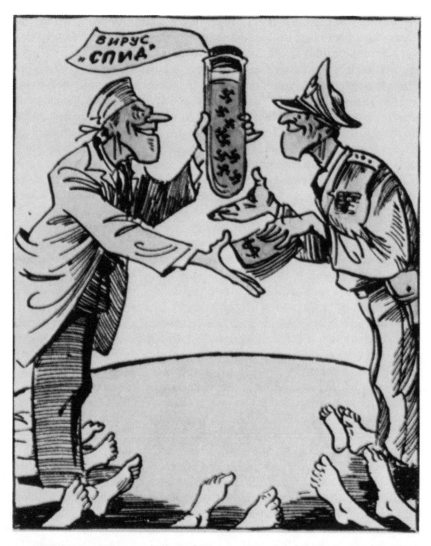

50. AIDS as an American biological weapon. Drawing by D. Agaeva (*Pravda*, 1 November 1986).

was to be found in Haiti in a heterosexual community. Heterosexual transmission was labeled by the investigators as a more primitive (or, to use the good nineteenth-century term, atavistic) stage of the development of AIDS. It was understood to be unlike the pattern of infection in the United States, where it existed only among marginal groups (which would include blacks).

It was only in the "higher" cultures, such as the United States, that the disease was limited to such specific groups that were immediately and visually identifiable. This creation of the boundary between the infected and the healthy rested on the need to see a clear boundary existing between the heterosexual, non–IV drug using, white community and those at risk. Thus as Anthony Pinching so cogently observed in his essay of September 1986, concerning the Western fantasies of a perverted and diseased black population that served as the necessary "originator" of AIDS: "Rumours have circulated about the use of anal intercourse as a common means of birth control in Africa; this idea represents a carry-over from the initial perceptions of AIDS as something intrinsically to do with homosexual behavior. The widespread acceptance of these alternative explanations seems to indicate a remarkable ignorance about the countries in question; more disturbingly they have shown that many observers are unwilling to accept the obvious, if unpleasant, conclusion that AIDS, or rather HIV, is heterosexually transmitted."[30] While heterosexual transmission is the primary means of the spread of the disease, another irony is that one of the minor means for the transmission of the HIV viruses in black Africa has its roots in the imposition (and acceptance) of models of Western medicine. The status of Western medicine, especially through its central icon, inoculation, is so high, that no medical treatment, even by indigenous medical practitioners, is complete without an injection.[31] Because of the prohibitive cost of needles and syringes, blood is passed from patient to patient as the needle is used and reused. It is not the fantasized perverted nature of black sexuality which is at the core of the transmission of the disease in Africa, but the results of a wholesale importation of a Western model of medicine without sensitivity to local circumstances.

The geography of AIDS in the United States, that is, the drawing of the boundaries of risk, has had yet another dimension. AIDS is perceived as an urban disease, a disease of cities, the traditional harbors of disease and degeneration.[32] It is the plague of cities after the biblical icon of Sodom and Gomorrah. Righteous Abraham, who dwells in a tent, is contrasted in Genesis with the sinful dwellers in the city. Thus arises the seemingly natural association among three quite distinct groups of those perceived as city-dwellers: homosexuals, IV drug users, and Haitians. For we know where corruption lives, in the city. And purity lives where our fantasy has it that nature (and therefore goodness) dominates: on the farm and in the small town. This Rousseauian image of the city has joined with the image of the AIDS patient to give us an image of the AIDS patient as black, drug-using, homosexual, and urban—a geography of difference which is now part of the American iconography of the AIDS patient.

The Borders of the Image

Now, the evident question that remains is what would have happened if AIDS had appeared in a much different context. What if it had first been identified among IV drug users, or among hemophiliacs? Among hemophiliacs, it would have been seen as an iatrogenic illness, not the fault of the patient but of the system. And there the group stigma would have been less. Among IV drug users, AIDS would still have been stigmatized, as a disease of a marginal group, but it would have been seen as an artifact of a sociopathic act associated with a specific class and race. And it would, therefore, be limited in its perceived locus. For in 1981 it was not the yuppies with their drug of choice, cocaine, who would have been infected, but the blacks of Harlem and the South Bronx, mainlining heroin with shared needles. But these were not the groups that defined the illness.

What did happen is that these two groups inherited the stigmatization of the sexually transmitted disease patient: the IV drug users continued to be defined through this paradigm as even more dangerous sociopaths, and the hemophiliacs as a marginalized, genetically disordered minority. This stigmatization became so widespread that it permeated categories of social organization, such as childhood, which would otherwise seem to be generally immune to such stigmatization. In the 1985 Queens School Board Case, two community school boards sued the City Board of Education in order to exclude a seven-year-old child, diagnosed as having AIDS, from the school system. (At the time the case was brought, there were about 78 children under the age of twelve in New York City who were diagnosed as having AIDS, and 52 had already died.) The child in question had most probably contracted the disease *in utero*.

The attorney for the local school board, Robert Sullivan, observed that "in many instances children who have AIDS are the children . . . of parents who are not as responsible as we would like them to be. . . . They may be the children of an IV drug user or a victim of sexual abuse." They are, in short, "not in the best family setting a child should be in . . . not a recommended family setting."[33] Even the dying child, the exemplary innocent within our pantheon of images of disease (think of the death of Dickens's Little Nell or Harriet Beecher Stowe's Little Eva), has become infected with the unclean image of the sexually transmitted disease patient. Nowhere is this often subconscious pollution of the image of the child clearer than in the caption to an Associated Press photograph of the central figure in a parallel court case, Ryan White, whose attempts to enter the Kokomo, Indiana, school system led to a massive boycott by parents of his schoolmates afraid of the potential for infection. In the

Ithaca Journal of 1 May 1986 a photograph of Ryan White showed him and "his sister Andrea . . . [meeting] cast members of 'Cats' at a star-studded gala in New York Tuesday night to raise money for AIDS research." According to the caption, "Ryan . . . is a homophiliac [*sic*] who contracted AIDS through a blood transfusion." The typographical conflation of the hemophiliac and the homosexual is an extraordinarily simple one to make given our construction of the image of the AIDS patient. To work against this conflation, many images of the child AIDS patient show the child in the family context. Such a juxtaposition contrasts radically with the imposed isolation of the homosexual or IV drug user AIDS patient. The presence of the family serves to signal the "normality" of the child and the low risk of transmission, in spite of the child's radical stigmatization. The media wish to maintain society's image of the pure, dying child. But such an iconographic device is rarely sufficient to overcome the stigma of AIDS.

The irrational reaction to the child living with AIDS has had disastrous consequences for children and family alike. The hysteria recently crescendoed in the much publicized case of the Ray family in Arcadia, a small town in southern Florida. In 1986 the three Ray hemophiliac sons, aged eight, nine, and ten, tested positive for the HIV virus and were promptly barred from the local elementary school. The following year, on 24 August, the children were readmitted to the school by court order. The community registered little compassion and reacted instead with a blind fear of infection. A boycott of the school was quickly organized. And on 28 August, just four days after the children reentered their school, the Ray house was burned down. Yet the children were not even ill: they only had the potential to become ill. The irony that these events happened the week before Labor Day weekend, the traditional time for Jerry Lewis's annual telethon to aid children suffering from muscular dystrophy, is especially acute. For the power of this telethon has been in the appearance of the impaired children as the object of the viewer's sympathy and concern. It is not unlikely that the same people who ignited the Ray home in Arcadia sat before their television sets a week later, feeling compassion for "Jerry's kids."

To understand the need for the continuation of this stigmatization after it has become evident that AIDS is not solely a sexually transmitted disease, it is important to note that there is a powerful secondary effect to the stigma. It clearly defines the boundaries of pollution, limiting the risk of pollution to the homosexual (and those other groups now stigmatized), and thus confined the fears the heterosexual community had about its vulnerability to the spread of sexually transmitted disease. But recently we have seen the appearance of the disease among heterosexuals. If the disease remains attributed to individuals associated with categories traditionally perceived as being different, its locus remains strictly defined—it is "over there," not "over here." The more heterosexual transmission of AIDS becomes "media" fact, the greater the need for heterosexuals to retain its image as a disease of socially marginal groups.

There were attempts in the media to make the public aware of the general risk run by all members of society, homosexual and heterosexual, of contracting AIDS. But the implied association of AIDS with homosexuality and sexually transmitted disease is unimaginably powerful. And this association was quite often captured in the image of the AIDS patient. In the *Newsweek* essay published in the summer of 1986, cited at the beginning of this chapter, there was the stated editorial intent to alter the image of individuals living with AIDS, in order to stress that all readers of the essay might be at risk. Accompanying this essay were three images of AIDS patients. All are male and all are represented in the traditional iconography of the male sufferer as isolated patient. Moreover, the first image—the first individual living with AIDS which the reader sees upon opening to this cover story—is not only male, he is black (Plate 51). The black male homosexual is still the archetype of the individual suffering from AIDS even in the context of an essay that explicitly stresses the potential for widespread heterosexual transmission of the disease. This contrast points toward the power of the initial stereotyping of the individual living with AIDS as a marginal member of society.

By the spring of 1987 the public understanding of AIDS as a disease not limited to specific marginal groups had begun to grow. The statement of the Surgeon-General of the United States, Everett Koop, in support of the general extension of information about condoms and the increased media attention to heterosexual transmission meant that by March 1987, a majority of those being tested in the public AIDS clinics in New York and San Francisco were heterosexuals. But even this awareness of the recategorization of AIDS from a disease of specific marginal groups to the "majority," to the heterosexual community, did not mitigate the need for strict boundaries to be maintained. In a cartoon of mid-March 1987, J. D. Crowe of the San Diego *Tribune* presents the source for the heterosexual transmission of AIDS in the form of a group of prostitutes represented as the threat of death (Plate 52). This shift, from the male sufferer to the female source of pollution, clearly parallels the history of the iconography of syphilis. Here a new group is labeled as the source of disease, women—but not of course all women, only those who are beyond the social pale of respectability. Even in the acknowledgment of the heterosexual transmission of the disease the attempt is made to maintain clear and definite boundaries so as to limit the "majority's" anxiety about their own potential risk.

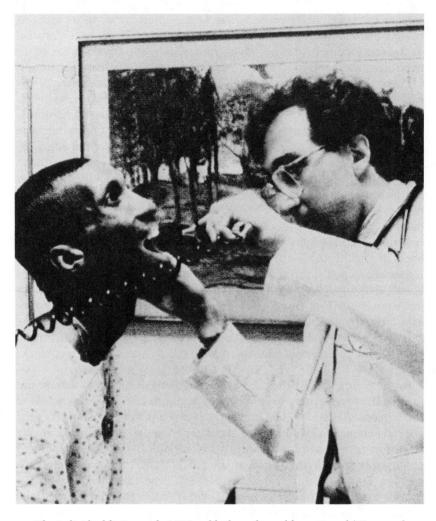

51. The individual living with AIDS as black, male, and homosexual (*Newsweek*, 21 July 1986).

It is evident that the study of the images, both verbal and visual, of the sufferer of a disease reveals many of the often contradictory structures of our understanding of disease. With society's attempt to categorize and limit AIDS still in its first decade, the construction of the image of the AIDS patient can already be seen to be both paralleling and deviating from earlier models of disease. While the powerful iconography of the sexually transmitted disease patient haunts our understanding of AIDS, other images, such as those of depression, have begun to enter into the

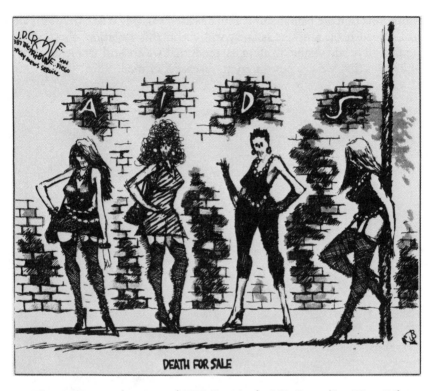

52. The prostitute as the source of AIDS. Drawing by J. D. Crowe (*San Diego Tribune,* 14 March 1987).

construction of the image of the person living with AIDS as it did that of the syphilitic. With the representation of AIDS, as with other images of disease, it is the historically determined variations that mark the function and place of the sufferer in relation to the society in which he or she dwells. From such images we can begin to understand how such models of disease evoke the most deep-seated sense of the self's fragility. Those suffering the very diseases about which such fantasies are spun are themselves not immune; they respond to the isolation and stigmatization that is the social boundary of their disease, not part of the disease itself. The necessary constraints placed on our dealing with fantasies of disease by our need to create a boundary between ourselves and the afflicted, our image of the patient as the container and transmitter of the disease, and, indeed, our sense of our own selves as mortal beings are all embedded in our need to distance and isolate those we designate as ill. And one locus for these fantasies is the work of art, whether the paintings of Goya or the illustrations in our popular weekly magazines. It is in this world of representations that we banish our fear of disease, isolating it as surely as if we had placed it on a desert island. And yet in this isolation, these icons remain alive and visible to all of us, proof that we are still whole, healthy, and sane; that we are not different, diseased, or mad.

NOTES

1. Depicting Disease: A Theory of Representing Illness

1. Manfred Bleuler, "What Is Schizophrenia?" *Schizophrenia Bulletin* 10 (1984): 8.

2. Mary Douglas, *Purity and Danger: An Analysis of the Concepts of Pollution and Taboo* (London: Routledge & Kegan Paul, 1966), p. 162.

3. I am using the term *icon* in the sense suggested by C. S. Peirce, *Collected Papers of Charles Sanders Peirce,* ed. Charles Hartshorne, Paul Weiss, and Arthur W. Burks, 8 vols. (Cambridge, Mass.: Harvard University Press, 1931–58). An icon is a sign that represents its object by being similar to it in some respect in that it exemplifies some property associated with the object (2:282). But the properties of the sign which underlie its iconic nature are intrinsic; that is, they are independent of the actual existence of the object (4:447). As a result, Peirce argues (and I agree with him in this), icons cannot represent particular individuals but only general classes of things (3:434). Therefore, the very representation of a patient suffering from a disease, even if the patient and disease are "real," i.e., existing separate from the icon in time and space, has iconic character, and it shall be so treated in the present study.

4. W. J. T. Mitchell, *Iconology: Image, Text, Ideology* (Chicago: University of Chicago Press, 1986), p. 38. On the general question of the representation of science, see the introduction to L. J. Jordanova, ed., *Languages of Nature: Critical Essays on Science and Literature* (London: Free Association Books, 1986), pp. 15–50. While Jordanova does not stress the representation of the pathological, it is clear that her general comments are applicable to the question of the representation of illness.

5. This concept is taken from Mikhail Bakhtin, *Rabelais and His World,* trans. Hélène Iswolsky (Cambridge, Mass.: M.I.T. Press, 1965). Much of the discussion of competing concepts of discourse is also taken from Bakhtin's essays, translated by Caryl Emerson and Michael Holquist, *The Dialogic Imagination* (Austin: University of Texas Press, 1981).

6. Lillian Feder, *Madness in Literature* (Princeton, N.J.: Princeton University Press, 1980).

7. See the discussion by Robert Scott Root-Bernstein, "On Paradigms and Revolutions in Science and Art: The Challenge of Interpretation," *Art Journal* 44 (1984): 109–18.

8. For a more detailed discussion of this view of stereotypes, see the introductory chapter of my *Difference and Pathology: Stereotypes of Sexuality, Race, and Madness* (Ithaca, N.Y.: Cornell University Press, 1985), pp. 15–35.

9. L. A. Nordholm, "Beautiful Patients Are Good Patients: Evidence for Physical Attractiveness Stereotype in First Impressions of Patients," *Social Science and Medicine* 14A (1980): 81–83.

10. Shirley M. Johnson, Margot E. Kurtz, Thomas Tomlinson, and Kenneth R. Howe, "Students' Stereotypes of Patients as Barriers to Clinical Decision-making," *Journal of Medical Education* 61 (1986): 727–35, and J. P. Trachtman, "Socio-economic Class Bias in Rorschach Diagnosis: Contributions to Psychosocial Attitudes of the Clinicians," *Journal of Personality Assessment* 35 (1971): 229–40. For an indication of the

complexities of this problem, see V. A. Braithwaite, "Old Age Stereotypes: Reconciling Contradictions," *Journal of Gerontology* 41 (1986): 353–60.

11. P. Franks, L. Culpepper, and J. Dickinson, "Psychosocial Bias in the Diagnosis of Obesity," *Journal of Family Practice* 14 (1982): 745–50.

12. Without a doubt the most revealing (and well-documented) case is that of the Fore of New Guinea and their attempts to understand (and therefore to control) kuru. See Shirley Lindenbaum, *Kuru Sorcery* (Palo Alto, Calif.: Mayfield, 1979).

13. Sander L. Gilman, *Jewish Self-Hatred: Anti-Semitism and the Hidden Language of the Jews* (Baltimore: Johns Hopkins University Press, 1986).

14. See the general discussion by Otto Kernberg in my *Introducing Psychoanalytic Theory* (New York: Brunner / Mazel, 1982), pp. 126–38.

15. Anna Freud, *The Ego and the Mechanisms of Defense* (New York: International Universities Press, 1966), pp. 109–21.

16. See Roy Porter, ed., *Patients and Practitioners: Lay Perceptions of Medicine in Pre-Industrial Society* (Cambridge: Cambridge University Press, 1986), for a first-rate introduction to this general problem.

17. For the general bipolar model of disease and health, see H. T. Engelhardt, Jr., "The Concepts of Health and Disease," in H. T. Engelhardt, Jr., and S. F. Spicker, eds., *Evaluation and Explanation in the Biomedical Sciences* (Dordrecht: Reidel, 1975), pp. 125–41.

18. Miriam Siegler and Humphry Osmond, *Models of Madness, Models of Medicine* (New York: Macmillan, 1974), p. xviii. The models that Siegler and Osmond describe in some depth are the "medical," the "moral," the "impaired," the "psychoanalytic," the "social," the "psychedelic," the "conspiratorial," and the "family interactional."

19. Paul R. McHugh and Phillip R. Slavney, *The Perspectives of Psychiatry* (Baltimore: Johns Hopkins University Press, 1983).

20. On the debate in philosophy concerning "realism" versus "antirealism," see the recent book by Anthony Appiah, *For Truth in Semantics* (Oxford: Blackwell, 1986).

21. Certainly the major works in this recent tradition are Michel Foucault, *Histoire de la folie à l'âge classique* (Paris: Gallimard, 1972); Thomas Szasz, *The Manufacture of Madness* (New York: Harper & Row, 1970); and Klaus Dörner, *Bürger und Irre* (Cologne: Europäische Verlagsanstalt, 1969). All of these works subscribe to the overall view that one can "explain" the "errors" of contemporary psychoanalytic and psychiatric practices through their history. Recent work has been undertaken to correct these positions. See esp. the collected work by William F. Bynum, Roy Porter, and Michael Shepherd, eds., *The Anatomy of Madness: Essays in the History of Psychiatry*, 2 vols. (London: Tavistock, 1985). Recently the Paris-based school devoted to the study of group response (*mentalité*), which had from the 1930s marginally dealt with the question of disease in society, has discovered the problem of the social construction of disease. See Claudine Herzlich and Janine Pierret, *Illness and Self in Society*, trans. Elborg Forster (Baltimore: Johns Hopkins University Press, 1987).

22. Why is it that the image of the "bag-lady" is feminized? There are indeed a large number of men who have been discharged by mental hospitals onto the street and yet our image of the street person is as a female. And, indeed, this has also been the media image, as can be seen by the portrayal of "bag-ladies" on television. Is it not a conflation of the images of the violent insane with the traditional Western image of the female as the sign of the irrational? On this topic, see the brilliant book by Elaine Showalter, *The Female Malady: Women, Madness, and English Culture, 1830–1980* (New York: Pantheon, 1985).

23. H. W. Dunham, *Community and Schizophrenia* (Detroit: Wayne State University Press, 1965).

24. On the nature of violence and mental illness, see E. D. Tanke and J. A. Yesavage, "Characteristics of Assaultive Patients Who Do and Do Not Provide Visible Cues of Potential Violence," *American Journal of Psychiatry* 142 (185): 1409–13.

25. See the more detailed discussion in my *Difference and Pathology*, pp. 59–76.

26. Alvin V. Sellers, *The Loeb-Leopold Case with Excerpts from the Evidence of the Alienists . . .* (Brunswick, Ga.: Classic Publishing, 1926), p. 180.

27. Renzo Villa, *Il deviante ei suoi segni: Lombroso e la nascita dell'antropologia criminale* (Milan: Angeli, 1985).

28. On the general context of the Hinckley case, see D. Shore et al., "White House Cases: Psychiatric Patients and the Secret Service," *American Journal of Psychiatry* 142 (1985): 308–12 and Lincoln Caplan, *The Insanity Defense: And the Trial of John W. Hinckley, Jr.* (New York: Laurel / Dell, 1987).

29. On the background to the testimony, see Peter Low, *The Trial of John W. Hinckley, Jr.* (Mineola, N.Y.: Foundation Press, 1986).

30. See André Mayer and Michael Wheeler, *The Crocodile Man: A Case of Brain Chemistry and Criminal Violence* (Boston: Houghton Mifflin, 1982).

2. Madness and Representation:
Toward a History of Visualizing Madness

1. This chapter summarizes the general history of psychiatric illustration which is presented in much greater detail in my *Seeing the Insane* (New York: Wiley, 1982; paperback, 1985). Until that work the literature on medical illustration all but ignored the question of psychiatric illustration. Robert Herrlinger does not touch on it in the first volume of his *Geschichte der medizinischen Abbildung* (Munich: Moos, 1967–72), and the posthumous second volume, compiled by M. Putscher, mentions only Géricault. Other works that touched on this topic are *Kunst und Medizin* (Cologne: DuMont / Schauberg, 1966); Rudolf Lemke, *Psychiatrische Themen in Malerei und Graphik* (Jena: Fischer, 1958); Rene Fülöp-Miller, *Kampf gegen Schmerz und Tod: Kulturgeschichte der Heilkunde* (Berlin: Süd-Ost, 1938); Hermann August Adam, *Über Geisteskrankheit in alter und neuer Zeit: Ein Stück Kulturgeschichte in Wort und Bild* (Regensburg: Rath, 1928); Eugen Holländer, *Die Karikatur und Satire in der Medizin* (Stuttgart: Enke, 1935); Jean Martin Charcot and Paul Richer, *Démoniaques dans l'art* (Paris: Delahaye et Lecrosnier, 1887).

2. Translation from Leonard Forster, ed., *The Penguin Book of German Verse* (Baltimore: Penguin, 1959), p. 22. See the background outlined by Raymond Klibansky, Erwin Panofsky, and Fritz Saxl, *Saturn and Melancholy: Studies in the History of Natural Philosophy, Religion, and Art* (London: Nelson, 1964); Moshe Barasche, *Gestures of Despair in Medieval and Early Renaissance Art* (New York: New York University Press, 1976); and André Chastel, *Fables, Formes, Figures* (Paris: Flammarion, 1978), 1:149–59.

3. William Schupbach, "A New Look at 'The Cure of Folly,'" *Medical History* 22 (1978): 267–81.

4. Michel Foucault, in *Histoire de la folie* (Paris: Gallimard, 1972), outlines the background of this shift, but confuses the "reality" of confinement with the metaphors used to describe it, especially the "ship of fools." See Kathleen M. Grange, "The Ship Symbol as a Key to Former Theories of the Emotions," *Bulletin of the History of Medicine* 36 (1961): 512–23.

5. Ronald Paulson, *Hogarth's Graphic Works* (New Haven: Yale University Press, 1965), 1:169–70. Hogarth's plate of Bedlam was an important force in creating a tradi-

tion of the madhouse scene. The interpretation of this plate which appeared in the continuation of Lichtenberg's Hogarth interpretation (*G. C. Lichtenberg's ausführliche Erklärung der Hogarthischen Kupferstiche mit verkleinerten aber vollständigen Copien derselben* [Göttingen: Dieterich, 1808], 3:132–44) is quoted in Moreau de la Sarthe's appendix on the physiognomy of insanity. It also served as the model for Wilhelm von Kaulbach's *Das Narrenhaus* (1835), perhaps the most famous popular presentation of the physiognomy of insanity in the graphic art of the nineteenth century. Kaulbach's engraving was extensively interpreted in the tradition of the physiognomy of insanity in Guido Görres, *Das Narrenhaus von Wilhelm Kaulbach* (Regensburg: Pustet, 1836), and again in Johann August Schilling, *Psychiatrische Briefe oder die Irren, das Irresein und das Irrenhaus* (Augsburg: Schlosser, 1864), 32:387–473.

6. Innes and Gustav Herdan, trans., *Lichtenberg's Commentaries on Hogarth's Engravings* (London: Cresset, 1966), p. 263.

7. Numerous surveys of the theories of physiognomy have been made. The best are those that introduce the volume *Ausdruckspsychologie*, ed. R. Kirchhof, vol. 5 of *Handbuch der Psychologie* (Göttingen: Hogrefe, 1965): R. Kirchhof, "Zur Geschichte des Ausdrucksbegriffs," pp. 9–38, and K. Holzkamp, "Zur Geschichte und Systematik der Ausdrucktheorien," pp. 39–116. From the standpoint of the history of art the best introduction remains the discussion by Ernst Kris, "Die Charakterköpfe des Franz Zavier Messerschmidt," *Jahrbuch der Kunsthistorischen Sammlungen Wien*, n.f., 6 (1932): 169–228. The latter contains numerous illustrations from works on physiognomy.

8. Johann Caspar Lavater, *Physiognomische Fragmente zur Beförderung der Menschenkenntnis und Menschenliebe* (Leipzig: Weidmann, 1776), 2:181. Concerning Lavater, see Reinhard Kunz, *Johann Caspar Lavaters Physiognomielehre im Urteil von Haller, Zimmerman und anderen zeitgenössischen Ärzten*. Züricher Medizingeschichtliche Abhandlunge, n.f., 71 (Zurich: Juris, 1970); John Graham, *Lavater's Essays on Physiognomy: A Study in the History of Ideas* (Frankfurt: Lang, 1979); and Graeme Tytler, *Physiognomy in the European Novel: Faces and Fortunes* (Princeton, N.J.: Princeton University Press, 1982).

9. *Goethe und Lavater: Briefe und Tagebücher*, ed. Heinrich Funck. Schriften der Goethe-Gesellschaft 16 (Weimar: Goethe-Gesellschaft, 1901), p. 58. See also the *Corpus der Goethezeichnungen* (Leipzig: Seemann, 1958 ff.), 1:239; 3:52, 122, 127, 133, 139, 140, 170.

10. Immanuel Kant, *Werke*, ed. Wilhelm Weischedel (Wiesbaden: Insel, 1964), 10:638–39.

11. Vincenzo Chiarugi, *Della pazzia in genere e in specie tratto medico-analitico con una centuria de osservazioni* (Florence: Carlieri, 1793–94).

12. Philippe Pinel, *Traité médico-philosophique sur l'aliénation mentale, ou la manie* (Paris: Richard, Caille, et Ravier, 1801). Concerning Pinel, see Walther Riese, *The Legacy of Philippe Pinel: An Inquiry into Thought on Mental Alienation* (New York: Springer, 1969).

13. George Rosen, "The Philosophy of Ideology and the Emergence of Modern Medicine in France," *Bulletin of the History of Medicine* 20 (1946): 329–39.

14. *Encyclopédie méthodique*, 172 vols.: *Médecine* (Paris: Agasse, 1816), 9:136–219.

15. *L'art de connaître des hommes par Gaspard Lavater* (Paris: n.p., 1807), 8:224, 230.

16. Charles Bell, *Essays on the Anatomy of Expression in Painting* (London: Longman et al., 1806). Concerning Bell, see Gordon Gordon-Taylor, *Sir Charles Bell: His Life and Times* (Edinburgh: Livingstone, 1958), esp. pp. 17–26.

17. See Anthony Blunt, "Blake's Pictorial Imagination," *Journal of the Warburg and*

Courtauld Institutes 6 (1943): 203–4; Jean H. Hagstrum, *William Blake: Poet and Painter* (Chicago: University of Chicago Press, 1964), p. 38; Kathleen Raine, *William Blake* (London: Thames and Hudson, 1970), p. 85. Blake makes reference to the legend of Nebuchadnezzar in a letter to William Hayley of 23 October 1804 (*The Letters of William Blake*, ed. Geoffrey Keynes [Cambridge, Mass.: Harvard University Press, 1968], p. 106).

18. The atlas was published by Maze in Paris. Concerning the rise and spread of phrenology, see David De Guistino, *Conquest of Mind: Phrenology and Victorian Social Thought* (London: Croom Helm, 1975).

19. Johann Gaspard Spurzheim, *Observations on the Deranged Manifestations of the Mind, or Insanity* (London: Baldwin, Cradock, and Joy, 1817), pp. 132–37. A reprint of the observations, with a historical introduction by Anthony A. Walsh, appeared in 1970. Walsh also introduced the reprint of Andrew Combe, *Observations on Mental Derangement* (1831) (Delmar, N.Y.: Scholar's Facsimiles, 1972). See also P. S. Noel and E. T. Carlson, "The Origins of the Word 'phrenology,'" *American Journal of Psychiatry*, 127 (1970): 694–97.

20. Certainly the most influential German figure in the synthesis of phrenological theory and theories of expression was Goethe's friend Carl Gustav Carus. In his *Vorlesungen über Psychologie gehalten im Winter 1829–30*, ed. Edgar Michaëlis (Erlenbach-Zurich: Rotapfel, 1931), Carus discusses the question of madness as the disruption of the mind-body identity (*Vorlesungen*, vols. 11–13). In his atlas *Grundzüge einer neuen und wissenschaftlich begrüdeten Cranioscopie* (Stuttgart: Balz, 1841), he presents two plates of the skulls of mentally ill subjects. All of Carus's work is summarized in his *Symbolik der menschlichen Gestalt: Ein Handbuch der Menschen kenntnis* (Leipzig: Brockhaus, 1853). See also Gerhard Kloos, *Die Konstitutionslehre von Carl Gustav Carus mit besonderer Berücksichtigung seiner Physiognomik*, *Bibliotheca psychiatrica et neurologica*, 90 (Basel: Karger, 1951).

21. Jean Etienne Dominique Esquirol, *Des maladies mentales, considérées sous les rapports médical, hygienique, et médico-legal* (Paris: Baillière, 1838), 2:167.

22. The tradition of the full-length symbolic portrait of the madwoman is found throughout English art of the period. Mortimer's *Britannia* is based on a poem by Thomson, and Richard Reinagle's *Fair Maria* on a character in Stern's *Sentimental Journey*. See Peter Tomory, *The Life and Art of Henry Fuseli* (London: Thames and Hudson, 1972), plates 190–93. The tradition continues into the mid-nineteenth century. The Belgian painter Antoine Wiertz painted his *Faim, Folie, Crime* in 1864; while this painting is symbolic, it is also rooted in the tradition of psychiatric illustration. See the catalogue *Antoine Wiertz, 1806–1865* (Paris: Damase, 1974).

23. Etienne Jean Georget, *De la folie* (Paris: Crevot, 1820), p. 133. The central essay on Georget and Géricault remains Margaret Miller, "Géricault's Paintings of the Insane," *Journal of the Warburg and Courtauld Institutes* 4 (1940–41): 151–63. Like Géricault, Goya too went into the asylum to paint the inmates. His paintings and drawings from the asylum at Saragossa reveal the contemporary concern with types of insanity which reappear in many of his other works. See August L. Mayer, *Francisco de Goya*, trans. Robert West (London: Dent, 1924), plates 115, 401, 402.

24. Charles Clément, *Géricault* (Paris: Didier, 1879), plate 37a.

25. Alexander Morison, *Outlines of Lectures on Mental Diseases*, 2d ed. (London: Longman et al., 1826), pp. 125–26, and his *The Physiognomy of Mental Diseases* (London: by the author, 1840), with much of the same introduction. A German translation/reprint of the atlas appeared in 1853. See also Vieda Skultans, ed., *Madness and Morals: Ideas of Insanity in the Nineteenth Century* (London: Routledge & Kegan Paul, 1975), pp. 71–98.

26. Karl Heinrich Baumgärtner, *Kranken-Physiognomik, Zweite Auflage* (Stuttgart: Rieger, 1842), p. 22; and Karl Wilhelm Ideler, *Biographieen Geisteskranker in ihrer psychologischen Entwicklung dargestellt* (Berlin: Schröder, 1841). Cf. Hermann Oppenheim, "Beiträge zum Studium des Gesichtsausdrucks der Geisteskranken," *Allgemeine Zeitschrift für Psychiatrie* 40 (1884): 840–63.

27. See my *The Face of Madness: Hugh W. Diamond and the Origin of Psychiatric Photography* (New York: Brunner and Mazel, 1976), pp. 19–24.

28. "The First Principle of Physiognomy," *Cornhill Magazine* 4 (1861): 570. On the general background, see Renata Taureck, *Die Bedeutung der Photographie für die medizinische Abbildung im 19. Jahrhundert*. Arbeiten der Forschungsstelle des Instituts für Geschichte der Medizin der Universität zu Köln, 15 (Cologne: Forschungsstelle des Instituts für Geschichte der Medizin der Universität zu Köln, 1980).

29. Bénédict-Auguste Morel, *Traité des dégénérescences physiques, intellectuelles, et morales de l'espèce humaine et des causes qui produisent ces variétés maladies. Atlas de XII. Planches* (Paris: Baillière, 1857), p. 5: "Les caractères de l'ordre intellectuel, physique et moral qui distinguent les variétés maladises des variétés naturelles dans l'espèce, ont été l'objet de mes recherches dans le *Traité* qui accompagne cet Atlas. La description de toutes les variétés qui s'éloignent du type normal de l'humanité ne pourra être complétée, je le sais, que par la généralisation de cette étude. Toutefois, je pense avoir déjà accumulé assez de faits pour établir d'une manière irréfragable qu'il existe entre *les races naturelles et les variétés dégénérées* des caractères distinctifs, fixes et invariables."

30. H. G. Wright, "On the Medical Uses of Photography," *Photographic Journal* 9 (1867): 204.

31. John Conolly, "The Physiognomy of Insanity," *Medical Times and Gazette*, n.s., 16 (1858): 3.

32. Published by Hunt in Philadelphia.

33. The first edition appeared in 1845 from Krabbe (Stuttgart), the second in 1861, the third in 1871, the fourth in 1876, and the fifth in 1892. An English edition was published in New York in 1867.

34. Published in Erlangen by Enke, 2d ed., 1865. Other contemporary illustrated handbooks are Dietrich von Kieser, *Elemente der Psychiatrik* (Breslau: Kaiserl. L. C. Akademie, 1855), with eleven plates, and A. Tebaldi, *Fisonomia ed espressione* (Padua: Drucker e Tedeschi, 1884), with plates taken from Morison and Leidesdorf.

35. For a general survey of the question, see Jerome Shaffer's essay "Mind-Body Problem," in *The Encyclopedia of Philosophy*, ed. Paul Edwards (New York: Macmillan, 1967), 5:336–46.

36. Charles Darwin, *The Expression of the Emotions in Man and Animals* (London: Murray, 1872).

37. In three volumes (Paris: Progrès médical, 1877–80). On the tradition of photographing the insane, see Aaron H. Esman, "Henri Dagonet: Pioneer of Psychiatric Photography," *New York State Journal of Medicine* 84 (1984): 79–81, and Georges Didi-Huberman, *Invention de l'hystérie: Charcot et l'iconographie photographique de la Salpêtrière* (Paris: Macula, 1982).

38. Theodor Reik, *Listening with the Third Ear* (New York: Farrar, Straus, 1949), pp. 144–45.

39. Immanuel Kant, *Critique of Practical Reason*, trans. L. W. Beck (Indianapolis: Liberal Arts Press, 1956), p. 14.

40. Alfred Freedman, Harold Kaplan, and Benjamin Sadock, *Modern Synopsis of Comprehensive Textbook of Psychiatry*, Student Edition (Baltimore: Williams and Wilkins, 1967), pp. 349, 444, 446–47, 492.

41. For a survey of the recent literature, see H. Brengelmann, "Expressive Movements and Abnormal Behavior," in *Handbook of Abnormal Psychology*, ed. H. J. Eysenck (New York: Basic Books, 1961), pp. 62–107.

42. See Robert Hughes, "Pictures at an Institution," *Time*, 23 January 1978, p. 91. For the context, see Allan Sekula, "On the Invention of Photographic Meaning," *Artforum*, January 1975, pp. 37–45.

43. Sara Facio, Alicia D'Amico, and Julio Cortázar, *Humanario* (Buenos Aires: La Azotea, 1976).

44. Thomas E. Hansen, Daniel E. Casey, and Ronald M. Weigel, "TD Prevalence: Research and Clinical Differences," *Proceedings of the American Psychiatric Association Annual Meeting* (1986): 113.

45. Thomas E. Hansen, Daniel E. Casey, and W. M. Vollmer, "Is There an Epidemic of Tardive Dyskinesia?" *Proceedings of the American Psychiatric Association Annual Meeting* (1985): 85–86.

3. The Rediscovery of the Body: Leonardo's First Image of Human Sexuality and Disease

1. There are numerous biographies of Leonardo which document this accusation. I rely here on the discussion by Giuseppina Fumagalli, *Eros di Leonardo* (Milan: Garzanti, 1952). Her view, stated against Freud's view of Leonardo, is used since she has taken the diametrically opposed position to my analysis concerning the interpretation of the anatomical drawings. Her discussion of this matter as well as of the anatomical drawings is to be found on pp. 98–126.

2. See Sigmund Freud, "Leonardo da Vinci and a Memory of His Childhood," *The Standard Edition of the Psychological Works of Sigmund Freud* (London: Hogarth, 1957), 11:59–138. It is clear that I have attempted to cover some of the same ground that Meyer Schapiro did in his two seminal essays "Two Slips of Leonardo and a Slip of Freud," *Psychoanalysis* 4 (1955–56): 3–8, and "Leonardo and Freud: An Art-Historical Study," *Journal of the History of Ideas* 27 (1956): 147–78, while trying to place the iconographic and historical reading within a psychological matrix. It is thus with some care that I have used K. R. Eissler, *Leonardo da Vinci: Psychoanalytic Notes on the Enigma* (New York: International Universities Press, 1961), which attempts to counter Schapiro, as Eissler's lack of understanding of the usefulness of Schapiro's method for a deeper reading of Leonardo is evident. I have also used the contemporary terms "gay" and "homosexual" to describe the internalized response as well as the social prejudice concerning same-sex erotic activity. While there are certainly differences in the perceptions of same-sex eroticism in the Renaissance and in contemporary use, the opprobrium associated with the term "sodomite" would slant the rhetoric of my presentation.

3. I am grateful for the background of Leonardo's potential fine to the work of Michael Rocke of the State University of New York at Binghamton, who is at present completing a dissertation on homosexuality in Renaissance Florence with the working title "Homosexuality in Late Medieval Florence."

4. Ludwig Freiherr von Pastor, *The History of the Popes from the Close of the Middle Ages*, trans. Ralph Francis Kerr (London: Kegan, Paul, 1924), 14:238–39, 266–68. Compare this with James M. Saslow, *Ganymede in the Renaissance* (New Haven: Yale University Press, 1986), in which the myth-making about as well as the practice of homosexuality during the Renaissance, especially in Florence, is examined in great

detail; cf. also Guido Ruggiero, *The Boundaries of Eros: Sex Crime and Sexuality in Renaissance Venice* (New York: Oxford University Press, 1985), pp. 109–45.

5. I am indebted to Mary Jacobus for making her chapter "Motherhood according to Kristeva" available to me in advance of the publication of her *Reading Woman* (New York: Columbia University Press, 1986).

6. Private, of course, only in the sense that diaries are private. Leonardo knew the representational value of these works even though he shielded them with his own "code," his mirror writing. He did will them to Francesco Melzi, who viewed them as one of the most valuable parts of Leonardo's estate. And these notebooks had immediate and constant value on the art market.

7. All references to this plate and to the translations have been checked against Kenneth S. Keele and Carlo Pedretti, eds., *Leonardo da Vinci, Corpus of the Anatomical Studies in the Collection of Her Majesty the Queen at Windsor Castle*, 3 vols. (New York: Johnson Reprint / Harcourt, Brace, Jovanovich, 1979), hereafter referred to as *K/P.* I do not always agree with the translations in this edition, but it is the most accurate reproduction of all of the extant anatomical materials. On the general background, see Heidi Lenssen, *Art and Anatomy* (New York: Augustin, 1944); Mario Senaldi, *L'anatomia e la fisologia di Leonardo da Vinci,* vol. 8 (Milan: Il Museo Nazionale della Scienza e della Tecnica, n.d.); Otto Baur, *Leonardo da Vinci, Anatomie, Physiognomik, Proportion und Bewegung* (Cologne: Forschungsstelle des Instituts für Geschichte der Medizin der Universität zu Köln, 1984); Moriz Holl, *Ein Biologe aus der Wende des XV. Jahrhunderts, Leonardo da Vinci* (Graz: Leuschner & Lubensky, 1905). The literature on Leonardo's anatomical drawings is summarized in Heinz Ladendorf, *Leonardo da Vinci und die Wissenschaft: Eine Literaturübersicht,* 2 vols. (Cologne: Forschungsstelle des Instituts für Geschichte der Medizin der Universität zu Köln, 1984).

8. Charles D. O'Malley and J. B. de C. M. Saunders, eds., *Leonardo on the Human Body* (New York: Dover, 1983), p. 460.

9. Rudolf Reitler, "Eine anatomisch-künstlerische Fehlleistung Leonardos da Vinci," *Internationale Zeitschrift für Psychoanalyse* 4 (1917): 205–7. Reitler's views are not unique; see Gabriel Peillon, *Etude historique sur les organes génitaux de la femme* (Paris: Berthier, 1891), pp. 131–73. On the complex question of Freud's reading of Leonardo's image of sexuality, see Jacqueline Rose, "Sexuality in the Field of Vision," in her *Sexuality in the Field of Vision* (London: Verso, 1986), pp. 224–33.

10. See Freud's source, Dmitri Mereschkowski, *Leonardo da Vinci: Ein biographischer Roman aus der Wende des 15. Jahrhunderts,* trans. Carl von Goetschow (Leipzig: Schulz, 1903). I am grateful to the Freud Museum, Hampstead, for granting me access to the volumes on Leonardo in Freud's London library.

11. Edmund Solmi, *Leonardo da Vinci,* trans. Emmi Hirschberg (Berlin: Hofmann, 1908). In his copy, Freud made a marginal note on the page where the dream is related with the mistranslation of the bird's name.

12. Ludwig Choulant, *Geschichte und Bibliographie der anatomischen Abbildung nach ihrer Beziehung auf anatomische Wissenschaft und bildende Kunst* (Leipzig: Weigel, 1852), translated and updated by M. Frank as *History and Bibliography of Anatomical Illustration* (Chicago: University of Chicago Press, 1945), pp. 23–27.

13. Ernest Wickersheimer, *Anatomie de Mondino dei Luzzi et de Guido de Vigevano* (Paris: Droz, 1926), and Lino Sighinolfi and Giacinto Viola, eds., *Mondino dei Luzzi, Anatomia* (Bologna: Cappelli, 1930). The former is a reproduction of the first printed edition, the latter, of a manuscript version with a contemporary Italian translation. See also Charles Singer, ed. and trans., *The Fasciculo de Medicina Venice, 1493* (Florence: Leier, 1925), 1:75–79, for an English translation of the relevant passages from Mon-

dino; also his "Notes of Renaissance Artists and Practical Anatomy," *Journal of the History of Medicine* 5 (1950): 156–62; and G. Rath, "Prevesalian Anatomy in the Light of Modern Research," *Bulletin of the History of Medicine* 35 (1961): 142–48.

14. William G. Eberhard, *Sexual Selection and Animal Genitalia* (Cambridge, Mass.: Harvard University Press, 1985), pp. 19–20.

15. But even more specifically, the sexual imagery of the "key and lock" haunts the description of the "cave of the lovers" in Gottfried von Strassburg's *Tristan*. See the clear reference to this in the text as translated by A. T. Hatto (Baltimore: Penguin, 1960), pp. 264–66.

16. Kenneth D. Keele, *Leonardo da Vinci's Elements of the Science of Man* (New York: Academic Press, 1983), pp. 243–45. See also the general introduction in his *Leonardo da Vinci and the Art of Science* (Hove, East Sussex: Wayland Publishers, 1977).

17. Edith Hamilton and Huntington Cairns, eds., *The Collected Dialogues of Plato*, Bollingen Series 71 (New York: Pantheon, 1961), p. 1210.

18. See Luigi Messedaglia, *Vita e costume della Rinascenza in Merlin Cocai* (Padua: Antenore, 1973), 2:419–25. It is important to note that Leonardo's page is undated, but even if the earliest date (1493) is taken, the potential for the knowledge of the disease was present. If a slightly later date is accepted (1495), such knowledge is a certainty.

19. Bernadette Boucher, *La sauvage aux seins pendants* (Paris: Hermann, 1977).

20. Erwin Panofsky, "Homage to Fracastoro in a Germano-Flemish Composition of about 1590?" *Nederlands Kunsthistorisch Jaarboek* 12 (1961): 14.

21. For a more detailed discussion of this figure and its implications, see Chapter 14.

22. The signification of this position for Leonardo and his contemporaries can be seen in the very fact that when Michelangelo chooses to portray his *Leda* after Leonardo he places his figures in a much more conventional supine position. See the discussion of this in Robert S. Liebert, *Michelangelo: A Psychoanalytic Study of His Life and Images* (New Haven: Yale University Press, 1983), pp. 256–57, and Bernard Schultz, *Art and Anatomy in Renaissance Italy* (Ann Arbor: UMI Research Press, 1985), pp. 69–109.

23. Aristotle, *Parts of Animals*, trans. A. L. Peck (Cambridge, Mass.: Harvard University Press, 1968), p. 297. Cf. Kenneth Keele, "Leonardo da Vinci's Studies of the Alimentary Tract," *Journal of the History of Medicine and Allied Sciences* 27 (1972): 133 ff., K/P 72r.

24. K/P 72r. See also Bernard Schultz, *Art and Anatomy in Renaissance Italy* (Ann Arbor: UMI Research Press, 1985), pp. 69–109.

25. Cited in the best and most detailed study of early attitudes toward homosexuality, John Boswell, *Christianity, Social Tolerance, and Homosexuality: Gay People in Western Europe from the Beginning of the Christian Era to the Fourteenth Century* (Chicago: University of Chicago Press, 1980), p. 357.

26. Jean Paul Richter, ed., *The Literary Works of Leonardo da Vinci* (London: Oxford University Press, 1939), 2:265.

27. The alternate view also existed. It saw homosexuality, as well as all forms of sexuality which did not lead to conception, as a human fault, which could not exist among the lower animals. Matteo Ricci, in commenting on the widespread practice of homosexuality in sixteenth-century China, observed: "Even the wild animals only make their bonds between female and male, none of them overturn the nature heaven gave them." Cited by Jonathan D. Spence, *The Memory Palace of Matteo Ricci* (New York: Penguin, 1984), p. 229.

28. Boswell, *Christianity, Social Tolerance, and Homosexuality*, pp. 303–32.

29. It is clear that the views of homosexuality present in the Middle Ages and the

Renaissance cannot be perfunctorily summarized. In addition to Boswell, I have relied on Vern L. Bullough and James Brundage, eds., *Sexual Practices and the Medieval Church* (Buffalo, N.Y.: Prometheus Books, 1982), and Michael Goodich, *The Unmentionable Vice: Homosexuality in the Late Medieval Period* (Santa Barbara, Calif.: ABC-Clio, 1979), esp. pp. 28–30.

30. Jacopo Berengario da Carpi, *A Short Introduction to Anatomy*, trans. L. R. Lind (Chicago: University of Chicago Press, 1959), p. 76. His relationship to Leonardo's anatomical illustration has been described by A. Hyatt Mayor, *Artists and Anatomists* (New York: Artists' Limited Edition / Metropolitan Museum of Art, 1984), pp. 90–93.

31. Guido Biagi, ed., *La Divina Commedia nella figurazione artistica e nel secolare commento*, 3 vols. (Turin: Unione Tipografico–Editore Torinese, 1924–39), and Peter Brieger, Millard Meiss, and Charles S. Singleton, eds., *Illuminated Manuscripts of the Divine Comedy*, 2 vols. (Princeton, N.J.: Princeton University Press, 1969). The parallels between human beings and the rest of the animal kingdom rests on an age-old set of analogies. See Otto Baur, *Bestiarum Humanum. Mensch-Tier-Vergleich in Kunst und Karikatur* (Munich: Moos, 1974).

32. Richard Kay, "The Sin of Brunetto Latini," *Mediaeval Studies* 31 (1969): 262–86.

33. Thomas Okey, trans., and H. Oelsner, ed., *Dante's Purgatorio* (London: Dent, 1962), p. 325.

34. On the shift in the tradition of reading the "Sodom" passage from Genesis 19, see Boswell, *Christianity, Social Tolerance, and Homosexuality*, pp. 92–95.

35. Galen, *On the Usefulness of the Parts of the Body*, ed. and trans. Margaret May, 2 vols. (Ithaca, N.Y.: Cornell University Press, 1968), 2:628–29.

36. Boswell, *Christianity, Social Tolerance, and Homosexuality*, pp. 234–35.

37. *K/P* 143r, pp. 115–16. On this passage Marie Bonaparte observes, in the introduction to her translations of Freud's essay on Leonardo (*Freud, Un souvenir d'enfance de Léonard de Vinci* [Paris: Gallimard, 1927], p. 30): "From the psychoanalytic point of view it is conceivable that this contiguity is not accidental and that there existed an unconscious connection between his undoubtedly extreme repression of infantile masturbation and his subsequent disgust of sexuality. This may even be true also of the fact that he was left-handed, or at least preferred the left hand for drawing, painting, and writing. For it is remarkable that the hands Leonardo drew on the page on which he set down his thoughts about the disgust prompted in him by the sexual act are *all right hands*."

38. Carlo Pedretti, *The Literary Works of Leonardo da Vinci: A Commentary to Jean Paul Richter's Edition*, 2 vols. (London: Phaidon, 1977), 2:280.

4. Masturbation and Anxiety: Henry Mackenzie, Heinrich von Kleist, William James

1. See Michel Foucault, *The History of Sexuality*, vol. 1: *An Introduction*, trans. Robert Hurley (New York: Vantage, 1980).

2. All references to the novel are to the edition edited by Brian Vickers, Henry Mackenzie, *The Man of Feeling* (London: Oxford University Press, 1931), but also of interest is W. F. Wright, *Sensibility in English Prose Fiction, 1760–1814: A Reinterpretation*, Illinois Studies in Language and Literature (Urbana: University of Illinois Press, 1937), pp. xxii, 3–4, and the essay by A. M. Kinghorn, "Literary Aesthetics and the Sympathetic Emotions—A Main Trend in Eighteenth-Century Scottish Criticism," *Studies in Scottish Literature* 1 (1963): 35–47. More generally on the present topic the following studies are of interest: Max Byrd, *Visits to Bedlam: Madness and*

Literature in the Eighteenth Century (Columbia: University of South Carolina Press, 1974); Michael V. DePorte, *Nightmares and Hobbyhorses: Swift, Sterne, and Augustan Ideas of Madness* (San Marino, Calif.: Huntington Library, 1974); Mervyn James Jannetta, "'The Predominant Passion and Its Force': Propensity, Volition, and Motive in the Works of Swift and Pope" (diss.: University of York, 1975).

3. A detailed description of the plate can be found in Ronald Paulson, *Hogarth's Graphic Works* (New Haven: Yale University Press, 1970, rev. ed.), 1:169–70. Concerning the lasting reputation of Hogarth in the nineteenth century and his influence on Wilhelm Kaulbach's asylum scene of 1835, see Fritz von Ostini, *Wilhelm von Kaulbach*, Künstler Monographien 84 (Bielefeld: Velhangen und Klasing, 1906), pp. 58–66.

4. *The Poems of Jonathan Swift*, ed. Harold Williams (Oxford: Clarendon Press, 1958), 3:837–39.

5. Concerning this section two major interpretations exist: Heinz Ide, *Der junge Kleist: ". . . in dieser wandelbaren Zeit. . .,"* (Würzburg: Holzner, 1961), pp. 224–27, and Heinz Politzer, "Auf der Suche nach Identität: Zu Heinrich von Kleists Würzburger Reise," *Euphorion* 61 (1967): 383–99. Also of interest is Hans Joachim Kreutzer, *Die dichterische Entwicklung Heinrichs von Kleist. Untersuchungen zu seinen Briefen und zur Chronologie und Aufbau seiner Werke*. Philologische Studien und Quellen 41 (Berlin: Erich Schmidt, 1968), esp. pp. 45–105.

6. All references to Kleist's letter to his fiancée, Wilhelmine von Zenge, are to the edition by Helmut Sembdner, *Heinrich von Kleist: Sämtliche Werke und Briefe* (Munich: Carl Hanser, 1961), 2:559–62.

7. Anton Müller, *Die Irren-Anstalt in dem Königlichen Julius-Hospital zu Würzburg und die sechs und zwanzigjährigen ärztlichen Dienstverrichtungen an derselben* (Würzburg: Stahel, 1824), p. 167. See Anke Bennholdt-Thomsen, "Die Tradierung einer unbewiesenen Behauptung in der Kleist-Forschung," *Euphorion* 76 (1982): 169–73. The older philological literature on the Würzburg trip provides much of this background: Max Morris, *Heinrich von Kleists Reise nach Würzburg* (Berlin: Conrad Skopnik, 1899); S. Rahmer, *Das Kleist-Problem auf Grund neuer Forschungen zur Charakteristik und Biographie Heinrich von Kleists* (Berlin: Georg Reimer, 1903), esp. pp. 2575–93; and Berthold Schulze, *Neue Studien über Heinrich von Kleist* (Heidelberg: Carl Winter, 1904).

8. The question of the role played by the problem of masturbation in Kleist's early life has been discussed in depth. Politzer provides an excellent summary of the earlier discussion. Of this earlier literature, J. Sadger, *Heinrich von Kleist: Eine pathographisch-psychologische Studien* (Wiesbaden: Bergmann, 1910), first raised the question. Most influential was Stefan Zweig's essay on Kleist in *Der Kampf mit dem Dämon* (Leipzig: Insel, 1925), pp. 153–224. A little-known work that provides admirable material for understanding the context of Kleist's work is Karl Birnbaum, *Psychopathologische Dokumente: Selbstbekenntnisse und Fremdzeugnisse aus dem seelischen Grenzlande* (Berlin: Springer, 1920), esp. the chapter "Visionäre und phantastische Veranlagungen," pp. 72–84.

9. On the complex bibliographical problem of *Onania*, see René A. Spitz, "Authority and Masturbation: Some Remarks on a Bibliographical Investigator," *Yearbook of Psychoanalysis* 9 (1953): 116. The standard studies of masturbatory insanity are E. H. Hare, "Masturbatory Insanity: The History of an Idea," *Journal of Mental Science* 108 (1962): 1–25, and H. T. Engelhardt, Jr., "The Disease of Masturbation: Values and the Concept of Disease," *Bulletin of the History of Medicine* 48 (1974): 234–48. Of use is Karl-Felix Jacobs, *Die Entstehung der Onanie-Literatur im 17. und 18. Jahrhundert* (diss.: University of Munich, 1963), and R. P. Neuman, "Masturbation, Madness, and the Modern Concepts of Childhood and Adolescence," *Journal of Social History* 8

(1975): 1–26. None of these studies treats the eighteenth-century literature on masturbation printed in German. On the more general background, see Jean-Paul Aron and
Roger Kempf, *La pénis et la démoralisation de l'occident* (Paris: Grasset & Fasquelle,
1978), which attempts to place this question in the general problem of the nature of
class development.

10. See esp. Gudrun Burggraf, *Christian Gotthilf Salzmann im Vorfeld der fran-
zösischen Revolution* (Germering near Munich: Stahlmann, 1966).

11. Of importance in this context is the essay by Maria M. Tatar, "Psychology and
Poetics: J. C. Reil and Kleist's *Prinz Friedrich von Homburg*," *Germanic Review* 48
(1973): 21–34.

12. Benjamin Rush, *Medical Inquiries and Observations upon the Diseases of the
Mind* (1812), facsimile edition (New York: Hafner, 1962), pp. 349–50.

13. In the German version, it is to be found in *Onania, oder die Sünde der Selbst-
Befleckung, mit allen ihren schädlichen Folgen . . .* (Leipzig: Jacobäer, 1765), pp. 52–
53.

14. G. W. Becker, *Verhütung und Heilung der Onanie mit allen ihren Folgen bey
beyden Geschlechten* (Leipzig: Tauchnitz, 1803), pp. 250–51.

15. *Onania*, p. 23.

16. Rush, *Medical Inquiries*, p. 182.

17. Voltaire, "Onan, Onanisme," *Oeuvres complètes 20: Dictionnaire philoso-
phique* (Paris: Garnier, 1879), 4:133–35.

18. *Onania*, p. 13. See also Rush, *Medical Inquiries*, p. 350.

19. Becker, *Verhütung und Heilung der Onanie*, pp. 245–46. The ramification of this
text for Kleist's later works is clear. The question of emotional states and their representation could be reexamined in the light of this earlier model of the presentation of
madness. See Joachim Müller, *"Verwirrung des Gefühls": Der Begriff des "Pa-
thologischen" im Drama Goethes und Kleists*. Sitzungsberichte der Sächischen
Akademie der Wissenschaften zu Leipzig. Philologisch-historische Klasse, Band 117,
Heft 2 (Berlin: Akademie Verlag, 1974).

20. The standard discussion of James's vision is Ralph Barton Perry, *The Thought
and Character of William James* (Boston: Little, Brown, 1935), vol. 1: *Inheritance and
Vocation*, pp. 320–23. Perry is extremely careful not to assume the literal dating of
James's vision to be the winter of 1870. Quite independently of this chapter, Cushing
Strout, "William James and the Twice-Born Sick Soul," in his *The Veracious Imagina-
tion: Essays in American History, Literature, and Biography* (Middletown, Conn.:
Wesleyan University Press, 1981), pp. 199–222, sought a "French" source for James's
representation of his illness. Also of interest is Maurice Le Breton, *La personnalité de
William James* (Bordeaux: Imprimerie de l'Université, 1928), esp. pp. 238–44.

21. All quotations from the text are from William James, *The Varieties of Religious
Experience* (New York: Collier, 1961), pp. 137–39, which is the most accessible edition; in the first edition this passage is found on pp. 160–61. The evidence for James's
linking of his own experience to older examples of melancholy (primary affective
disorder) is tenuous. See Bridget Gellert Lyons, *Voices of Melancholy: Studies in Literary Treatments of Melancholy in Renaissance England* (London: Routledge & Kegan
Paul, 1971), for comparative examples.

22. Gay Wilson Allen, *William James: A Biography* (New York: Viking, 1967), pp.
164–67.

23. Cited from James's diaries by Allen, ibid., p. 164.

24. Henry James, *Society, the Redeemed Form of Man* (Boston: Houghton, Osgood,
1879), pp. 44–49. See also Frederic Harold Young, *The Philosophy of Henry James, Sr.*
(New York: Bookman Associates, 1951).

25. Jean Etienne Dominique Esquirol, *Des maladies mentales, considérées sous les rapports médical, hygienique, et médico-legal* (Paris: Baillière, 1838), 2:93–94.

26. The standard study has been C. Hartley Grattan, *The Three Jameses: A Family of Minds* (London: Longmans, Green, 1932), esp. pp. 122–25. It has recently been replaced by Howard Feinstein, *Becoming William James* (Ithaca, N.Y.: Cornell University Press, 1984).

27. Cited by Perry, *Thought and Character*, p. 165.

28. For a very good summary of the late nineteenth- and early twentieth-century literature on masturbation, see Wilhelm Stekel, *Auto-Erotism: A Psychiatric Study of Onanism and Neurosis*, trans. James S. Van Teslaar (New York: Liveright, 1950). Stekel argues (against Freud) that "masturbatory illnesses" are the internalization of a culture's prohibition against masturbation.

29. Henry Maudsley, *Body and Mind* (London: Macmillan, 1873), pp. 86–87.

30. Karen Horney, *Our Inner Conflicts: A Constructive Theory of Neurosis* (New York: Norton, 1945), pp. 115–30.

5. Images of the Asylum: Charles Dickens and Charles Davies

1. All references to this essay are to the edition of Harry Stone, ed., *Charles Dickens' Uncollected Writings from "Household Words," 1850–1859* (Bloomington: Indiana University Press, 1968), 2:381–91. Stone (p. 381) describes the state of the preserved manuscript of the essay and supplies editorial comment to it. The literature on the essay, as well as on the question of Dickens's knowledge of nineteenth-century psychiatric theories and practice, is not great. The major essays are: Richard A. Hunter and Ida Macalpine, "A Note on Dickens's Psychiatric Reading," *The Dickensian* 53 (1957): 49–51, and Leonard Manheim, "Dickens' Fools and Madmen," *Dickens Studies Annual* 2 (1971): 69–97, 357–59. Also of interest are H. P. Sucksmith, "The Identity and Significance of the Mad Huntsman in *The Pickwick Papers*," *The Dickensian* 68 (1972): 109–14; A. and P. Plichet, "Charles Dickens et ses observations neuro-psychiatriques," *Presse médicale* 64 (1956): 2230–33; L. Schotte, "La médecine et les médecins dans la vie et l'oeuvre de Charles Dickens (1812–1870)," *Chronique médicale* 19 (1912): 97–105; Isaak Oehlbaum, *Das pathologische Element bei Dickens* (diss.: University of Zurich, 1944); *Dickens and Medicine*, Exhibition Catalogue No. 5 (London: Wellcome Institute of the History of Medicine, 1970), pp. 9–10; and Fred Kaplan, *Dickens and Mesmerism: The Hidden Springs of Fiction* (Princeton, N.J.: Princeton University Press, 1975), pp. 4–26.

2. Richard Hunter and Ida Macalpine, *Three Hundred Years of Psychiatry, 1535–1860* (London: Oxford University Press, 1963), pp. 998–99.

3. A parallel walk through an asylum is described in chapter 4 of Dickens's joint novel with Wilkie Collins, "The Lazy Tour of Two Idle Apprentices," *Nonesuch Dickens* (Bloomsbury [London]: Nonesuch Press, 1938), 21:822–23.

4. Conolly was attacked in Charles Reade's novel *Very Hard Cash*, which was published by Dickens in his journal *All the Year Round* (1863). The personal embarrassment this caused Dickens is reflected in his correspondence of the time. See Richard A. Hunter and Ida Macalpine, "Dickens and Conolly: An Embarrassed Editor's Disclaimer," *Times Literary Supplement*, 11 August 1961, pp. 534–35, and the letter by Philip Collins, "Dickens and Conolly," *Times Literary Supplement*, 18 August 1961, p. 549. On Conolly, see Andrew Scull, "A Victorian Alienist: John Conolly, FRCP, DCL (1794–1866)," in W. F. Bynum, Roy Porter, and Michael Shepherd, eds., *The*

Anatomy of Madness: Essays in the History of Psychiatry (London: Tavistock, 1985), 1:103–50.

5. Vieda Skultans, ed., *Madness and Morals: Ideas of Insanity in the Nineteenth Century* (London: Routledge & Kegan Paul), p. 9. Cf. Andrew Scull, ed., *Madhouses, Mad-Doctors, and Madmen: The Social History of Psychiatry in the Victorian Era* (Philadelphia: University of Pennsylvania Press, 1981), as well as his major study *Museums of Madness: The Social Organization of Insanity in Nineteenth-Century England* (New York: St. Martin's Press, 1979).

6. The text is quoted in Harvey Peter Sucksmith, *The Narrative Art of Charles Dickens* (Oxford: Clarendon Press, 1970), pp. 37–38. Sucksmith, in an otherwise accurate book, reflects the conventional knowledge of Dickens's understanding of insanity. He makes a fleeting reference to Conolly (pp. 39–40), misspelling his name.

7. Cited by Skultans, *Madness and Morals*, p. 172.

8. Reprinted by Stone, *Dickens' Uncollected Writings*, 2:497. Stone does not mention that Harriet Martineau published a sequel to Dickens's and Wills's essay entitled "Idiots Again," *Household Words* 9 (15 April 1854): 197–200. Comparison of Ann Lohrli, comp., *Household Words: A Weekly Journal, 1850–1859* (Toronto: University of Toronto Press, 1973), pp. 357–60, would be a valuable exercise.

9. This essay, which later appeared in Taine's history of English literature, first appeared in his *Essais de critique et d'histoire* (Paris: Hachette, 1858), p. 76.

10. Taine, *Essais*, p. 86.

11. The description of an unpublished letter, cited in *The Letters of Charles Dickens*, ed. Walter Dexter (Bloomsbury [London]: Nonesuch Press), 2:321.

12. John Conolly, "The Physiognomy of Insanity," *Medical Times and Gazette*, n.s., 16 (1858): 3.

13. Ibid., 17 April 1858, p. 397.

14. Dickens, *Letters*, 3:3.

15. Richard A. Hunter and Ida Macalpine, *Psychiatry for the Poor: 1851 Colney Hatch Asylum—Friern Hospital 1973: A Medical and Social History* (London: Dawons, 1974), p. 86.

16. Described in *Dickens and Medicine*, p. 31.

17. Printed in Rene Fülöp-Miller, *Kampf gegen Schmerz und Tod: Kulturgeschichte der Heilkunde* (Berlin: Süd-Ost, 1938), p. 286.

18. Jacques Lavalleye, comp., *Lucas van Leyden / Pieter Breughel d. Ä: Das gesamt graphische Werk* (Vienna: Schroll, n.d.), plates 55, 59, 120–24. A comment on the nature of the dance in Breughel's work is to be found in Carl Gustav Stridbeck, *Breughelstudien: Untersuchungen zu den ikonologischen Problemen bei Pieter Breughel d. Ä sowie dessen Beziehungen zum niederländischen Romanismus.* Stockholm Studies in the History of Art (Stockholm: Almqvist & Wiksell, 1956), 2:218–19.

19. The traditions of the various types of frenetic dances in the Middle Ages have been traced by Justus Friedrich Karl Hecker, *Die Tanzwuth: Eine Volkskrankheit im Mittelalter* (Berlin: Enslin, 1832), and *Die grossen Volkskrankheiten des Mittelalters* (Berlin: Enslin, 1865). A parallel study of interest is Stephan Cosacchi, *Makabertanz: Der Totentanz in Kunst, Poesie und Brauchtum des Mittelalters* (Meisenheim am Glan: Anton Hain, 1965). The history of the use of music in psychotherapy has been well summarized in J. Opper, *Science and the Arts: A Study in Relationships from 1600 to 1900* (Rutherford, N.J.: Fairleigh Dickinson University Press, 1973), H. J. Möller, *Musik und "Wahnsinn": Geschichte und Gegenwart musiktherapeutischer Vorstellungen* (Munich: Fink, 1971), and Rudolf Schumacher, *Die Musik in der Psychiatrie des 19. Jahrhunderts* (Frankfurt: Lang, 1982).

20. A popular understanding of the origin of the St. Vitus's myth is given by Johannes

Agricola von Eisleben in his proverb collection of 1534. Agricola emphasizes that the belief that chorea can be cured by St. Vitus is related to the belief that Vitus could grant good health to those who danced before his image on his saint's day. See my edition of the proverbs, Johannes Agricola von Eisleben, *Die Sprichwörtersammlungen* (Berlin: De Gruyter, 1971), 1:384.

21. Penelope B. R. Doob, *Nebuchadnezzar's Children: Conventions of Madness in Middle English Literature* (New Haven: Yale University Press, 1974), pp. 45–48. See also Judith Neaman, *Suggestions of the Devil: The Origins of Madness* (New York: Anchor, 1975), and Richard Bernheimer, *Wild Men in the Middle Ages: A Study in Art, Sentiment, and Demonology* (Cambridge, Mass.: Harvard University Press, 1952).

22. The basic study remains Erwin Rohde, *Psyche: Seelencult und Unsterblichkeits-glaube der Griechen* (Tubingen: Mohr, 1903), 2:44–55. See also *Pauly Real-Encyclopädie der classischen Altertumswissenschaft* (Stuttgart: Metzler, 1922), 11: cols. 1441–46. For an alternate view, see E. R. Dodds, *The Greeks and the Irrational* (Berkeley: University of California Press, 1951), esp. chap. 3, "The Blessings of Madness," and Bennett Simon, *Mind and Madness in Ancient Greece* (Ithaca, N.Y.: Cornell University Press, 1978), pp. 43–52, 180–99.

23. *Politics*, 1340b4. Cited in the edition of Richard McKeon, ed., *The Basic Works of Aristotle* (New York: Random House, 1941), p. 1312.

24. *Laws*, vii, 790.3–791b. Cited in the edition of Edith Hamilton and Huntington Cairns, eds., *Plato: The Collected Dialogues*. Bollingen Series No. 71 (New York: Pantheon, 1961), p. 1363.

25. The literature on the image of the fool is summarized in the chapter "The Feast of Fools," in my study *The Parodic Sermon in European Perspective* (Wiesbaden: Steiner, 1974).

26. Biographical information on Davies is available in Joseph McCabe, *A Biographical Dictionary of Modern Rationalists* (London: Watts, 1920), col. 198. All references to the essay are from Charles Maurice Davies, *Mystic London; or, Phases of Occult Life in the British Metropolis* (New York: Lovell, Adam, Wesson, 1884), pp. 31–41.

6. The Insane See the Insane: Richard Dadd

1. Prinzhorn's work *Bildnerei der Geisteskranken* (Berlin: Springer, 1922) is available in translation as *Artistry of the Mentally Ill*, trans. Eric von Brockdorff (New York: Springer, 1972). On the general background, see my essay "The Mad as Artist: Medicine, History, and Degenerate Art," *Journal of Contemporary History* 20 (1985): 575–97.

2. Hans Gercke and Inge Jarchov, eds., *Die Prinzhornsammlung* (Königstein: Athenäum, 1980).

3. For an overview, see Johann Glatzel, "Über die sogenannte Antipsychiatrie," in U. H. Peters, ed., *Psychiatrie 2* (Weinheim: Beltz, 1984), pp. 534–42.

4. D. Locker, *Symptoms and Illness: The Cognitive Organization of Disorder* (London: Tavistock, 1981).

5. Mary Frances Wack, "The Measure of Pleasure: Peter of Spain on Men, Women, and Lovesickness," *Viator* 17 (1986), 191.

6. All of the references to Dadd are from Patricia Allderidge, *The Late Richard Dadd, 1817–1886* (London: Tate Gallery, 1974). See also Marina Vaizey, "Dadd in the Desert," *Country Life* 180 (25 June 1987): 134–35, on Dadd's trip to the Near East.

7. W. P. Frith, *My Autobiography and Reminiscences* (London: Bentley, 1888), 3:182.

8. William Wood, *Remarks on the Plea of Insanity* (London: n.p., 1851), pp. 41–42. All of Dadd's comments on his paranoia are taken from this source.

9. *Quarterly Review* 101 (1857): 361–62.

10. On the implications of Egyptian images as a sign of the "hidden" powers that are exorcised in Dadd's system, see Liselotte Dieckmann, *Hieroglyphics: The History of a Literary Symbol* (St. Louis: Washington University Press, 1970).

11. Wood, *Remarks on the Plea of Insanity*, p. 42.

12. *Art Union*, 1 May 1844, p. 122.

13. I am here paralleling the reading of the Schreber case by C. Barry Chabot, *Freud on Schreber: Psychoanalytic Theory and the Critical Act* (Amherst: University of Massachusetts Press, 1982).

14. See Louis A. Sass, "Schreber's Panopticism: Psychosis and the Modern Soul," *Social Research* 54 (1987): 101–47.

7. The Insane See the Insane: Vincent Van Gogh

1. For the present study the following works were of value: Victor Doiteau and Edgard Leroy, *La folie de Vincent Van Gogh* (Paris: Editions Aesculape, 1928); Edgard Leroy, "L'art et la folie de Vincent Van Gogh," *Journal des practiciens* 29 (21 July 1928): 1558–63; Karl Jaspers, *Strindberg und Van Gogh* (Berlin: Springer, 1926); C. Mauron, "Vincent et Theo," *L'arc* 2 (1959): 3–12; J. Hulsker, "Vincent's Stay in the Hospitals at Arles and St.-Rémy: Unpublished Letters from the Reverend Mr. Salles and Doctor Peyron to Theo Van Gogh," *Vincent* 1 (1971): 224–44, and his "Van Gogh's Threatened Life in Saint-Rémy and Auvers," *Vincent* 2 (1972): 21–39; Ronald Pickvance, *Van Gogh in Saint-Rémy and Auvers* (New York: Abrams, 1986).

2. All references to Van Gogh's works refer to J. B. de la Faille, *L'oeuvre de Vincent Van Gogh: Catalogue raisonné* (Paris: Van Oest, 1928), 5 vols.

3. All references to the letters are to *The Complete Letters of Vincent Van Gogh* (Greenwich, Conn.: New York Graphic Society, n.d.), here, 3:323.

4. J. Seznec, "Literary Inspiration in Van Gogh," in B. Welsh-Ovcharov, ed., *Van Gogh in Perspective* (Englewood Cliffs, N.J.: Prentice-Hall, 1971), pp. 126–33. See also C. Nordenfalk, "Van Gogh and Literature," *Journal of the Warburg and Courtauld Institutes* 10 (1947): 132–47.

5. See V. Skultans, ed., *Madness and Morals: Ideas on Insanity in the Nineteenth Century* (London: Routledge & Kegan Paul, 1975), esp. pp. 1–30.

6. There is one landscape of Van Gogh's from March 1884 (F 1130) which presents an evocative scene under the title *Melancholy*.

7. Another influence on Van Gogh may have been the passive figures in Charles Green's illustration "Hospital" for the *Graphic* [London], which he mentions in a letter of February 1883 (3:364).

8. See Chapter 5 for a detailed discussion of Dickens's image of the insane.

9. B. Bramwell, *Atlas of Clinical Medicine* (Edinburgh: Constable, 1892), plate 25.

10. Alexander Morison, author of *Outlines of Lectures on Mental Diseases* (1825) and *Physiology of Mental Diseases* (1840), postulated that the facial expressions of mental patients were the result of the acquisition of patterns through constant repetition. He thus followed the example of Philippe Pinel and his school (see the detailed discussion in Chapter 2).

8. The Science of Visualizing the Insane: Charles Darwin

1. Paul Ekman, ed., *Darwin and Facial Expression* (New York: Academic Press, 1973), pp. 261–62. Ekman also supplies the most detailed bibliography of secondary studies on Darwin's theory of expression.

2. Charles Darwin, *The Descent of Man* (London: Murray, 1871), and his *The Expression of the Emotions in Man and Animals* (London: Murray, 1872). There is a first-rate presentation of some of the problems dealing with this text, based upon this chapter, in the essay by Janet Browne, "Darwin and the Face of Madness," in W. F. Bynum, Roy Porter, and Michael Shepherd, eds., *The Anatomy of Madness: Essays in the History of Psychiatry* (London: Tavistock, 1985), 1:151–65.

3. Biographical information on Sir James Crichton Browne can be found in the *Dictionary of National Biography Supplement for 1931–40* (London: Oxford University Press, 1949), pp. 106–7. See also Richard Hunter and Ida Macalpine, eds., *Three Hundred Years of Psychiatry, 1535–1860* (London: Oxford University Press), p. 882; and Sir James Crichton Browne, *What the Doctor Thought* (London: Benn, 1930), *The Doctor's Second Thoughts* (London: Benn, 1931), *The Doctor's Afterthoughts* (London: Benn, 1932), *From the Doctor's Notebook* (London: Duckworth, 1937), and *The Doctor Remembers* (London: Duckworth, 1938).

4. Dickson's book was published in London by Lewis in 1874 and has photographs by Diamond opposite pp. 87, 112, 314, and 406.

5. Arthur Schopenhauer, *Parerga and Paralipomena*, trans. E. F. J. Payne (Oxford: Clarendon Press, 1974), 2:634. The complex backgrounds to this view in nineteenth-century thought are well stated in Allan Sekula, "The Traffic in Photographs," *Art Journal* 41 (1981): 15–25.

6. See the frontispiece to John Charles Bucknill and Daniel H. Tuke, *A Manual of Psychological Medicine* (Philadelphia: Blanchard and Lea, 1858). There is an extensive discussion of the physiognomy of insanity on pp. 282–89.

7. See Francis Wey's review of Piot's *L'Italie monumentale* in *La lumière* (1851): 74–75, reprinted by Heinz Buddemeier, *Panorama, Diorama, Photographie: Entstehung und Wirkung neuer Medien im 19. Jahrhundert. Theorie und Geschichte der Literatur und der schönen Künste* (Munich: Wilhelm Fink, 1970), pp. 115–18, 284–85.

8. See Edwin Clarke and Kenneth Dewhurst, *An Illustrated History of Brain Function* (Berkeley: University of California Press, 1972), esp. pp. 101–13.

9. To place Darwin's study in the overall scope of his work, see Sir Gavin de Beer, *Charles Darwin: Evolution by Natural Selection* (Garden City, N.Y.: Doubleday, 1967), pp. 220–25.

10. Darwin, *Expression of the Emotions*, pp. 13–14.

11. Darwin also cites unpublished contributions by Patrick Nicoll of Sussex Lunatic Asylum. Darwin, *Expression of the Emotions*, p. 14.

12. Ibid., pp. 155, 185.

13. Ibid., p. 199.

14. Boyd's paper "General Paralysis of the Insane" appeared in the *Journal of Mental Sciences* 17 (1871): 1–24; Browne's discussion is in the same issue on pp. 147–49.

15. Darwin, *Expression of the Emotions*, p. 203.

16. Ibid., p. 245. Here Darwin again cites parallel cases provided by Patrick Nicoll.

17. Ibid., p. 246; Henry Maudsley, *Body and Mind* (London: Macmillan, 1873).

18. Darwin, *Expression of the Emotions*, p. 264.

19. Ibid., p. 293.

20. Ibid., pp. 295–97.

21. Ibid., p. 296.

22. I am indebted to Mr. P. J. Gautrey of the Cambridge University Library for making this material available to me. The Browne letters to Darwin are preserved in their original holograph form. Darwin's letters to Browne, however, are preserved only in Francis Darwin's transcriptions. None of the correspondence was published in the collections of Darwin's letters. Francis Darwin mentions Browne in passing in his *Life and Letters of Charles Darwin* (New York: Appleton, 1896), 2:314. For the context of the Browne-Darwin exchange, see pp. 310–24 of that volume, and Francis Darwin and A. C. Seward, eds., *More Letters of Charles Darwin* (New York: Appleton, 1903), pp. 98–111.

23. Guillaume Benjamin Amand Duchenne, *De l'électrisation localisée et de son application à la pathologie et à la thérapeutique* (Paris: Baillière, 1861), and his *Mécanisme de la physionomie humaine* (Paris: Renouard, 1862). See Emanuel B. Kaplan, "Duchenne of Boulogne and the Physiologie des Mouvements," in *Victor Robinson Memorial Volume*, ed. Solomon R. Kagan (New York: Froben, 1948), pp. 177–92.

24. See Francis X. Dercum, ed., *Text-Book on Nervous Diseases* (Philadelphia: Lea Brothers, 1895), p. 636.

25. In this regard, see Peter Pollack, *The Picture History of Photography* (New York: Abrams, 1958), p. 175. Also Cecil Beaton and Gail Buckland, *The Magic Image: The Genius of Photography from 1839 to the Present Day* (Boston: Little, Brown, 1975), pp. 51–53.

9. Medical Colonialism and Disease: Lam Qua and the Creation of a Westernized Medical Iconography in Nineteenth-Century China

1. Joseph Needham, *Science and Civilization in China*, 5 vols. in 8 (Cambridge: Cambridge University Press, 1954–76). For this chapter I have relied on A. Chamfrault, *Traité de médecine chinoise*, 5 vols. (Angoulême: Editions Coquemard, 1957–64), and the more recent survey by S. M. Hillier and J. A. Jewell, *Health Care and Traditional Medicine in China, 1800–1982* (London: Routledge & Kegan Paul, 1983). See also Ilza Veith, ed., *The Yellow Emperor's Classic of Internal Medicine* (Baltimore: Williams and Wilkins, 1949), her introduction.

2. Joseph Needham, *China and the Origin of Immunology* (Hong Kong: Centre of Asian Studies, 1980), and his (together with Lu Gwei-djen), *Celestial Lancets: History and Rationale of Acupuncture and Moxa* (Cambridge: Cambridge University Press, 1980). Needham's major interest, in the latter volume, in the tradition of medical illustration lies in tracing the reception of Chinese studies of acupuncture in the West (pp. 269–302). What is striking is the redrawing of the Chinese images to fit Western ideas of what would be appropriate medical illustration. In one case, a study on acupuncture by Andreas Cleyer published in 1682, the author is pressed to label the images he expropriates with terms from the contemporary theory of primogenital moisture, a version of the temperaments. Since these stood within a specific iconographic tradition in the West, that of representing the humors, he was able to draw on the analogies between the Chinese and Western systems based on the very notion of the existence of iconographic representations in the West. The source of Cleyer's images, the *Lei Ching* (1624) of Chang Chieh-Pin, contains no such specific iconographic parallel between representations of the correct positioning of the needles for various illnesses and the abstract nature of the disease. Needham reproduces images

from Cleyer's source that represent both the schematic model (figure 5) as well as the symbolic model (figures 17–18).

3. See Claude Philibert Dabry de Thiersant, *La médecine chez les chinois* (Paris: Henri Plon, 1863).

4. See Ralph C. Crozier, *Traditional Medicine in Modern China: Science, Nationalism, and The Tensions of Cultural Change* (Cambridge. Mass.: Harvard University Press, 1968), p. 4.

5. Wu Lien-te, "A Hundred Years of Modern Medicine in China," *Chinese Medical Journal* 50 (1936): 152–54.

6. William R. Morse, *Chinese Medicine* (New York: Hoeber, 1938), pp. 137–61. See the plates on p. 147 (for the schematic model) and p. 151 (for the symbolic model). See also Manfred Porkert, *Die chinesische Medizin* (Düsseldorf: Econ, 1982), plates on p. 147 (schematic) and p. 144 (symbolic).

7. J. W. S. Johnsson, *L'anatomie mandchoke et les figures Th. Bartholin: Etude d'iconographie comparée* (Copenhagen: Høst & Son, 1928).

8. Shih Fan, *Ming chi hsi-i yang ch'uan ju chih i hsüeh* [On the influence of Western medicine at the end of the Ming], 4 vols. ([Shanghai]: Chinese Academy of the History of Medicine, 1943).

9. On the background of Lam Qua, see Henry and Sidney Berry-Hill, *George Chinnery, 1774–1852, An Artist of the China Coast* (Leigh-on-Sea: Lewis, [1963]), p. 39; Carl L. Crossman, *The China Trade* (Princeton, N.J.: Pyne Press, 1972), pp. 31–35; Edward V. Gulick, *Peter Parker and the Opening of China* (Cambridge, Mass.: Harvard University Press, 1973), pp. 153–56; Robin Hutcheon, *Chinnery, The Man and the Legend* (Hong Kong: South Chinese Morning Post, 1975), pp. 78–79; Hillier and Jewell, *Health Care*, pp. 3–27. Of the 115 paintings, 86 are at the Yale Medical College; 23 at the Gordon Museum, Guy's Hospital, London; 5 at the Johnson Art Museum, Cornell University; and 1 at the Countway Medical Library, Boston. They represent portraits of 80 patients.

10. See the contemporary discussion by "Old Nick," i.e., P. E. D. Forgues, *La Chine ouverte* (Paris: Fournier, 1845), p. 56.

11. Crossman, *China Trade*, p. 34.

12. Cited by Albert Ten Eyck Gardiner, "Cantonese Chinnerys: Portraits of How-Qua and Other China Trade Paintings," *Art Quarterly* 16 (1953): 316.

13. William Fane de Salis, *Reminiscences of Travel in China and India in 1848* (London: Waterlow & Sons, 1892), p. 12.

14. Osmond Tiffany, Jr., *The Canton Chinese, or The American Sojourn in the Celestial Empire* (Boston: Monroe, 1849), p. 85.

15. Gulick, *Peter Parker*, p. 115; an engraving of Chinnery's portrait of Thomas Colledge is reproduced in Hillier and Jewell, *Health Care*, plate 7(a).

16. See Robert Herrlinger and Marielene Putscher, *Geschichte der medizinischen Abbildung*, 2 vols. (Munich: Moos, 1967–72). Herrlinger, in the first volume of his study, points toward the potential origin of medieval Western European medical illustration in the schematic medical illustration of China. If this is the case, the interrelationship between the two systems of medical representation is much older than the seventeenth century and works in both directions even at this very early stage. They base their comments on the observations of Ludwig Choulant, *Geschichte und Bibliographie der anatomischen Abbildung nach ihrer Beziehung auf anatomische Wissenschaft und bildende Kunst* (Leipzig: Weigel, 1852). What little information is available on this is documented by Herrlinger and Saburo Miyasita, "A Link in the Westward Transmission of Chinese Anatomy in the Later Middle Ages," *Isis* 58 (1967):

486–90. For documentation on the image of the somatic patient, see Helmuth Vogt, *Das Bild des Kranken* (Munich: Lehmann, 1969).

17. Quoted from the 1888 obituary of Parker by Hillier and Jewell, *Health Care*, p. 11.

18. Gulick, *Peter Parker*, p. 154.

19. Rudolf Virchow, *Die krankenhafte Geschwülste* (Berlin: Hirschwald, 1863), vol. 1.

20. On the creation of textbooks of Western medicine in China, see Hillier and Jewell, *Health Care*, pp. 11–12. The first drawings that Hobson commissioned are reproduced in the reprint of his 1851 *Ch'üan t'i hsin lun*, 2 vols. (Taipei: I-wen yin shu kuan, 1968).

21. Rudolf G. Wagner, *Reenacting the Heavenly Vision: The Role of Religion in the Taiping Rebellion*, Chinese Research Monograph 25 (Berkeley: Institute of East Asian Studies, 1982), reproduces the illustrations.

10. Opera, Homosexuality, and Models of Disease: Richard Strauss's *Salome* in the Context of Images of Disease in the Fin de Siècle

1. This phrase is taken from Strauss's 1942 memoir "Reminiscences of the First Performance of My Operas," in *Richard Strauss, Recollections and Reflections*, ed. Willi Schuh, trans. L. J. Lawrence (London: Boosey & Hawkes, 1953), here p. 150. On the differences between Wilde's text and the libretto (though with no attempt at analysis), see Ernst Krause, *Richard Strauss: The Man and His Work*, trans. John Coombs (London: Collet, 1964), pp. 296–98.

2. While I will not follow Fish's mode of reading, I believe that the question of the presuppositions of the author in regard to his or her idealized audience does focus many of the questions I pose. See Stanley Fish, *Is There a Text in This Class? The Authority of Interpretive Communities* (Cambridge, Mass.: Harvard University Press, 1980), pp. 303 ff.

3. This essay is indebted to the work of Norbert Kohl, *Oscar Wilde: Das literarische Werk zwischen Provokation und Anpassung* (Heidelberg: Winter, 1982), and J. E. Chamberlin, *Ripe Was the Drowsy Hour: The Age of Oscar Wilde* (New York: Seabury, 1977), on Oscar Wilde and his *Salome*.

4. See the beginning of Strauss's "The History of *Die schweigsame Frau*," in which he praises Lindner for having recognized *Salome* as a "covert opera text," published as an appendix to *A Confidential Matter: The Letters of Richard Strauss and Stefan Zweig, 1931–35*, ed. Edward E. Lowinsky, trans. Max Knight (Berkeley: University of California Press, 1977), p. 107. On the general background to the composition of the opera, see Ludwig Kusche, *Richard Strauss im Kulturkarussell der Zeit 1864–1964* (Munich: Süddeutscher Verlag, 1964), pp. 129–50 (with many contemporary illustrations), and Roland Tenschert, *7 × 7 Variationen über das Thema Richard Strauss* (Vienna: Frick, 1944), pp. 91–101.

5. George R. Marek, *Richard Strauss: The Life of a Non-Hero* (New York: Simon and Schuster, 1967), pp. 99, 138.

6. See the discussion by Erwin Panofsky on the erotic Salome in his *Problems in Titian, Mostly Iconographic* (New York: New York University Press, 1969), pp. 42–47. (This corrects his earlier view in his *Early Netherlandish Painting* [Cambridge, Mass.: Harvard University Press, 1953], p. 281.) On the popularity of this motif at the turn of the century, see the monographs by E. W. Bredt, "Die Bilder der Salome," *Die Kunst* 7

(1903–4): 249–54; Hugo Daffner, *Salome: Ihre Gestalt in Geschichte und Kunst* (Munich: Schmidt, 1912); and Reimarus Secundus, *Geschichte der Salome von Cato bis Oscar Wilde*, 3 vols. (Leipzig: Wigand, [1907–9]). More recent overviews are to be found in Helen Grace Zagona, *The Legend of Salome and the Principle of Art for Art's Sake* (Geneva: Droz, 1960), and Mechthilde Hatz, "Frauengestalten des alten Testaments in der bildenenen Kunst von 1850 bis 1918: Eva, Dalila, Judith, Salome" (diss.: University of Heidelberg, 1972).

7. The references to Lindner, Grünfeld, and Eysolt (but not to Reinhardt, a nonperson at the time of Strauss's writing) are in Strauss's 1942 *Recollections*, pp. 150–54.

8. Cited from *Strauss, Recollections*, p. 150. The German text is in Richard Strauss, *Betrachtungen und Erinnerungen*, ed. Willi Schuh (Zurich: Atlantis, 1949), pp. 224–29. See the further discussion in Norman Del Mar, *Richard Strauss: A Critical Commentary on His Life and Works* (London, 1962; reprint, Ithaca, N.Y.: Cornell University Press, 1986), 1:243.

9. Shlomo Avineri, *The Making of Modern Zionism: The Intellectual Origins of the Jewish State* (New York: Basic Books, 1981).

10. See my essay "The Mad as Artists," in my *Difference and Pathology: Stereotypes of Sexuality, Race, and Madness* (Ithaca, N.Y.: Cornell University Press, 1985), pp. 217–38, and Peter Gay's discussion of the Jews' "Encounter with Modernism" in his *Freud, Jews, and Other Germans: Master and Victims in Modernist Culture* (New York: Oxford University Press, 1978), pp. 93–168.

11. The term *Jew* here is a precise usage. When I apply it to any individual, I use it only within the strict limits set by the anti-Semites of the period. My reference is the standard anti-Semitic reference tool, Theodor Fritsch, *Handbuch der Judenfrage*, 38th ed. (Leipzig: Hammer, 1935).

12. Peter Funke, *Oscar Wilde in Selbstzeugnissen und Bilddokumenten* (Reinbek: Rowohlt, 1969), p. 7.

13. There are over a hundred reviews and articles on this production preserved in the Max Reinhardt Archive of the State University of New York at Binghamton.

14. *Die Zeit* (15 June 1895), signed by "Dr. Handl"; Eduard Bernstein, "Aus Anlass eines Sensationsprozess" and "Die Beurteilung des widernormalen Geschlechtsverkehrs," *Die neue Zeit* 2 (1894–95): 171–76, 228–33. On the image of Wilde before the trials, see the discussion in Max Nordau, *Degeneration* (New York: Appleton, 1895), pp. 318–22, in which Nordau speaks of Wilde as an aesthete, mentions "his buffoon mummery," but does not see him as exemplary a figure for his conservative attack on "degeneration" as were Nietzsche or Ibsen.

15. The general background to the homosexual emancipation movement is provided in James D. Steakley, *The Homosexual Emancipation Movement in Germany* (New York: Arno Press, 1975).

16. Reprinted in Moeller van den Bruck, *Die Zeitgenossen: Die Geister—Die Menschen* (Minden: Bruns, 1906), pp. 238–56. Cf. the later discussion by Ernst Schultze, "Englische Sexualprüderie," *Zeitschrift für Sexualwissenschaft* 4 (1917–18): 199–203, which repeats, during World War I, many of the same charges. In the same issue of the *Zeitschrift* there is also a long, positive essay on Wilde by L. Hamilton (pp. 307–20), which includes in German the suppressed extracts from Wilde's "De Profundis."

17. Barbara W. Tuchman, *Bible and Sword: England and Palestine from the Bronze Age to Balfour* (New York: Ballantine Books, 1984), p. 212.

18. Friedrich Nietzsche, *Sämtliche Werke: Kritische Studienausgabe* (Berlin: de Gruyter, 1980), 6:192–93. Cited in Walter Kaufmann's translation from my essay "Nietzsche, Heine, and the Otherness of the Jew," in James C. O'Flaherty, Timothy F. Sellner, and Robert M. Helm, eds., *Studies in Nietzsche and the Judaeo-Christian*

Tradition (Chapel Hill: University of North Carolina Press, 1985), pp. 206–25 (with extensive notes on Nietzsche and contemporary attitudes toward the Jews).

19. Oscar Sero, *Der Fall Wilde und das Problem der Homosexualität: Ein Prozeß und ein Interview* (Leipzig: Spohr, 1896).

20. Numa Prätorius, "Oscar Wilde," *Jahrbuch für sexuelle Zwischenstufen* 3 (1901): 265–74.

21. Reprinted in his *Die prosaischen Schriften gesammelt* (Berlin: Fischer, 1917), 2:85–94. For the general context, see Thomas A. Kovach, *Hofmannsthal and Symbolism: Art and Life in the Work of a Modern Poet* (New York: Lang, 1985).

22. *Hugo von Hofmannsthal—Richard Beer-Hofmann: Briefwechsel*, ed. Eugene Weber (Frankfurt: Fischer, 1972), p. 59.

23. Erich Mühsam, "Boehme" (1906), reprinted in his *Ausgewählte Werke* (Berlin: Aufbau, 1978), 2:30.

24. The only essay on this topic is the narrowly focused piece by Hugh Salvesen, "Zu den Wilde-Übersetzungen in der 'Fackel,'" *Kraus Hefte* 24 (1982): 5–11.

25. *Die Fackel* 148 (2 December 1903): 19–20.

26. Ibid.: 31.

27. Ibid. 150 (23 December 1903): 1–14.

28. See my *Jewish Self-Hatred: Anti-Semitism and the Hidden Language of the Jews* (Baltimore: Johns Hopkins University Press, 1986), esp. pp. 209–60.

29. See Jacob Katz, *Richard Wagner: Vorbote des Antisemitismus* (Königstein in the Tannus: Jüdischer Verlag, 1985), and my *Jewish Self-Hatred*, pp. 209–11.

30. F[riedrich] Sch[ütz], "Oskar Wilde: Zur Aufführung seiner "Salome" im Deutschen Volkstheater," *Neue freie Presse*, 15 December 1903, pp. 1–3.

31. "Das Bildnis Dorian Gray's (Zum Bildnis des Friedrich Schütz)," *Die Fackel* 151 (4 January 1904): 18–23.

32. On the political background to the homosexual scandals of the day and their close association with images of Jewish discourse (esp. the idea of journalism as a form of Jewish discourse), see Isabel V. Hull, *The Entourage of Kaiser Wilhelm II, 1888–1918* (Cambridge: Cambridge University Press, 1982), pp. 57–145, and James D. Steakley, "Iconography of a Scandal: Political Cartoons and the Eulenberg Affair," *Studies in Visual Communication* 9 (1983): 20–51.

33. *Richard Strauss—Willi Schuch: Briefwechsel* (Zurich: Atlantis, 1969), p. 153.

34. *Strauss, Recollections*, p. 151.

35. The entire review is cited in Friedrich von Schuch, *Richard Strauss / Ernst von Schuch und Dresdens Opera* (Leipzig: Breitkopf & Härtel, n.d.), pp. 72–73.

36. Cited in Clemens Höslinger, " 'Salome' und ihr österreiches Schicksal 1905 bis 1918," *Österreichische Musikzeitschrift* 32 (1977): 301.

37. Eugen Schmitz, *Richard Strauss als Musikdramatiker* (Munich: Lewy, 1907), p. 45.

38. Oscar Bie, *Die moderne Musik und Richard Strauss* (Berlin: Marquardt, 1906), p. 69.

39. Cited here from the translation by Rollo Myers, *Richard Strauss and Romain Rolland: Correspondence* (Berkeley: University of California Press, 1968), pp. 37, 83.

40. H. Ernstmann, *Salomé an den deutschen Hofbühnen* (Berlin: Walter, 1906), pp. 16–17, 23–27.

41. My reference is, of course, to Freud and Breuer's 1895 *Studies in Hysteria*.

42. See my essay "The Madness of the Jews," in my *Difference and Pathology*, pp. 150–62, and Jan Goldstein, "The Wandering Jew and the Problem of Psychiatric Anti-Semitism in Fin-de-Siècle France," *Journal of Contemporary History* 20 (1985): 521–52.

43. Cited in his discussion of Jews and hysteria by Alexander Pilcz, *Beitrag zur vergleichenden Rassen-Psychiatrie* (Leipzig: Deuticke, 1906), p. 18.

44. See the discussion (and refutation) of the charges of "moral crimes" in the following pamphlets: Anon., *Der Juden Antheil am Verbrechen: Auf Grund der amtlichen Statistik über die Thätigkeit der Schwurgerichte, in vergleichender Darstellung mit den christlichen Confession* (Berlin: Hentze, 1881); Ludwig Fuld, *Das jüdische Verbrecherthum: Eine Studie über den Zusammenhang zwischen Religion und Kriminalität* (Leipzig: Huth, 1885); and S. Löwenfeld, *Die Wahrheit über der Juden Antheil am Verbrechen: Auf Grund amtlicher Statistik* (Berlin: Stuhr, 1881).

45. Cited from Wilde's text in *The Complete Works of Oscar Wilde* (Garden City, N.Y.: Doubleday, Page, 1923), 9:106.

46. Stendhal, *The Life of Rossini*, trans. Richard N. Coe (Seattle: University of Washington Press, 1972), p. 113.

47. *Confidential Matter*, p. 90.

48. See my discussion of this view in *Difference and Pathology*, pp. 33–35.

49. All citations are from the English translation, Otto Weininger, *Sex and Character* (London: Heinemann, 1906), pp. 195, 324.

50. This citation is from the Nazis' child's introduction to Jew hatred, *The Poison Mushroom*, published by Julius Streicher in 1938, but it represents a tradition that reaches back into the representation of the stage Jew during the late nineteenth century. See my *Jewish Self-Hatred*, p. 312.

51. See the discussion in my *Jewish Self-Hatred*, p. 292. "Perversion" is also associated with the cultural elite, but with Wagner. Romain Rolland pointed out to Strauss that "the incest in the *Walküre* is a thousand times more healthy than the conjugal and legitimate love in such and such a dirty Parisian comedy, which I don't want to name," Myers, *Richard Strauss and Romain Rolland*, p. 83. And Wilde's play is little better than that comedy. Oskar Panizza also ironically pointed toward the homoeroticism of Wagner and its relationship to actual homosexual practices; his "Bayreuth und die Homosexualität," *Die Gesellschaft* 11 (1895): 88–92.

52. See Breuer's notes to the case of "Anna O." in Albrecht Hirschmüller, *Physiologie und Psychoanalyse in Leben und Werk Josef Breuers* (Bern: Huber, 1978).

53. On the medical literature, see, for example, the case studies of homosexuality reported in Richard von Krafft-Ebing, *Psychopathia Sexualis mit besonderer Berücksichtigung der conträren Sexualempfindung: Eine klinisch-forensische Studien* (Stuttgart: Enke, 1893), which regularly record the nature of the patient's voice. On the popular signs of degeneration, see Nordau, *Degeneration*, pp. 17–18. For an overview of the problem of the signs and symptoms of degeneration, see *Degeneration: The Dark Side of Progress* (New York: Columbia University Press, 1985), edited by J. E. Chamberlin and myself.

54. Nordau, *Degeneration*, p. 16.

55. See Rathenau's essay "Höre, Israel!" in *Die Zukunft* (6 March 1897), pp. 454–62.

56. Max Nordau, *Zionistische Schriften* (Cologne: Jüdischer Verlag, 1909), pp. 379–81.

57. See Hjalmar J. Nordin, "Die eheliche Ethik der Juden zur Zeit Jesu," trans. W. A. Kastner and Gustave Lewié in *Beiwerke zum Studium der Anthropophyteia* 4 (1911): 99–104, for a rebuttal of the general discussions of the Levirate marriage which were circulating at the turn of the century.

58. K. W. F. Grattenauer, *Über die physische und moralische Verfassung der heutigen Juden* (Leipzig, 1791). On the general background, see Jacob Katz, *From Prejudice to Destruction: Anti-Semitism, 1700–1933* (Cambridge, Mass.: Harvard University Press, 1980), pp. 51–62.

59. This tradition is documented in great detail and with a good deal of critical acumen in Tuchman's *Bible and Sword*, which can be read as the British parallel to Katz's history of anti-Semitism.

60. Cited by Anne Fremantle, *This Little Band of Prophets: The British Fabians* (New York: Mentor, 1959), p. 204 (with a discussion of left-wing anti-Semitism in Britain).

61. Houston Stewart Chamberlain, *Foundations of the Nineteenth Century*, trans. John Lees, 2 vols. (London: Lane, 1910), 1:388–89.

62. I am playing with Strauss's own repudiation of the Nazi concept of the "Volk" in the famous letter to the "Jewish" poet Stefan Zweig of 17 June 1935, which was seized and delivered to the Gestapo. There Strauss ironically attacks Zweig's solidarity with other victims of anti-Semitism as "Jewish obstinacy" and "pride of race," while condemning the Nazi view that true art must be "'Aryan.'" In that letter he comments: "The people [*Volk*] exist for me only at the moment they become audience," *Confidential Matter*, p. 99.

63. On Strauss and Wagner, see Strauss's early letter to Cosima Wagner printed under the title "Erlebnis und Bekenntnis des jungen Richard Strauss," in *Internationale Mitteilungen: Richard-Strauss-Gesellschaft* 30 (1961): 1, and A. A. Abert, "Richard Strauss und das Erbe Wagners," *Musikforschung* 27 (1974): 165–71.

64. On the question of Jews and the Wagner circle, see Peter Gay's essay on Levi in his *Freud, Jews, and Other Germans*, pp. 189–231.

65. Cited by Herta Blaukopf, ed., *Gustav Mahler—Richard Strauss: Briefwechsel 1888–1911* (Munich: Piper, 1980), p. 211.

66. Ibid., p. 152.

67. Egon Gartenberg, *Mahler: The Man and His Music* (New York: Schirmer, 1978), p. 47.

68. Cited from Nicolas Slonimsky, ed., *Lexikon of Musical Invective. Critical Assaults on Composers since Beethoven's Time* (Seattle: University of Washington Press, 1965), p. 121. My emphasis.

69. Alma Mahler Werfel, *Gustav Mahler: Erinnerungen und Briefe* (Amsterdam: de Lange, 1940), p. 360.

70. Klaus Pringsheim, "Zur Uraufführung von Mahlers Sechster Symphonie," *Musikblätter des Anbruch* 2 (1920): 497.

71. "Is There an Avant-Garde in Music?" (1907), in *Strauss, Recollections*, pp. 12, 16.

72. See the discussion in Fritsch, *Handbuch der Judenfrage*, p. 325: "man erinnere sich, daß der größte Vertreter der Vorkriegsmusik, Richard Strauß, 'an den Geist der Zersetzung verlorengegangen ist' (Eichenauer), daß er nicht nur von der jüdischen Presse gelobhudelt wurde, sondern daß seine Textdichter (Hofmannsthal, Stefan Zweig), sein Verleger (Fürstner) und sein Biograph (Specht) sämtlich Juden sind."

11. Constructing the Image of the Appropriate Therapist: The Struggle of Psychiatry with Psychoanalysis

1. The debate about the scientific status of psychoanalysis is summarized in Adolf Grünbaum, *The Foundations of Psychoanalysis: A Philosophical Critique* (Berkeley: University of California Press, 1984). On Grünbaum, see Barbara Von Eckardt, "Adolf Grünbaum: Psychoanalytic Epistemology," in J. Reppen, ed., *Beyond Freud: A Study of Modern Psychoanalytic Theorists* (Hillsdale, N.J.: Analytic Press, 1985), pp. 353–403. A brief historical overview of the nature of psychotherapeutic treatment is given by Sol

L. Garfield, "Psychotherapy: A Forty-Year Appraisal," *American Psychologist* 36 (1981): 174–83.

2. The historical background is outlined by Peter Amacher, *Freud's Neurological Education and Its Influence on Psychoanalytic Theory* (New York: International Universities Press, 1965); Kenneth Levin, *Freud's Early Psychology of the Neurosis: A Historical Perspective* (Pittsburgh: University of Pittsburgh Press, 1978); and polemically in Frank J. Sulloway, *Freud, Biologist of the Mind: Beyond the Psychoanalytic Legend* (New York: Basic Books, 1979).

3. On the history of psychiatry as a mode of control, see Michel Foucault, *Histoire de la folie à l'âge classique* (Paris: Gallimard, 1972), and, more recently, Andrew Scull, ed., *Madhouses, Mad-Doctors, and Madmen: The Social History of Psychiatry in the Victorian Era* (Philadelphia: University of Pennsylvania Press, 1981).

4. On the history of the psychiatric hospital, see Dieter Jetter, *Grundzüge der Geschichte des Irrenhauses* (Darmstadt: Wissenschaftliche Buchgesellschaft, 1981).

5. Immanuel Kant, *Werke,* ed. Wilhelm Weischedel, 6 vols. (Wiesbaden: Insel, 1956–64), 1:887–906.

6. William Bynum, "Time's Noblest Offspring: The Problem of Man in British Natural Historical Sciences" (diss.: Cambridge University, 1974).

7. Kant, *Werke,* 6:517–18.

8. On the general background of this debate, see Henri Ellenberger, *The Discovery of the Unconscious: The History and Evolution of Dynamic Psychiatry* (New York: Basic Books, 1970), Gerlof Verwey, *Psychiatry in an Anthropological and Biomedical Context: Philosophical Presuppositions and Implications of German Psychiatry, 1820–70* (Dordrecht: Reidel, 1985), and U. H. Peters, "Die Situation der deutschen Psychiatrie bei Beginn der psychiatrischen Emigrationsbewegung 1933," in Otto Baur and Otto Glandien, eds., *Zusammenhang: Festschrift für Marielene Putscher* (Cologne: Wienand, 1984), pp. 837–64.

9. J. G. Langermann, *De methodo cognoscendi curandique animi morbos stabilienda* (diss.: University of Jena, 1797).

10. Christian Heinrich Spiess, *Biographien der Wahnsinnigen,* ed. Wolfgang Promies (Cologne: Luchterhand, 1966).

11. Emil Kraepelin, "Hundert Jahr Psychiatrie," *Zeitschrift für die Neurologie und Psychiatrie* 38 (1919): 161–275.

12. Sulloway, in *Freud, Biologist,* claims that Freud's perception of anti-Semitism and the marginality of his own views were "myths." If indeed Sulloway is right, and there is little doubt about the force of this argument and the materials he has mustered to prove it, we must ask the evident next question: Why did Freud perceive the world in the manner in which he reported? It is the reconstruction of the fantasies about the world rather than the assumption that there are "realities" in history to be "discovered" which is the central undertaking, especially of the historian of psychoanalysis.

13. See my essay "Jews and Mental Illness: Medical Metaphors, Anti-Semitism, and the Jewish Response," *Journal of the History of the Behavioral Sciences* 20 (1984): 150–59.

14. See Hannah S. Decker, *Freud in Germany: Revolution and Reaction in Science, 1893–1907* (New York: International Universities Press, 1977).

15. Max Schur, "Some Additional 'Day Residues' of the Specimen Dream of Psychoanalysis," in Rudolph M. Löwenstein et al., eds., *Psychoanalysis, a General Psychology: Essays in Honor of Heinz Hartmann* (New York: International Universities Press, 1966), pp. 45–85.

16. Monika Richarz, *Der Eintritt der Juden in die akademische Berufe* (Tübingen:

Mohr, 1974), pp. 28–43, and Erna Lesky, *Die Wiener medizinische Schule im 19. Jahrhundert* (Graz: Böhlau, 1978).

17. See the introduction by Jeffrey Moussaieff Masson to his edition of *The Complete Letters of Sigmund Freud to Wilhelm Fliess, 1887–1904* (Cambridge, Mass.: Harvard University Press, 1985), pp. 1–14. See also Peter Heller, "A Quarrel over Bisexuality," in Gerald Chapple and Hans H. · Schulte, eds., *The Turn of the Century: German Literature and Art, 1890–1915* (Bonn: Bouvier, 1978), pp. 87–116.

18. G. Valentin, *Handbuch der Entwickelungsgeschichte der Menschen* (Berlin: Rücker, 1835).

19. Wilhelm His, *Anatomie menschlicher Embryonen*, 3 vols. (Leipzig: Vogel, 1880–85).

20. Ernst Mayr, *The Growth of Biological Thought: Diversity, Evolution, and Inheritance* (Cambridge, Mass.: Belknap Press, 1982).

21. See Jacob Katz, *From Prejudice to Destruction: Anti-Semitism, 1700–1933* (Cambridge, Mass.: Harvard University Press, 1980).

22. Judith Vogt, *Historien om et Image: Antisemitisme og Antizionisme i Karikaturer* (Copenhagen: Samieren, 1978).

23. Friedrich Nietzsche, *Beyond Good and Evil*, trans. Marianne Cowan (Chicago: Regnery, 1955), pp. 184–88.

24. Hanns Bächtold-Stäubli, ed., *Handwörterbuch des deutschen Aberglaubens* (Berlin: de Gruyter, 1934–35), 6:970–79.

25. Masson, *Complete Letters*, p. 256.

26. Ibid., p. 270.

27. Ibid., p. 199.

28. See, for example, F. A. Forel, "Cas de menstruation chez un homme," *Bulletin de la société médicale de la Suisse romande* (Lausanne), 1869: 53–61, and W. D. Halliburton, "A Peculiar Case," *Weekly Medical Review and Journal of Obstetrics* (St. Louis), 1885: 392.

29. Magnus Hirschfeld, *Sexualpathologie*, 2 vols. (Bonn: Marcus and Weber, 1917–18), 2:1–92.

30. Thomas de Cantimpré, *Miraculorum et exemplorum memorabilium sui temporis libro duo* (Duaci: Belleri, 1605), pp. 305–6.

31. Heinrich Kornmann, *Opera curiosa I: Miracula vivorum* (1st ed., 1614; Frankfurt: Genschiana, 1694), pp. 128–29; Thomas Calvert, *The Blessed Jew of Marocco; or, A Blackmoor Made White Being a Demonstration of the True Messias out of the Law and Prophets by Rabbi Samuel* (York: Broad, 1649), pp. 20–21.

32. On Franco da Piacenza, see Leon Poliakov, *The History of Anti-Semitism*, trans. Richard Howard, 3 vols. (New York: Vanguard Press, 1965–75), 1:143 n.

33. F. L. de la Fontaine, *Chirurgisch-Medicinische Abhandlungen verschiedenen Inhalts Polen betreffend* (Breslau: Korn, 1792). See also J. A. Elie de la Poterie, *Questo medica. An viris lex eadem quä mulieribus, periodicas evacuationes pati?* (diss.: University of Paris, 1764).

34. Theodor Fritsch, *Handbuch der Judenfrage* (Leipzig: Hammer, 1935), p. 409 (with a further discourse on psychoanalysis as a sign of Jewish degeneracy).

35. E. P. Eckholm, *The Picture of Health: Environmental Sources of Disease* (New York: Norton, 1977). The irony is that the image of male menstruation among the Jews probably has a pathological origin. Even today in parts of Africa "male menstruation," in the form of urethral bleeding, seems to be an indicator of "sexual maturation." What actually happens is that, for reasons not completely understood, a parasite, *Schistosoma haematoboum*, which lives in the veins surrounding the bladder, becomes active during the early teenage years. One can imagine that Jews infected with schistosomiasis,

giving the appearance of menstruation, would have reified the notion of difference that the Northern European, not prone to this snail-born parasite, would have sensed. On the symbolic value of this manifestation, see Herbert Ian Hogbin, *The Island of Menstruating Men: Religion in Wogeo, New Guinea* (Scranton, Pa.: Chandler, 1970).

36. On the implications of the attitudes of Christian Vienna toward the new "Jewish" science of psychoanalysis, see Dennis B. Klein, *Jewish Origins of the Psychoanalytic Movement* (New York: Praeger, 1981). Freud's ambiguous quest for status in science was paralleled by his fascination with Christianity. Just as the society he lived in never permitted him to become a full-fledged academic, at least in his own eyes, it also tantalized him with the promise of acceptance based on conversion. Freud remained on the outside also in terms of his relation to structures of power such as the Church, but was clearly fascinated by it. See Paul C. Vitz, "Sigmund Freud's Attraction to Christianity: Biographical Evidence," *Psychoanalysis and Contemporary Thought* 6 (1983): 73–183.

37. See the discussion in Robert S. Steele, *Freud and Jung: Conflicts of Interpretation* (London: Routledge & Kegan Paul, 1982).

38. See the discussion of this influence in my essay "Sexology, Psychoanalysis, and Degeneration: From a Theory of Race to a Race to Theory," in J. E. Chamberlin and Sander L. Gilman, eds., *Degeneration: The Dark Side of Progress* (New York: Columbia University Press, 1985), pp. 72–96.

39. Sigmund Freud, "The Question of Lay Analysis: Conversations with an Impartial Person," in *The Complete Psychological Works of Sigmund Freud*, trans. James Strachey (London: Hogarth, 1959), 20:177–258. See the contemporary newspaper discussion of the case in Vienna: "Dr. Reik und die Kurpfuschereifrage," *Neue freie Presse*, 18 July 1926; "Psychoanalyse und Kurpfuscherei," *Neue freie Presse*, 24 July 1926; "Der Fall des Dr. Reik und die Kurpfuscherei, *Neue freie Presse*, 15 July 1926; "Kurpfuscher," *Neues wiener Journal*, 18 July 1926; "Der Kampf gegen die Kurpfuscher," *Neues wiener Journal*, 14 July 1926; "Psychoanalyse und Kurpfuscherei," *Wiener allgemeine Zeitung*, 13 July 1926; "Psychoanalyse und Kurpfuscherei," *Wiener allgemeine Zeitung*, 17 July 1926. In general on the background to the case, see Harald Leupold-Löwenthal, "Zur Geschichte der 'Frage der Laienanalyse,'" *Psyche* 38 (1984): 97–120, and Karl Sablik, "Sigmund Freud und Julius Tandler: Eine rätselhafte Beziehung," *Sigmund Freud Haus Bulletin* 9 (1985): 12–19. On the debate in the United States, see Norman S. Greenfield and Gene M. Abroms, "The Role and Status of the Non-Medical Psychotherapist in the United States," *Human Context* 5 (1973): 657–58. In addition to the Reik case, a case was brought in 1927 against Alfred Adler, himself a physician, by the Viennese Physician's Association for awarding diplomas indicating the completion of a lay analysis. This case was adjudicated in October 1928, and Adler was forbidden to award such diplomas. See Manfred Skopec, "Zur Geschichte des österreichischen Vereins für Individualpsychologie," *Zeitschrift für Individualpsychologie* 9 (1984): 52–63.

40. Freud, "Question of Lay Analysis," p. 230.

41. Ibid., p. 231.

42. Ibid., pp. 253–54.

43. See the debate between Josef Gicklhorn and Renee Gicklhorn, *Sigmund Freuds akademische Laufbahn im Lichte der Dokumente* (Vienna: Urban & Schwarzenberg, 1960), and Kurt R. Eissler, *Sigmund Freud und die wiener Universität: Über die Pseudo-Wissenschaftlichkeit der jüngste wiener Freud-Biographik* (Bern: Huber, 1966).

44. See U. H. Peters, *Anna Freud: Ein Leben für das Kind* (Frankfurt: Fischer, 1984), pp. 68–71.

45. See Phyllis Grosskurth, *Melanie Klein: Her World and Her Work* (New York: Knopf, 1986), pp. 99–100.

46. See my *Difference and Pathology: Stereotypes of Sexuality, Race, and Madness* (Ithaca, N.Y.: Cornell University Press, 1985), pp. 150–62.

47. All of the material cited is from the archives of the American Psychoanalytic Society, now housed in the Archives of Psychiatry, Cornell Medical College, New York. See also Hendrick M. Ruitenbeek, *Freud and America* (New York: Macmillan, 1966).

48. Theodor Billroth, *The Medical Science in the German Universities: A Study in the History of Civilization*, trans. William H. Welch (New York: Macmillan, 1924), pp. 107–8. Billroth's view was developed in the added context of the growing professionalization of the physician in Vienna. One must remember that Vienna's medical establishment had, from its rejection of Mesmer and Gall to its attack on Reik, always defined itself in terms of what it was not. See the special issue of the *Österreichische Ärzte-Zeitung* 121–132 (1976) on "Medizin auf Ab- und Seitenwegen."

49. Robert Michels, "Psychoanalysis and Psychiatry—the End of the Affair," *Academy Forum* 25 (1981): 7–8. See also his more detailed discussion in his *The Evolution of Psychodynamic Psychotherapy* (Philadelphia: Institute of Pennsylvania Hospital, 1985), and I. F. Knight, "Paradigms and Crises in Psychoanalysis," *Psychoanalytic Quarterly* 54 (1985): 597–614.

50. Michels, "Psychoanalysis and Psychiatry," pp. 8–10.

51. *The New York Times*, 19 May 1985, p. 20E.

12. Constructing Schizophrenia as a Category of Mental Illness

1. There have been many attempts to sketch the history of the concept of schizophrenia, either independently or within broader contexts, all of which are helpful, but none of which provides any synthetic history of the concept.

For 1928 to 1941, see Adolf Meyer, "The Evolution of the Dementia Praecox Concept," in Charles L. Dana et al., eds., *Schizophrenia [Dementia Praecox]* (New York: Hoeber, 1928), pp. 3–15; H. W. Gruhle, "Die Schizophrenie. Geschichtliches," in O. Bumke, ed., *Handbuch der Geisteskranken*, vol. 9, special section 5 (Berlin: Springer, 1932), pp. 1–30; Gregory Zilboorg, *A History of Medical Psychology* (New York: Norton, 1941; rev. ed., 1954).

For 1956 to 1970, see J. Wyrsch, *Zur Geschichte und Deutung der endogenen Psychosen* (Stuttgart: Thieme, 1956); Erwin Ackerknecht, *Kurze Geschichte der Psychiatrie* (Stuttgart: Enke, 1957); Manfred Bleuler, "The Conception of Schizophrenia within the Last Fifty Years and Today," *International Journal of Psychiatry* 1 (1965): 501–23; Franz Alexander and Sheldon Selesnick, *The History of Psychiatry* (New York: Harper & Row, 1966); Dieter Wyss, *Depth Psychology: A Critical History, Development, Problems* (New York: Norton, 1966); N. D. Lewis, "The History of the Nosology and the Evolution of the Concepts of Schizophrenia," *Proceedings of the American Psychopathological Association* 54 (1966): 1–18; G. Tourney, "A History of Therapeutic Fashions in Psychiatry, 1800–1966," *American Journal of Psychiatry* 124 (1967): 784–96.

For 1970 to 1975, see Robert Cancro and Paul W. Pruyser, "A Historical Review of the Development of the Concept of Schizophrenia," in Robert Cancro, ed., *The Schizophrenic Reactions* (New York: Brunner / Mazel, 1970), pp. 3–12; Henri F. Ellenberger, *The Discovery of the Unconscious: The History and Evolution of Dynamic Psychiatry* (New York: Basic Books, 1970); Silvano Arieti, *Interpretation of Schizophrenia* (New

York: Basic Books, 1974), pp. 9–29; Werner Janzarik, *Themen und Tendenzen der deutschsprachigen Psychiatrie* (Berlin: Springer, 1974); A. D. Forrest, "Concepts of Schizophrenia: Historical Review," in A. D. Forrest and J. Affleck, eds., *New Perspectives in Schizophrenia* (Edinburgh: Livingstone, 1975), pp. 1–15.

For 1976 to 1979, see M. D. Altschule, "Historical Perspective: Evolution of the Concept of Schizophrenia," in Stewart Wolf and Beatrice Bishop Berle, eds., *The Biology of the Schizophrenic Process* (New York: Plenum Press, 1976), pp. 1–13; J. Ramano, "On the Nature of Schizophrenia: Changes in the Observer as Well as the Observed," *Schizophrenia Bulletin* 3 (1977): 532–59; Henry Werlinder, *Psychopathy: A History of the Concepts: Analysis of the Origin and Development of a Family of Concepts in Psychopathology* (Stockholm: Almqvist & Wiksell, 1978), pp. 100–27; Hannah S. Decker, "The Historical Evolution of *Dementia Praecox*," in William E. Fann et al., eds., *Phenomenology and Treatment of Schizophrenia* (New York: Spectrum, 1978), pp. 301–9; Manfred Bleuler, "On Schizophrenic Psychoses," *American Journal of Psychiatry* 136 (1979): 1403–9.

For 1980 to 1983, see Peter Berner, "Schizophrenie: Überblick und Geschichte," in U. H. Peters, ed., *Psychiatrie* (Zurich: Kindler, 1980), 1:353–70; John M. Neale and Thomas F. Oltmanns, *Schizophrenia* (New York: Wiley, 1980), pp. 2–16; Seymour S. Kety, "The Syndrome of Schizophrenia: Unresolved Questions and Opportunities for Research," *British Journal of Psychiatry* 136 (1980): 421–36; Sue A. Shapiro, *Contemporary Theories of Schizophrenia: Review and Synthesis* (New York: McGraw-Hill, 1981), pp. 7–23; Kenneth Kendler and Ming T. Tsuang, "The Nosology of Paranoid Schizophrenia and Other Paranoid Psychoses," *Schizophrenia Bulletin* 7 (1981): 594–610; S. P. Fullinwider, *Technicians of the Finite: The Rise and Decline of the Schizophrenic in American Thought, 1840–1960* (Westport, Conn.: Greenwood Press, 1982); Ph. Van Meerbeck, "D'où nous viennent la démence précoce et la schizophrénie?" *Acta psychiatrica belgica* 82 (1982): 243–76; R. D. Chandresna, "Phenomenology and Nosology of Schizophrenia: Historical Review," *Psychiatric Journal of the University of Ottawa* 8 (1983): 17–24; William N. Goldstein, "DSM-III and the Diagnosis of Schizophrenia," *American Journal of Psychotherapy* 37 (1983): 168–81.

2. Quoted from the Student Edition of Alfred M. Freedman, Harold I. Kaplan, and Benjamin J. Sadock, eds., *Modern Synopsis of Comprehensive Textbook of Psychiatry* (Baltimore: Williams & Wilkins, 1976), p. 418.

3. On historical changes in the appearance of schizophrenia, see B. Mahendra, "Where Have All the Catatonics Gone?" *Psychological Medicine* 1 (1981): 669–71. Cf. J. R. Morrison, "Changes in Sub-Type Diagnosis in Schizophrenia: 1920–66," *American Journal of Psychiatry* 131 (1974): 674–77.

I am relying in this chapter on the accepted distinction between an "illness" as a social state created by human evaluation of problematic experiences and a "disease" as a variety of biological events existing independently of human knowledge and evaluation; see D. Locker, *Symptoms and Illness: The Cognitive Organization of Disorder* (London: Tavistock, 1981). The research in the area of schizophrenia is, in general, operating without a specific definition of the concept of schizophrenia. The standard American periodical that deals with this area, the *Schizophrenia Bulletin* (funded by the National Institute of Mental Health), has been running a series of guest columns under the title "What Is Schizophrenia?" Such openness about the difficulty of definition is rare in any medical subspeciality. See John S. Strauss and Thomas E. Gift, "Choosing an Approach for Diagnosing Schizophrenia," *Archives of General Psychiatry* 34 (1977): 1248–53.

4. Quoted in Richard Hunter and Ida Macalpine, eds., *Three Hundred Years of Psychiatry, 1535–1860* (London: Oxford University Press, 1963), p. 987.

5. Bleuler provides his own discussion of the history of the concept of schizophrenia,

which shall be discussed in detail below (see note 26). See Eugen Bleuler, *Dementia Praecox oder Gruppe der Schizophrenien. Handbuch der Psychiatrie* (Leipzig: Deuticke, 1911), pp. 1–5 (for the English translation from which all quotations are taken, see note 10).

6. On the problems of interpreting "signs" and symptoms historically, see Joel Wilbush, "Clinical Information: Signs, Semeions, and Symptoms," *Journal of the Royal Society of Medicine* 77 (1984): 766–73.

7. See Jane M. Murphy, "Psychiatric Labeling in Cross-Cultural Perspective," *Science* 191 (1976): 1019–28. See also Erwin H. Ackerknecht, *Medicine and Ethnology*, ed. H. H. Walser and H. M. Koelbing (Baltimore: Johns Hopkins University Press, 1971), and Arthur Kleinman, Leon Eisenberg, and Byron Good, "Culture, Illness, and Care: Clinical Lessons from Anthropologic and Cross-Cultural Research," *Annals of Internal Medicine* 88 (1978): 251–58.

8. H. Tristram Engelhardt, Jr., "The Concepts of Health and Disease," in Arthur L. Caplan, H. Tristram Engelhardt, Jr., and James J. McCartney, eds., *Concepts of Health and Disease* (Reading, Mass.: Addison-Wesley, 1981), p. 40.

9. See P. D'Estrube, "Diagnostic Labels in the History of Psychiatry," *Journal of the Canadian Psychiatric Association* 11 (1966): 356–57.

10. Bleuler's study was translated into English only after World War II: *Dementia Praecox; or the Group of Schizophrenias*, trans. Joseph Zinkin (New York: International Universities Press, 1950). For a more detailed discussion of the literature on Bleuler, see note 26.

11. Thomas Willis, *De anima brutorum . . . exercitationes duae.* (London: Dring et al., 1683). On the tradition of a "mental ailment during the teen-age years," see Ernest Harms's introduction to the reprint of Emil Kraepelin, *Dementia Praecox and Paraphrenia* (1919; Huntington, N.Y.: Krieger, 1971), p. xiii. All references to Kraepelin are to this translation.

12. Etienne Georget, *De la folie* (Paris: Crevot, 1820), p. 119; J. E. D. Esquirol, *Mental Madness: A Treatise on Insanity* (Philadelphia: Lea & Blanchard, 1845), pp. 417–18. In general on this topic, see P. J. Pichot, "The Diagnosis and Classification of Mental Disorders in French-speaking Countries: Background, Current Views, and Comparison with Other Nomenclatures," *Psychological Medicine* 12 (1982): 475–92, and his "The French Approach to Psychiatric Classification," *British Journal of Psychiatry* 144 (1984): 113–18.

13. Allen W. Hagenbach, "Masturbation as a Cause of Insanity," *Journal of Nervous and Mental Diseases* 6 (1879): 609. For the background to this concept, see H. Tristram Engelhardt, Jr., "The Disease of Masturbation: Values and the Concept of Disease," *Bulletin of the History of Medicine* 48 (1974): 234–48.

14. Patricia Meyer Spacks, *The Adolescent Idea: Myths of Youth and the Adult Imagination* (New York: Basic Books, 1981).

15. Bénédict-Auguste Morel, *Traité des maladies mentales* (Paris: Masson, 1860), pp. 1565–66 (translation from Altschule, "Historical Perspective," p. 7; see note 1).

16. J. T. Dickson, *The Science and Practice of Medicine in Relation to Mind* (New York: Appleton, 1874), pp. 290–92, and G. C. Gauthier, *De la démence précoce chez les jeunes aliénés héréditaires* (thesis: University of Paris [376], 1883).

17. Richard von Krafft-Ebing, *Textbook of Insanity*, trans. Charles Gilbert Chaddock (Philadelphia: Davis, 1904), p. 350.

18. Alois Pick, "Über primäre chronische Demenz (sog. Dementia Praecox) im jugendlichen Alter," *Prager medizinische Wochenschrift* 16 (1891): 312–15.

19. See George Mora's introduction to the translation of K. L. Kahlbaum, *Catatonia* (Baltimore: Johns Hopkins University Press, 1973), pp. viii–xviii.

20. See the discussion in Werner Leibbrand and Annemarie Wettley, *Der Wahnsinn:*

Geschichte der abendländischen Psychopathologie (Freiburg: Alber, 1961), pp. 582–86.

21. U. H. Peters, *Wörterbuch der Psychiatrie und medizinische Psychologie* (Munich: Urban & Schwarzenberg, 1984), p. 289.

22. Altschule, "Historical Perspective," p. 10.

23. See Albrecht Hirschmüller, *Physiologie und Psychoanalyse in Leben und Werk Josef Breuers* (Bern: Huber, 1978), p. 207 n.

24. On the destructive influence of this model, see E. M. Butler, *The Tyranny of Greece over Germany* (Boston: Beacon Press, 1958). For the turn of the century, see more specifically Wendelin Schmidt-Dengler, "Decadence and Antiquity: The Educational Preconditions of *Jung-Wien*," in Erika Nielsen, ed., *Focus on Vienna 1900: Change and Continuity in Literature, Music, Art, and Intellectual History* (Munich: Fink, 1982), pp. 32–45.

25. Kraepelin, *Dementia Praecox and Paraphrenia*, p. 243. On the contemporary reception of Kraepelin, see Louise Brink and Smith Ely Jelliffe, "Emil Kraepelin: Psychiatrist and Poet," *Journal of Nervous and Mental Diseases* 77 (1933): 134–52. For a more general background, see R. L. James and P. R. May, "Diagnosing Schizophrenia: Professor Kraepelin and the Research Diagnostic Criteria," *American Journal of Psychiatry* 138 (1981): 50–54; H. Hippius et al., eds., *Emil Kraepelin: Lebenserinnerungen* (Berlin: Springer, 1983). The editions of Emil Kraepelin's *Psychiatrie* which appeared during his lifetime were, first to eighth, all published in Leipzig: Abel, 1883, 384 pp.; Abel, 1887, 540 pp.; Abel, 1889, 584 pp.; Meiner, 1893, 707 pp.; Barth, 1896, 825 pp.; Barth, 1899, 969 pp.; Barth, 1903–4, 1369 pp.; Barth, 1909–13, 2500 pp.

26. Hans Stierlin, "Bleuler's Concept of Schizophrenia: A Confusing Legacy," *American Journal of Psychiatry* 123 (1967): 996–1001; David E. Raskin, "Bleuler and Schizophrenia," *British Journal of Psychiatry* 127 (1975): 231–34; David Rosenthal, "Eugen Bleuler's Thoughts and Views about Heredity in Schizophrenia," *Schizophrenia Bulletin* 4 (1978): 476–77; M. Menuck, "What Did Eugen Bleuler Really Say?" *Canadian Journal of Psychiatry* 24 (1979): 161–66; T. J. Crow and E. C. Johnstone, "Dementia Praecox and Schizophrenia: Was Bleuler Wrong?" *Journal of the Royal College of Physicians* (London) 14 (1980): 238–40; Mark Ast, "Kraepelin and Bleuler: A Comparison of Dementia Praecox and Schizophrenia" (diss.: Yeshiva University, 1984). On the World Health Organization's *International Pilot Study of Schizophrenia* and its findings, which seem to contradict those of Bleuler, see Norman Sartorius, Robert Shapiro, and Assen Jablensky, "The International Pilot Study of Schizophrenia," *Schizophrenia Bulletin* 11 (1974): 21–34; Assen Jablensky, "Multicultural Studies and the Nature of Schizophrenia: A Review," *Journal of the Royal College of Medicine* 80 (1987): 162–67.

27. Freud's works are cited to *The Standard Edition of the Complete Psychological Works of Sigmund Freud* (London: Hogarth Press, 1953–74), hereafter referred to as *SE*; here "The Neuro-Psychoses of Defence" (1894), *SE* 3:41–68. On Freud's understanding of the disease, see B. L. Boyer and P. C. Giovacchini, *Psychoanalytic Treatment of Characterological and Schizophrenic Disorders* (New York: Science House, 1967); P.-N. Pao, "Notes on Freud's Theory of Schizophrenia," *International Journal of Psycho-Analysis* 54 (1973): 469–76; T. Freeman, "On Freud's Theory of Schizophrenia," *International Journal of Psycho-Analysis* 58 (1977): 383–88.

28. Freud, "Further Remarks on the Defence Neuro-Psychosis" (1896), *SE* 3:157–85.

29. Bleuler, *Dementia Praecox*, p. 5.

30. For example, the Dadaist and Expressionist Hugo Ball wrote a series of poems called "Sieben schizophrene Sonette." See Thomas Anz, ed., *Phantasien über dem Wahnsinn: Expressionistische Texte* (Munich: Hanser, 1980), pp. 56–61, for the text, as

well as Wolfgang Rothe, "Der Geisteskranke im Expressionismus," *Confinia psychiatrica* 15 (1972): 195–211, for the popular reception of the idea of schizophrenia.

31. L. Bellak, *Dementia Praecox: The Past Decade's Work and Present Status: A Review and Examination* (New York: Grune, 1948); L. Bellak, *Schizophrenia: A Review of the Syndromes* (New York: Logos, 1957).

32. See Karl Jaspers, *Allgemeine Psychopathologie* (1913; Berlin: Springer, 1973, 9th ed.).

33. See the English translation, Kurt Schneider, *Clinical Psychopathology* (New York: Grune & Stratton, 1959). On Schneider's influence, see H. A. Fox, "Bleuler, Schneider, and Schizophrenia," *Journal of Clinical Psychiatry* 39 (1978): 703–8; J. Hoenig, "Kurt Schneider and Anglophone Psychiatry," *Comprehensive Psychiatry* 23 (1982): 391–400, and "The Concept of Schizophrenia: Kraepelin-Bleuler-Schneider," *British Journal of Psychiatry* 142 (1983): 547–56.

34. Freud, "Psychoanalytic Notes upon an Autobiographical Account of a Case of Paranoia (*Dementia Paranoides*)" (1911), *SE* 12:1–82.

35. Freud, "On Narcissism" (1914), *SE* 14:67–107.

36. A good interpretation of the Schreber case and an introduction to the problems that it presented to the early psychoanalysts can be found in C. Barry Chabot, *Freud on Schreber: Psychoanalytic Theory and the Critical Act* (Amherst: University of Massachusetts Press, 1982).

37. See my essay "The Mad as Artist: Medicine, History, and Degenerate Art," *Journal of Contemporary History* 20 (1985): 575–97.

38. Hans Prinzhorn, *Bildnerei der Geisteskranken: Ein Beitrag zur Psychologie und Psychopathologie der Gestaltung* (Berlin: Springer, 1923); Wilhelm Mayer-Gross, *Selbstschilderungen der Verwirrtheit: Die onairoide Erlebnisform* (Berlin: Springer, 1924). See Aubrey Lewis, "William Meyer-Gross," *Confrontations psychiatriques* 6 (1973): 109–25.

39. On the parallels and differences between Freud and Jung, see Robert S. Steele, *Freud and Jung: Conflicts of Interpretation* (London: Routledge & Kegan Paul, 1982).

40. *The Collected Works of C. G. Jung* (Princeton, N.J.: Princeton University Press, 1967 ff.), hereafter cited as *CW*. See his essays "The Psychology of Dementia Praecox" (1907), *CW* 3:1–151, and "On Dementia Praecox" (1910e / 1908), *CW* 18:335.

41. Jung, "A Contribution to the Study of Psychological Types," *CW* 6:499–509.

42. See the more detailed discussion in Chapter 7.

43. For the appropriate materials, see A. Lief, ed., *The Commonsense Psychiatry of Dr. Adolf Meyer* (New York: McGraw-Hill, 1948), and Eunice E. Winters, ed., *The Collected Papers of Adolf Meyer*, 4 vols. (Baltimore: Johns Hopkins University Press, 1951). On Meyer, see the essay by L. B. Ritvo in the *Dictionary of National Biography* 4 (1946–50): 569–72; Manfred Bleuler, "Early Swiss Sources of Adolf Meyer's Concepts," *American Journal of Psychiatry* 119 (1962): 193–96; Hans H. Walser, "Die wissenschaftlichen Anfänge von Adolf Meyer (1866–1950) und die Entstehung der 'Züricher psychiatrischen Schule,'" *Gesnerus* 23 (1966): 202–10; Hans H. Walser, "Adolf Meyer—Student of the Zurich Psychiatric School," *Gesnerus* 41 (1984): 49–51. Meyer's disappearance from the discussion of the concept of schizophrenia by the late 1970s (following the publication of *DSM-III*) can be judged by the absence of his name from Sue A. Shapiro's review (see note 1) of those theories still held to be important at the time of the publication of her overview (1981).

44. P. H. Hoch and P. Polatin, "Pseudoneurotic Forms of Schizophrenia," *Psychiatric Quarterly* 23 (1949): 248–76; P. H. Hoch and S. L. Dunaif, "Pseudoneurotic Schizophrenia," in P. H. Hoch and J. Zubin, eds., *Psychiatry and the Law* (New York: Grune & Stratton, 1955).

45. See specifically Thomas Szasz, *Schizophrenia: The Sacred Symbol of Psychiatry* (New York: Basic Books, 1976) and his *Insanity: The Idea and Its Consequences* (New York: Wiley, 1987). On Szasz and the critics of contemporary psychiatry, see P. Sedgwick, *Psycho Politics: Laing, Foucault, Gofman, Szasz, and the Future of Mass Psychiatry* (New York: Harper & Row, 1982).

46. See Harry Stack Sullivan, *Clinical Studies in Psychiatry* (New York: Norton, 1956) and his *Schizophrenia as a Human Process* (New York: Norton, 1962), which comprise most of the early papers. On Sullivan, see the comprehensive biography by Helen Swick Perry, *Psychiatrist of America: The Life of Harry Stack Sullivan* (Cambridge, Mass.: Belknap Press, 1982).

47. Sullivan, "Schizophrenia: Its Conservative and Malignant Features" (1924), reprinted in his *Schizophrenia*, p. 20.

48. J. S. Kasanin, ed., *Language and Thought in Schizophrenia* (1944; New York: Norton, 1964). This volume presented papers read at a meeting of the American Psychiatric Association in 1939. For the most recent attempts to systematize the phenomenology of schizophrenic language, see R. E. Hoffman, S. Stopek, and N. C. Andreasen, "A Comparative Study of Manic vs. Schizophrenic Speech Disorganization," *Archive of General Psychiatry* 43 (1986): 831–38, and W. I. Fraser, K. M. King, P. Thomas, and R. E. Kendell, "The Diagnosis of Schizophrenia by Language Analysis," *British Journal of Psychiatry* 148 (1986): 275–78.

49. E. von Domarus, "The Specific Laws of Logic in Schizophrenia," in Kasanin, *Language*, pp. 104–14.

50. E. Hanfmann and J. Kasanin, "A Method for the Study of Concept Formation," *Journal of Psychology* 3 (1936): 521–40.

51. Harry Stack Sullivan, *Conceptions of Modern Psychiatry* (New York: William Alanson White Psychiatric Foundation, 1940).

52. See the appropriate papers in Frieda Fromm-Reichmann, *Psychoanalysis and Psychotherapy: Selected Papers* (Chicago: University of Chicago Press, 1959). On Fromm-Reichmann, see the essay by R. C. Powell and S. G. Hoff in *Notable American Women: The Modern Period* (Cambridge, Mass.: Belknap Press, 1980), 4:252–55; Alfred H. Stanton, "Frieda Fromm-Reichmann, M.D.: Her Impact on American Psychiatry," *Psychiatry* 45 (1982): 121–27; and U. H. Peters, "Frieda Fromm-Reichmann und die psychoanalytisch orientierte Psychotherapie der Schizophrenie," *Fundamenta Psychiatrica* 77 (1987): 184–91.

53. Hannah Green, *I Never Promised You a Rose Garden* (New York: Holt, Rinehart & Winston, 1964). See "Frieda Fromm-Reichmann Discusses the 'Rose Garden' Case," *Psychiatry* 45 (1982): 128–36.

54. See the appropriate essays in Melanie Klein, *Contributions to Psychoanalysis, 1921–45* (New York: McGraw-Hill, 1964). The best overview of this entire school is Jay R. Greenberg and Stephen A. Mitchell, *Object Relations in Psychoanalytic Theory* (Cambridge, Mass.: Harvard University Press, 1983). The best introduction to Klein's work is Phyllis Grosskurth, *Melanie Klein: Her World and Her Work* (New York: Knopf, 1986). See also P. H. King, "The Life and Work of Melanie Klein in the British Psycho-Analytic Society," *International Journal of Psycho-Analysis* 64 (1983): 251–60.

55. See Gregory Bateson, *Steps to an Ecology of the Mind* (New York: Ballantine, 1972).

56. See the appropriate essays in W. R. D. Fairbairn, *An Object-Relations Theory of the Personality* (New York: Basic Books, 1952).

57. See the appropriate essays in D. W. Winnicott, *Through Paediatrics to Psycho-Analysis* (London: Hogarth, 1958) and *The Maturational Process and the Facilitating Environment* (New York: International Universities Press, 1965).

58. R. D. Laing, *The Divided Self: An Existential Study in Sanity and Madness* (1959; Harmondsworth: Penguin, 1981).

59. On Laing, see Elaine Showalter, *The Female Malady: Women, Madness, and English Culture, 1830–1980* (New York: Pantheon, 1985), pp. 220–47, and Robert Boyers and Robert Orrill, eds., *Laing and Anti-Psychiatry* (Harmondsworth: Penguin, 1972).

60. Mary Barnes and Joe Berke, *Mary Barnes: Two Accounts of a Journey through Madness* (New York: Harcourt Brace Jovanovich, 1971).

61. U. H. Peters, "Mary Barnes. Psychopathologische Literaturinterpretation am Beispiel einer literarischen Gattung: Psychose-Fiktion," in Bernd Urban and Winfried Kudszus, eds., *Psychoanalytische und Psychopathologische Literaturinterpretation* (Darmstadt: Wissenschaftliche Buchgesellschaft, 1981), pp. 280–99.

62. All of the basic papers (including the later work of Laing and Wynne) are collected in Carlos E. Sluzki and Donald C. Ransom, eds., *Double Bind: The Foundation of the Communicational Approach to the Family* (New York: Grune & Stratton, 1976).

63. Theodore Lidz, *The Origin and Treatment of Schizophrenic Disorders* (New York: Basic Books, 1973).

64. Typical for this early stage is the paper by L. C. Wynne, I. M. Ryckoff, J. Day, and S. Hirsch, "Pseudomutuality in the Family Relations of Schizophrenics," *Psychiatry* 21 (1958): 205–20. See Wynne's own overview "Current Concepts about Schizophrenics and Family Relationships," *Journal of Nervous and Mental Disease* 169 (1981): 82–89.

65. See L. C. Wynne, M. Singer, and J. J. Bartko, "Schizophrenics and Their Families: Recent Research on Parental Communication," in J. M. Tanner, ed., *Psychiatric Research: The Widening Perspective* (New York: International Universities Press, 1975).

66. L. C. Wynne, R. L. Cromwell, and S. Matthysse, eds., *The Nature of Schizophrenia: New Approaches to Research and Treatment* (New York: Wiley, 1978).

67. See table 4, "Chronology of Major Psychoanalytic and Family Works on Schizophrenia," in Shapiro, *Contemporary Theories*, pp. 84–85.

68. In general on this question, see Hilary Putnam, "The Impact of Science on Modern Conceptions of Rationality," in his *Reason, Truth, and History* (Cambridge: Cambridge University Press, 1981), pp. 174–200.

69. I am indebted to the overviews of Shapiro, *Contemporary Theories*, and Neale and Oltmanns, *Schizophrenia*, for this segment. I do not, however, always agree with their interpretation of this data.

70. Ernst Rüdin, *Zur Vererbung und Neuentstehung der Dementia Praecox* (Berlin: Springer, 1916).

71. For a much more detailed criticism of Kallmann's work, see J. Richard Marshall, "The Genetics of Schizophrenia Revisited," *Bulletin of the British Psychological Society* 37 (1984): 177–81.

72. Cited by Marshall, ibid., p. 177.

73. Reported in Franz Kallmann, *The Genetics of Schizophrenia* (New York: Augustin, 1938).

74. Franz Kallmann, "The Genetic Theory of Schizophrenia," *American Journal of Psychiatry* 103 (1946): 309–22.

75. R. C. Lewontin, Steven Rose, and Leon J. Kamin, *Not in Our Genes: Biology, Ideology, and Human Nature* (New York: Pantheon, 1984), pp. 197–231.

76. Kallmann, *Genetics of Schizophrenia*, p. 3.

77. J. A. Böök, "A Genetic and Neuropsychiatric Investigation of a North-Swedish Population with Special Regard to Schizophrenia and Mental Deficiency," *Acta Genetica* 4 (1953): 1–139; S. S. Kety et al., "The Types and Prevalence of Mental Illness in the

Notes to Pages 228–233

Biological and Adoptive Families of Adopted Schizophrenics," in D. Rosenthal and S. S. Kety, eds., *The Transmission of Schizophrenia* (New York: Pergamon, 1968), pp. 345–62. On the background, see Kety, "The Syndrome of Schizophrenia," cited in note 1.

78. See the critique in Lewontin et al., *Not in Our Genes*, pp. 221–26.

79. P. E. Meehl, "Schizotaxia, Schizotypy, Schizophrenia," *American Psychologist* 17 (1962): 827–38.

80. S. S. Kety, "Biochemical Hypotheses and Studies," in L. Bellak and L. Loeb, eds., *The Schizophrenic Syndrome* (New York: Grune & Stratton, 1969), pp. 155–71.

81. E. Kretschmer, *Physique and Character*, trans. W. J. H. Sprott (London: Kegan Paul, Trench & Trubner, 1925); W. H. Sheldon, *The Varieties of Temperament* (New York: Harper, 1942). In this context, see esp. Davydd J. Greenwood, *The Taming of Evolution: The Persistence of Nonevolutionary Views in the Study of Humans* (Ithaca, N.Y.: Cornell University Press, 1985), pp. 86–96.

82. H. Osmond and J. Smythies, "Schizophrenia: A New Approach," *Journal of Mental Science* 98 (1952): 309–15.

83. J. E. Cooper, F. E. Bloom, and R. H. Roth, *The Biochemical Basis of Neuropharmacology* (New York: Oxford University Press, 1974).

84. A. J. Friedhoff and E. Van Winkle, "Isolation and Characterization of a Compound from the Urine of Schizophrenics," *Nature* 194 (1962): 897–98.

85. A. J. Friedhoff, S. Park, S. Schweitzer, E. I. Burdock, and M. Armour, "Excretion of 3,4-dimethoxphenylethylamine (DMPEA) by Acute Schizophrenics and Controls," *Biological Psychiatry* 12 (1977): 643–54.

86. W. Pollin, P. V. Cardon, and S. S. Kety, "Effects of Amino Acid Feedings in Schizophrenic Patients Treated with Iproniazid," *Science* 133 (1961): 104–5.

87. D. L. Murphy and R. J. Wyatt, "Reduced Monoamine Oxidase Activity in Blood Platelets from Schizophrenic Patients," *Nature* 238 (1972): 225–26; R. G. Heath and I. M. Krupp, "Schizophrenia as an Immunologic Disorder," *Archives of General Psychiatry* 16 (1967): 1–9.

88. Manfred Bleuler, "What Is Schizophrenia?" *Schizophrenia Bulletin* 10 (1984): 8.

13. Seeing the Schizophrenic: On the "Bizarre" in Psychiatry and Art

1. See the works of Michel Foucault on the history of medicine and madness, esp. his *Naissance de la clinique: Une archéologie du regard médical* (Paris: Presses universitaires de France, 1963). My selection of examples here is in no way exhaustive; rather, it reflects the various uses of the "bizarre" in modern psychiatry. A good introduction to the overall problem of diagnostic categories is Charles C. Hughes, "Culture-Bound or Construct-Bound? The Syndromes and DSM-III," in Ronald C. Simons and Charles C. Hughes, eds., *The Culture-Bound Syndromes* (Dordrecht: Reidel, 1985), pp. 1–24.

2. B. A. Morel, "Considérations générales sur les excentricités, les bizarreries de caractère et de goût, les passions violentes, dans leurs rapports avec la folie," *L'union médicale* 7 (1853): 417–18, 421–22, 425–27.

3. *DSM-III-R in Development. Second Draft. 1 August 1986* (Washington, D.C.: Work Group to Revise DSM-III, American Psychiatric Association, 1986), section D:1.

4. *Diagnostic and Statistical Manual of Mental Disorders*, 3d ed. (Washington, D.C.: American Psychiatric Association, 1980), p. 182.

5. *DSM-III Draft* (Washington, D.C.: American Psychiatric Association, 1978), section C:2, dated 10 December 1977.

6. Robert L. Spitzer et al., eds., *DSM-III Case Book* (Washington, D.C.: American

Psychiatric Association, 1981), p. 103; *Quick Reference to the Diagnostic Criteria from DSM-III* (Washington, D.C.: American Psychiatric Association, 1980), p. 6.

7. *Diagnostic and Statistical Manual of Mental Disorders* (Washington, D.C.: American Psychiatric Association, 1952), p. 27.

8. *Diagnostic and Statistical Manual of the Mental Disorders II* (Washington, D.C.: American Psychiatric Association, 1968), p. 33.

9. Hans Bürger-Prinz, "Über die künstlerischen Arbeiten Schizophrener," in *Handbuch der Geisteskranken*, vol. 9: *Die Schizophrenie* (Heidelberg: Springer, 1932), p. 690.

10. Walter Benjamin, "Bücher von Geisteskranken: Aus meiner Sammlung," in his *Gesammelte Schriften*, ed. Rolf Tiedemann (Frankfurt: Suhrkamp, 1972), pp. 2, 4, 619.

11. Eugen Bleuler, *Dementia Praecox oder Gruppe der Schizophrenien. Handbuch der Psychiatrie* (Leipzig: Deuticke, 1911), vol. 4, section 1:10.

12. Eugen Bleuler, *Dementia Praecox; or the Group of Schizophrenias*, trans. Joseph Zinkin (New York: International Universities Press, 1950), p. 14.

13. Carney Landis, *Varieties of Psychopathological Experience* (New York: Holt, Rinehart & Winston, 1964), p. 168.

14. David V. Forrest, "New Words and Neologisms with a Thesaurus of Coinages by a Schizophrenic Savant," *Psychiatry* 32 (1969): 45.

15. Harold J. Vetter, *Language Behavior and Psychopathology* (Chicago: Rand McNally, 1969), p. 142.

16. Silvano Arieti, *Interpretation of Schizophrenia* (New York: Basic Books, 1974), p. 251.

17. Alfred M. Freedman, Harold I. Kaplan, and Benjamin J. Sadock, eds., *Modern Synopsis of the Comprehensive Textbook of Psychiatry* (Baltimore: Williams & Wilkins, 1976), p. 438. This is identical to the essay in the third edition.

18. N. C. Andreasen and P. S. Powers, "Overinclusive Thinking in Mania and Schizophrenia," *British Journal of Psychiatry* 125 (1974): 452–56.

19. Richard Hunter and Ida Macalpine, eds. and trans., *Memoirs of My Nervous Illness by Daniel Paul Schreber* (London: Dawson, 1955), p. 408.

20. R. D. Laing, *The Divided Self: An Existential Study in Sanity and Madness* (1959; Harmondsworth: Penguin, 1981), p. 143.

21. Stephen N. Gerson, Frank Benson, and Shervert H. Frazier, "Differential Diagnosis: Schizophrenia vs. Posterior Aphasia," *American Journal of Psychiatry* 134 (1977): 966–69.

22. L. Kerschbaumer, "Poetry in Schizophrenia and Other Psychoses," *Journal of Nervous and Mental Disease* 91 (1940): 153.

23. Wilhelm Mayer-Gross, Eliot Slater, and Martin Roth, *Clinical Psychiatry* (London: Baillière, Tindall & Cassell, 1969), p. 276.

24. H. C. Rümke, "The Clinical Differentiation within the Group of the Schizophrenias," *Proceedings of the Second International Congress for Psychiatry*, ed. W. A. Stoll (Zurich: Angst, 1959), p. 305.

25. W. Th. Winkler, *Übertragung und Psychose* (Bern: Huber, 1971).

26. U. H. Peters, *Übertragung-Gegenübertragung* (Munich: Kindler, 1977), p. 74.

27. William A. White, "The Language of Schizophrenia," in *Schizophrenia*, ed. Charles L. Dana et al. (New York: Hoeber, 1928), p. 323.

28. E. von Domarus, "The Specific Laws of Logic in Schizophrenia," in J. S. Kasanin, ed., *Language and Thought in Schizophrenia* (1944; New York: Norton, 1964), pp. 104 ff.

29. Sherry Rochester and J. R. Martin, *Crazy Talk: A Study of the Discourse of Schizophrenic Speakers* (New York: Plenum, 1979), see esp. pp. 2–54.

30. John M. Neale and Thomas F. Oltmanns, *Schizophrenia* (New York: Wiley, 1980), pp. 102–61.

31. I have relied in the chapter on the basic study by Fritz Schalk, "Das Wort *bizarr* im Romanischen," in *Etymologica: Walther von Wartburg zum siebzigsten Geburtstag* (Tübingen: Niemeyer, 1953), pp. 655–79. In addition, the references in the *Oxford English Dictionary (OED)* and in Kluge's *Etymologisches Wörterbuch* (Berlin: de Gruyter, 1960) helped me to see parallels in the use of the term in non-Romance sources.

32. *The Inferno of Dante Alighieri* (London: Dent, 1962), pp. 82–85. (My emphasis.)

33. *Seneca I: Moral Essays*, trans. John W. Basore (Cambridge, Mass.: Harvard University Press, 1950), pp. 107–9.

34. Giovanni Boccaccio, *The Decameron*, trans. G. H. McWilliam (Baltimore: Penguin, 1972), pp. 718–20.

35. See Schalk, "Das Wort *bizarr*," pp. 666–67, for these references.

36. Schalk comments on the close relationship between the *caprichos* and the *bizarrias* in seventeenth-century Spain, ibid., p. 667.

37. Johann Lauremberg, *Niederdeutsche Scherzgedichte*, ed. Wilhelm Braune (Halle: Niemeyer, 1879), p. 47.

38. "Bizarre" in the citation given in the *OED* is often found in an aesthetic context, thus Dryden speaks of "the ornament of writing . . . in poesie" as "bizarre."

39. Condillac, *Dictionnaire des synonymes*, ed. Georges Le Rou in the Corpus Général des Philosophes Français (Paris: Presses Universitaires de France, 1951), 3„109.

40. Lois Boe Hyslop and Francis E. Hyslop, Jr., trans., *Baudelaire as a Literary Critic* (University Park: Pennsylvania State University Press, 1964), pp. 81–82.

41. In this regard, see the two review essays on the language of schizophrenia: Brendhan Maher, "The Language of Schizophrenia: A Review and Interpretation," *British Journal of Psychiatry* 120 (1972): 3–7, and Peter F. Ostwald, "Language and Communication Problems with Schizophrenic Patients—A Review, Commentary, and Synthesis," in W. E. Fann et al., *Phenomenology and Treatment of Schizophrenia* (New York: Spectrum, 1978), pp. 163–91. See also Richard Haier, "The Diagnosis of Schizophrenia," in *Schizophrenia 1980* (Washington, D.C.: U.S. Government Printing Office, 1980), pp. 2–13. The relative importance of the label "bizarre" in contemporary psychiatry can be judged in the volume edited by Lyman C. Wynne, Rue L. Cromwell, and Steven Matthysse, *The Nature of Schizophrenia: New Approaches to Research and Treatment* (New York: Wiley, 1978). The book concludes with an essay by Loren R. Mosher, "Can Diagnosis Be Non-Pejorative?" (pp. 690–95), which avoids any discussion of the language of diagnosis, even though in a preceding essay Rue L. Cromwell boldly states: "I also would suggest that psychopathology is described and defined primarily in terms of how it deviates from the norms and expectancies of society in general. Certain manifestations of schizophrenia deviate enough to be viewed as bizarre, intolerable, or threatening. Other manifestations do not and they are often overlooked" (p. 219). Needless to say, the first category contains language and behavioral disruptions.

42. Manfred Bleuler, "What Is Schizophrenia?" *Schizophrenia Bulletin* 10 (1984): 8.

43. *World Health Organization: Report of the International Pilot Study of Schizophrenia*, vol. 1 (Geneva: WHO Press, 1973).

14. Seeing the AIDS Patient

1. *Newsweek*, 21 July 1986. On the general background of the image of the AIDS patient, see Caspar G. Schmidt, "The Group-Fantasy Origins of AIDS," *Journal of*

Psychohistory 12 (1984): 37–78; Dennis Altman, *AIDS in the Mind of America: The Social, Political, and Psychological Impact of a New Epidemic* (New York: Anchor / Doubleday, 1986); David Black, *The Plague Years: A Chronicle of AIDS, the Epidemic of our Times* (New York: Simon & Schuster, 1986); Graham Hancock and Enver Carim, *AIDS: The Deadly Epidemic* (London: Gollanz, 1986); Richard Liebmann-Smith, *The Question of AIDS* (New York: New York Academy of Sciences, 1985); Eve K. Nicols, *Mobilizing against AIDS: The Unfinished Story of a Virus* (Cambridge, Mass.: Harvard University Press, 1986); Lon G. Nungasser, *Epidemic of Courage: Facing AIDS in America* (New York: St. Martin's, 1986); Earl E. Shelp, Ronald H. Sunderland, and Peter W. H. Mansell, *AIDS: Personal Stories in Pastoral Perspective* (New York: Pilgrim Press, 1986); Barbara Peabody, *The Screaming Room: A Mother's Journal of Her Son's Struggle with AIDS / A True Story of Love, Dedication, and Courage* (San Diego: Oak Tree, 1986); Randy Shilts, *And the Band Played On: Politics, People, and the AIDS Epidemic* (New York: St. Martin's, 1987). More important, see George L. Mosse's brilliant study *Nationalism and Sexuality: Respectability and Abnormal Sexuality in Modern Europe* (New York: Fertig, 1985) for a sense of the cultural context of much of this literature.

2. Michael S. Gottlieb and Jerome E. Groopman, eds., *Acquired Immune Deficiency Syndrome: Proceedings of a Schering Corporation–UCLA Symposium* (held in Park City, Utah, 5–10 February 1984) (New York: Liss, 1984).

3. See H. Schwartz, "AIDS in the Media," in the Twentieth Century Fund's *Science in the Streets* (New York: Priority Press, 1984), pp. 30 ff., and Andrea J. Baker, "The Portrait of AIDS in the Media: An Analysis of the *New York Times*," in Douglas A. Feldman and Thomas M. Johnson, eds., *The Social Dimension of AIDS: Method and Theory* (New York: Praeger, 1986), pp. 179–97.

4. A detailed chronology of the scientific findings about AIDS has now been worked out between Robert C. Gallo and Luc Montagnier, scientists who were both involved in many of the initial discoveries concerning the disease. It details the disease from 1981 to 1985. See *The Chronicle of Higher Education*, 8 April 1987, p. 8, for that chronology.

5. A. Friedman-Kien et al., "Kaposi's Sarcoma and *Pneumocystis* Pneumonia among Homosexual Men—New York City and California," *Morbidity and Mortality Weekly Report* 30 (1981): 305–8.

6. M. S. Gottlieb et al., "*Pneumocystis* Pneumonia—Los Angeles," *Morbidity and Mortality Weekly Report* 30 (1981): 250–52, and S. M. Friedman et al., "Follow-up on Kaposi's Sarcoma and *Pneumocystis* Pneumonia," *Morbidity and Mortality Weekly Report* 30 (1981): 409–10.

7. See the initial editorial by J. A. Sonnabend, "The Etiology of AIDS," in *AIDS Research* 1 (1983/4): 1–12.

8. See Liebmann-Smith, *Question of AIDS*, pp. 84–86, and M. M. Lederman, "Transmission of the Acquired Immunodeficiency Syndrome through Heterosexual Activity," *Annals of Internal Medicine* 104 (1986): 115–17.

9. See Jacques Leibowitch, *A Strange Virus of Unknown Origin*, trans. Richard Howard (New York: Ballantine, 1985), pp. 3–9, as well as J. W. Curran, W. M. Morgan, E. T. Starcher, A. M. Hardy, and H. W. Jaffe, "Epidemiological Trends of AIDS in the United States," *Cancer Research* 45 (1985): 4602s–4s.

10. June E. Osborn, "The AIDS Epidemic: An Overview of the Science," *Issues in Science and Technology* 2 (1986): 56–65.

11. J. Seale, "AIDS and Hepatitis B Cannot Be Venereal Diseases," *Journal of the Canadian Medical Association* 130 (1984): 109–10. See further L. D. Grouse's editorial

"HTLV-III Transmission," *Journal of the American Medical Association* 254 (1985): 2130–31. It is not, as Helen Mathews Smith notes, that "syphilis presents a paradigm for our latest venereal epidemic," but rather that AIDS is not a sexually transmitted disease but has been so categorized. Helen Mathews Smith, "AIDS: Lessons from History," *MD Magazine* 30 (1986): 43–51.

12. Allan Brandt, *No Magic Bullet: A Social History of Venereal Disease in the United States since 1880* (New York: Oxford University Press, 1985), p. 134.

13. On the general history of syphilis, see Iwan Bloch, *Der Ursprung der Syphilis*, 2 vols. (Jena: Fischer, 1901–11). While Bloch supports the "Columbian" thesis, he does summarize the other literature as well. On the modern history of the disease, see Brandt, *No Magic Bullet*, as well as H. L. Arnold, Jr., "Landmark Perspective: Penicillin and Early Syphilis," *Journal of the American Medical Association* 251 (1984): 2011–12.

14. Erwin Panofsky, "Homage to Fracastoro in a Germano-Flemish Composition of about 1590," *Nederlands Kunsthistorisch Jaarboek* 12 (1961): 1–33. On the iconographic significance of the scorpion as a sign of perverse sexuality, see Luigi Aurigemma, *Le signe zodiacal du scorpion dans les traditions occidentales de l'antiquité gréco-latine à la renaissance* (Paris: Mouton, 1976), p. 92. On the more general problem of disease and art in the Renaissance, see Millard Meiss, *Painting in Florence and Siena after the Black Death* (Princeton, N.J.: Princeton University Press, 1951).

15. Karl Sudhoff, *Zehn Syphilis-Drucke aus den Jahren 1495–98* (Milan: Lier, 1924), p. xxii.

16. Ibid., p. 71.

17. Reproduced in the *Archiv für die Geschichte der Medizin* 1 (1907), plate 8.

18. See Moshe Barasch, *Gestures of Despair in Medieval and Early Renaissance Art* (New York: New York University Press, 1976).

19. Jean-Louis Alibert, *Description des maladies de la peau . . .* (Paris, n.p.: 1806–14). See the general discussion of Alibert in Susanne Dahm, *Frühe Krankenbildnisse: Alibert, Esquirol, Baumgärtner* (Cologne: Arbeiten der Forschungsstelle des Instituts für Geschichte der Medizin der Universität zu Köln, 1981). On the image of the prostitute as the source of pollution in terms of a nineteenth-century model of public health, see Charles Bernheimer, "Of Whores and Sewers: Parent-Duchatelet, Engineer of Abjection," *Raritan* 6 (1987): 72–90.

20. *Discover*, September 1986.

21. See Edwin H. Zeydel's translation of *The Ship of Fools* (New York: Dover, 1962), pp. 220–23. Brant's is the first German text to indicate the source of the disease in the New World. It quickly becomes a commonplace, partially because the "cure" proposed for the disease in early sixteenth-century German tractates such as that by Ulrich von Hutten also is seen to come from the New World. The cure, said to be found in the wood and bark of the *guaiacum* tree, becomes an important import into Germany through the efforts of the German trading family the House of Fugger. The view is that, given the inherent balance of nature, if the disease comes from the New World, so too must its cure. It is an attempt to recreate a sense of balance lost with the opening of the New World and the spread of syphilis. Many contemporary writers, among them Paracelsus, reject this analogy as spurious.

22. Liebowitch, *Strange Virus*, pp. 77–80.

23. Sander L. Gilman, *Difference and Pathology: Stereotypes of Sexuality, Race, and Madness* (Ithaca, N.Y.: Cornell University Press, 1985), pp. 131–49.

24. James H. Jones, *Bad Blood: The Tuskegee Syphilis Experiment—A Tragedy of Race and Medicine* (New York: Free Press, 1981). Compare the iconography of syphilis

and AIDS, with their perceived sudden onset, with the long history of the iconography of diseases such as cholera. On the iconography of cholera (and its comparison to AIDS), see Patrice Bourdelais and André Dodin, *Visages du choléra* (Paris: Belin, 1987), esp. pp. 146–47.

25. S. Piomelli, "Chronic Transfusions in Patients with Sickle Cell Disease: Indications and Problems," *American Journal of Pediatric Hematology and Oncology* 7 (1985): 51–55.

26. Gilman, *Difference and Pathology*, pp. 76–108.

27. Leibowitch, *Strange Virus*, p. 5.

28. J. Seale, "AIDS Virus Infection: A Soviet View of Its Origin," *Journal of the Royal Society of Medicine* 79 (1986): 494–95.

29. On the Haitian question, see J. W. Pape et al., "The Acquired Immunodeficiency Syndrome in Haiti," *Annals of Internal Medicine* 103 (1985): 774–78. On the "African" connection see the exchange of letters in the *British Medical Journal [Clinical Research]* 290 (1985): 932, 1006, 1284–85; 291 (1986): 216.

30. Anthony J. Pinching, "AIDS and Africa: Lessons for Us All," *Journal of the Royal Society of Medicine* 79 (1086): 501–3.

31. John R. Seale and Zhores A. Medvedev, "Origin and Transmission of AIDS: Multi-Use Hypodermics and the Threat to the Soviet Union: Discussion Paper," *Journal of the Royal Society of Medicine* 80 (1987): 301–4.

32. On theories of degeneration and the city, see Sander L. Gilman and J. Edward Chamberlin, eds., *Degeneration: The Dark Side of Progress* (New York: Columbia University Press, 1985).

33. Dorothy Nelkin and Stephen Hilgartner, "Disputed Dimensions of Risk: A Public School Controversy over AIDS," *Milbank Memorial Fund Quarterly* 64, Supplement 1 (1986): 118–42. Cf. K. M. Shannon and A. J. Amman, "Acquired Immune Deficiency Syndrome in Childhood," *Journal of Pediatrics* 106 (1985): 332–42.

INDEX

Page numbers in bold type refer to illustrative plates.

Library of Congress Cataloging-in-Publication Data

Gilman, Sander L.
  Disease and representation: images of illness from madness to AIDS /
Sander L. Gilman.
    p.   cm.
  Includes index.
  ISBN 0-8014-2119-5 (alk. paper). ISBN 0-8014-9476-1 (pbk.)
  1. Mental illness—History. 2. Mental illness in art. 3. Diseases in art. I.
Title.
  [DNLM: 1. Disease—psychology. 2. Medicine in Art—history. 3. Mental
Disorders—history. 4. Sick Role. WM 49 G487d]
RC438.G54 1988
306'.46—dc19
DNLM/DLC   87-47864